Handbook of Clinical Massage

To Annette, with love.

For Churchill Livingstone:

Editorial Director: Mary Law
Project Development Manager: Claire Wilson
Project Manager: Ailsa Laing
Designer: Judith Wright
Illustrations Manager: Bruce Hogarth
Illustrators: Zoë Harrison and Marie Cornall

Handbook of Clinical Massage

A Complete Guide for Students and Professionals

SECOND EDITION

Mario-Paul Cassar ND DO
Senior Lecturer and Faculty Member, College of Osteopaths, London
Principal, Massage and Bodywork Institute
Private Practitioner in Massage and Osteopathy

Foreword by

Clare Maxwell-Hudson
Founder, The Clare Maxwell-Hudson School of Massage, London, UK
Affiliate of the GCMT

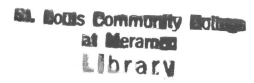
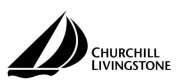
CHURCHILL
LIVINGSTONE

EDINBURGH   LONDON   NEW YORK   OXFORD   PHILADELPHIA   ST LOUIS   SYDNEY   TORONTO   2004

CHURCHILL LIVINGSTONE
An imprint of Elsevier Limited

First edition 1999
Reprinted 2000
Second edition 2004

ISBN 0443 07349 X

British Library Cataloguing in Publication Data
A catalogue record for this book is available from the British
Library

Library of Congress Cataloging in Publication Data
A catalog record for this book is available from the Library of
Congress

Note
Medical knowledge is constantly changing. Standard safety
precautions must be followed, but as new research and clinical
experience broaden our knowledge, changes in treatment and drug
therapy may become necessary or appropriate. Readers are
advised to check the most current product information provided
by the manufacturer of each drug to be administered to verify the
recommended dose, the method and duration of administration,
and contraindications. It is the responsibility of the practitioner,
relying on experience and knowledge of the patient, to determine
dosages and the best treatment for each individual patient.
Neither the Publisher nor the editors assumes any liability for any
injury and/or damage to persons or property arising from this
publication.

The Publisher

ELSEVIER
SCIENCE
your source for books,
journals and multimedia
in the health sciences
www.elsevierhealth.com

The
publisher's
policy is to use
**paper manufactured
from sustainable forests**

Printed in China

Contents

Foreword

The message of massage is universal: you can use your hands to help literally anyone. Massage is one of the simplest ways to help us achieve and maintain good health, to show someone that we care, to comfort and soothe.

In the 1960s, when I started as a professional therapist, massage was barely used in this country. At that time massage, in many people's minds, was connected with the pampered rich or with burly footballers. Nowadays that picture is transformed and massage is in the mainstream. Massage therapy is now one of the fastest growing professions, with reports that at least 20% of the population now use complementary medicine. Massage is to be found in hospitals and hospices, in offices and in sports and health centres. With this growing interest in massage, and the increased use of massage in the medical setting, comes a need for increased professionalism and knowledge. Mario-Paul Cassar's book addresses this need.

Massage is probably one of the oldest healing therapies known to mankind. It is an extension of a basic instinct seen in animals and humans alike; apes groom each other, animals lick their wounds, humans rub away their aches and pains. The basis of massage is touch – the most fundamental of human needs. Touch is so essential that if it is absent or withdrawn all sorts of problems can ensue, ranging from a failure to thrive in babies to irritability and bad behaviour in children and depression in adults. One of the many reasons for its increased popularity is that massage allows us to reach out and touch each other. Massage is formalized touch; giving us a licence to touch within clearly defined boundaries.

I am often asked where massage fits into the overall picture of complementary therapies, but the fact is that massage is *sui generis* (of its own kind). Massage is an independent therapy. For thousands of years it has been a central factor in medical and psychological practice around the world. In this it is surely unique. We in the profession do not ally it to, or divorce it from, any other procedure or practice. However, with the trend of integration of massage and other complementary therapies into mainstream healthcare, the benefits are being scrutinized. The fact that (almost without exception) people feel better after a massage is not enough. There is now a need for research-based evidence that these therapies work. Examples of research are given throughout the book, addressing this need and giving credibility to the use of massage.

Massage is a generic term for a wide variety of techniques and this book has been designed to ensure that the techniques are easy to follow. They are well illustrated and clearly described, with explanations of how and when the different techniques should be used.

In addition to the well-known effects of relaxation and emotional support that massage offers, its benefits influence a number of body processes. In this book, Mario-Paul Cassar has described the application of massage as it relates to the various systems of the body, and deals in depth with the application of massage for common disorders and malfunctions. He also looks at ways to help the practitioner assess the suitability of the massage treatment and guidance is given on the use of the appropriate techniques for each region of the body, and their use as an adjunct to conventional treatment. Contraindications to massage treatment are highlighted throughout the text, emphasizing the need for safe and effective treatment.

It is a common mistake to assume that a good massage requires only that the massage therapist has strong hands and considerable physical strength. In reality, the most significant requisite for an effective massage is good technique applied with the minimum of effort. To achieve this it is essential that the therapist uses the correct posture and uses body-weight instead of strength. A good posture is one in which the therapist feels well grounded while having the free-dom to move. In this book the author discusses the various postures for massage and throughout the text there are examples of the correct posture for the technique described.

I have known Mario-Paul Cassar for many years and was delighted to be asked to write this Foreword. I read every chapter of this book with great interest and imagine that it will become a well-thumbed reference for practising massage therapists, as well as an excellent text-book for those learning the art of massage. In short, this book is a cornucopia of information, to be used as thoroughly as a favourite cook-book. It should inspire and encourage all of us for whom massage is more than just a job, but is a way of life.

Claire Maxwell-Hudson
London 2004

Preface

In this volume I have retained the theme of my previous text, *Handbook of Massage Therapy,* and continued to explore the application of clinical massage. The particular utilization of clinical massage is, of course, its specific application in the treatment of disease, dysfunctions and musculoskeletal imbalances, whether it is carried out as an adjunct to conventional or complementary medicine or as a holistic treatment by itself. Taking a medical approach does not undermine the benefits of the primary effect of massage, i.e. relaxation. Indeed relaxation through massage is often used very effectively (as some of the current research shows) to instigate a therapeutic response, such as the lowering of stress hormones and promoting parasympathetic activity.

The history of massage is always of interest and frequently included in most massage books, however, this subject has become extensive due to the magnitude of data now available. I have consequently narrowed the history to a short section on the clinical use of massage and given examples when it was of significant interest in the past.

Massage movements and techniques have been developed over many years and there are now a great number of methods that are very similar or even identical in implementation, but which are described in differing terms. Petrissage, for example, is used by some authors to describe kneading, wringing, rolling, picking up and shaking, while in other texts these movements are classified under soft-tissue and compression techniques. In an attempt to simplify this array of terminology, I have given an introduction and a simple classification of the massage techniques in Chapter 2. This is by no means comprehensive and may vary from other categorizations. It is worth pointing out that while opinions may differ about the terminology, the effect and safety of massage movements take precedence over their classification.

As in other fields of complementary medicine, the efficacy of clinical massage has to be backed by research. I have cited research material in support of the discussions on the effects of massage on the systems of the body (Chapter 3). The value of research is that it provides information on the physiological effects of massage at the biochemical or tissue level, for example effects on the peripheral circulation or changes in hormonal activity. Research data had been rather limited in the past and this has meant that, in some instances, the only available material was published some years ago and, in some cases, lacked any conclusive evidence. Some of the investigative information from the past does, however, serve the purpose of identifying the connections between the nerves, organs, muscles and soft tissues. Updated research into the effects of massage is now more widely available and references from this data have been quoted accordingly throughout the text. For instance, The Touch Research Institutes (University of Miami School of Medicine and Nova Southeastern University, Florida, USA), headed by Tiffany Field PhD, have carried much valuable and detailed research into the effects of massage.

The clinical application of massage considers the most common conditions pertaining to each of the body systems (Chapter 4). Support for its efficacy has been based on research material and clinical experience. My intention is not to present massage as a complete cure but rather to highlight its beneficial effects and indeed its contraindications. In the absence of research data on the efficacy of massage for a specific disorder, its appropriateness of application can be based on the studies carried out into its effects at the biochemical or tissue level. For instance, as massage has been shown to improve the circulation, it can be applied in a condition where enhancing the circulation would be of benefit, for example in the region of arthritic joints. This is only one hypothesis of course, among many others. As in any other therapy, there are many differing viewpoints on the application of clinical massage. Treatment of a 'reflex zone' with massage is discouraged by some authors for instance, as it is postulated that it would stimulate reflex activity. Others would argue that it helps to normalize reflex activity without over-stimulating the organs. What matters most in the end is that the patient benefits and that the treatment is professional and safe. As noted earlier, the contraindications to the massage are of equal importance to its benefits. Accordingly, I have listed the general contraindications in Chapter 1 and wherever appropriate throughout the text, including those precautions that apply to the regions of the body (Chapters 5–10).

As with my previous publication, this book is aimed at students and practitioners of massage, bodywork and associated manipulative therapies. However, it is assumed that the reader, at whatever level of learning, is already familiar with anatomy and physiology, basic pathology and regional anatomy of muscles. These subjects are essential to massage therapy and yet too vast to include in this text. I hope that this book will stimulate as well as inform, and that it will encourage both students and practitioners to carry out research, to discuss the many aspects of this modality, to experiment and develop their own techniques, and to further the accomplishments of clinical massage.

Mario-Paul Cassar
London 2004

Acknowledgements

During the many years I have been teaching I have met many wonderful students from England, America, Japan, Canada, Australia and many other countries. Many have established themselves as highly regarded practitioners, some have also turned out to be excellent tutors, while others still, I am happy to say, have become colleagues and friends. Furthermore, they have been a great source of information, support and much appreciated critique of my work. I would therefore like to show my appreciation to, among others: Dr Patrick Lincoln, Carol Jordan, Indrajit Garai and James Earles (my apologies go to all the others I have left out).

Contributors I would like to thank are Marie Cornall for some of the illustrations, Paul Forrester for his excellent photography, Penny King, and the models Nick Wooley, Hazel Stratton, April Martin, Ruth Adams, Jocelyn Banks, Alison Peggs and Trevor Wicks.

I am extremely grateful for the cooperation and encouragement I have received from the production office at Elsevier; so many thanks to Mary Emerson Law, Katrina Mather, Claire Wilson, Sarah Beanland, Ailsa Laing, Barbara Muir and the rest of the production team. I would also like to express my gratitude to my friends who have supported me in my work and who kindly propped up my personal life in time of need. They include Judith Kane, Hazel Stratton, Pam and Tony Parkinson, Leslie Cuozzo, Chris Hanson, Alan Jones, Liz Hunt and Ken Gallichan.

Finally I would like to thank all my family for their continuous support that is sincerely appreciated.

The massage treatment

THE HISTORY OF MASSAGE

The history of massage is extensive and has generated a profusion of literature. Some of the historical facts are common knowledge, and the need to repeat them could almost be contested. None the less, the history of massage remains an important subject for students and practitioners alike and, accordingly, merits a mention in every book on massage therapy. In keeping with the theme of this book, the history of massage in this section gives a brief account of the application of massage for 'medical' conditions. It is by no means comprehensive but the aim of this section is merely to highlight some of the early pioneers and concepts of massage therapy.

The practice of massage dates back to prehistoric times, with origins in India, China, Japan, Greece and Rome. Massage has been mentioned in literature dating back to the ancient times, with the earliest recorded reference appearing in the *Nei Ching*, a Chinese medical text written before 2500 BC. Later writings on massage came from scholars and physicians such as Hippocrates in the fifth century BC and Avicenna and Ambroise Pare in the 10th and 16th (some say 17th) centuries AD, respectively. A very famous book on massage, *The Book of Cong-Fou*, was translated by two missionaries named Hue and Amiot, and this created great interest and influenced the thinking of many massage practitioners.

The word *therapeutic* is defined as 'of or relating to the treatment or cure of a disorder or disease'. It comes from the Greek *therapeutikos*, and relates to the effect of the medical treatment (*therapeia*). The word *massage* also comes from the Greek *masso*, meaning to knead. Hippocrates (480 BC) used the term *anatripsis*, meaning to rub down, and this was later translated into the Latin *frictio*, meaning friction or rubbing. This term prevailed for a long time, and was still in use in the USA until the middle of the 1870s. The expression for massage in India was *shampooing*; in China it was known as *Cong-Fou*, and in Japan as *Ambouk*. It is usual to record the history of massage chronologically, but rather than follow this format it is of interest to consider some of its historical applications as a therapeutic medium.

Relaxation

Relaxation, which itself has a therapeutic value, is perhaps the effect most freely associated with massage. As long ago as 1800 BC the Hindus in India used massage for weight reduction and to help with sleep, fatigue and relaxation. Over the centuries the relaxation aspect of massage has been used to treat many conditions, such as hysteria and neurasthenia (a form of postviral syndrome).

General health

Massage, in combination with exercise, has always been advocated for general health. Artifact discoveries indicate that prehistoric man used ointments and herbs to promote general wellbeing and to protect against injury and infection. The potions that were rubbed into the body would also have had a healing effect, especially if the 'rubbing' was carried out by a religious or medical 'healer'. In the Indian art of *Ayurveda* medicine, the patient was expected to undergo a process of shampooing or massage every morning after bathing. The health-promoting properties of massage, exercise and hydrotherapy were mentioned in the writings of the Arabic physician and philosopher Ali Abu Ibn Szinna (Avicenna) in the 10th century AD.

Exercises, or '*gymnastics*', were again endorsed for health in the 18th and early 19th centuries. Francis Fuller in England and Joseph-Clement Tissot in France advocated an integrated system of exercises and movement for the preservation and restoration of health. Fuller died in 1706, but his work on gymnastics was in print until 1771. A similar system of medical gymnastics was developed by Tissot, who used very little massage except for some friction movements, and a book on his work was published in 1780 (Licht and Licht, 1964). These two pioneers preceded the Swedish physician, Per Henrik Ling, and very probably influenced his thinking on gymnastics.

Per Henrik Ling (1776–1839) developed the science of '*gymnastics*', which was a form of treatment combining massage and exercise. The massage component of the therapy was not particularly emphasized by Ling as it was only part of the overall treatment, and he placed more importance on the exercises that were carried out by the patient and the '*gymnast*' (massage practitioner). Ling's system was known as the Swedish Movement, or the Movement Cure. Years later, after his death, the massage aspect was taken out of context and practised on its own as Swedish massage. Similarly, changes took place concerning the goals of the treatment. Ling had also advocated the Swedish Movement to improve hygiene and to prevent ill health, but by the late 19th century physicians were only interested in Ling's method as a treatment for disease. Ling's system of massage was introduced to England in 1840, soon after his death.

In 1850, Dr Mathias Roth wrote the first book in English on the Swedish Movement. He also translated an essay by Ling on the techniques and their effects. Between 1860 and 1890, George H. Taylor MD of New York published many articles on the Swedish Movement Cure, which he had learned from Per Henrik Ling. His brother, Charles Fayette Taylor, was also an ardent writer on the subject (Van Why, 1994). During the latter years of the 19th century, when massage was widely used, it was claimed that the Swedish Movement Cure had many positive effects on general health and in the treatment of disease. These claims were described and supported by case histories in the writings of George Taylor. Some of them, as mentioned here, continue to be valid today.

Blood circulation

There was a positive improvement in the blood circulation following the gymnastics and massage application, and this benefit was said to be systemic as well as specific to a region. With the increased circulation the tissues were nourished and the secretions of the glands increased. The venous return was also enhanced, thereby reducing congestion.

Respiration

The expansion of the chest was considerably increased as a result of the exercise and massage. Respiration improved as a consequence of this change and served as effective prevention against diseases such as consumption (tuberculosis). Furthermore, the improved respiration created a more efficient elimination of toxins and, accordingly, the level of fatigue was reduced and the overall condition of the body improved. Deformities of the rib cage were also corrected with the system of exercises and massage.

Digestive organs

Diseases of the digestive organs could be treated by means of suitable exercises together with the necessary dietary changes and correct hygiene. Improving the flow of blood to the skin and extremities helped to reduce congestion, and appropriate movements and massage were used to stimulate elimination.

Fitness and joint function

Claims for the effects of massage date back to physicians such as Herodicus (fifth century BC), who professed to have great success in prolonging lives with a combination of massage, herbs and oils. One of his pupils, Hippocrates (the father of medicine, who lived around 480 BC), followed suit and claimed he could improve joint function and increase muscle tone with the use of massage. He also stated that the strokes of massage should be carried out towards the heart and not towards the feet. This must have been an intuitive statement or a wild guess, since there was no knowledge of the blood circulation at the time.

During the Renaissance (1450–1600), massage was very popular with royalty. In France, for example, physician Ambroise Pare (1517–1590) was sought after by the royal household for his massage treatments. His main interest was the use of massage, and especially friction movements, in the treatment of dislocated joints.

John Grosvenor (1742–1823), an English surgeon and professor of medicine at Oxford, was extremely enthusiastic about the results that were being achieved with massage and took on the work of Per Henrik Ling and his contemporary, Dr Johann Mezger of Amsterdam. Grosvenor demonstrated the benefits of massage in the relief of stiff joints, gout and rheumatism. However, he did not include exercise as part of his treatment because he was mostly interested in the healing of tissues and joints by the action of friction or rubbing. He claimed that this technique abolished the need to conduct operations in many diseases. William Cleobury MD, a member of the Royal College of Surgeons, also used massage for the treatment of joints. He followed the practice of John Grosvenor MD, and used friction and rubbing to treat contraction of joints and fluid in the knee.

In New York, Charles Fayette Taylor (1826–1899) published volumes of material on the Swedish Movement throughout the 1860s. His writings covered many topics of medicine, but he wrote a great deal about the treatment of spinal curvatures. Charles Taylor had studied the Swedish Movement in London under the guidance of Dr Mathias Roth, who was a prominent homeopathic orthopod and a great believer in Ling's system of treatment. Although Taylor returned to New York after only 6 months he was very committed to the Swedish Movement system. His brother, George Taylor, was also keen to show the effects of the system for curvatures of the spine, and gave sample case histories in his writings.

Rheumatism

In 1816, Dr Balfour successfully treated rheumatism using percussion, friction and compression.

However, the full recognition of massage in the treatment of rheumatism came much later in the same century. Like many other members of royalty, Queen Victoria benefited a great deal from the Swedish Movement Cure and consequently gave the reputation of massage a boost in the late 1880s. Ling had founded the Central Gymnastics Institute of Berlin in 1813, and had appointed Lars Gabriel Branting as his successor. One of Branting's students, Lady John Manners, Duchess of Rutland, arranged for Branting to treat Queen Victoria for her rheumatic pains, and the much publicized success of Branting's treatment by 'gymnastics' created a new demand for the Swedish Massage Cure.

Writer's cramp

In the 1880s, a calligrapher from Frankfurt-am-Main, Germany, found fame as a masseur. Julius Wolff become known in medical circles for his treatment of the spasmodic form of writer's cramp by using gymnastics, calligraphic exercises and massage. He claimed a success rate of 57%, and his reputation and work spread to France and London. The treatment was observed and approved by Dr de Watteville (de Watteville, 1885), physician in charge of the Electrotherapeutical Department of St Mary's Hospital, London.

Paralysis

Tiberius (42 BC–37 AD), a Roman physician, made great claims for massage, declaring that it cured paralysis. Much later, in the early 19th century, an American doctor, Cornelius E. De Puy MD (Van Why, 1991), used massage techniques to treat palsy and apoplexy (paralysis). De Puy was a founder member of the Physico-Medical Society of New York and, during his short life (he died in a shipwreck at the age of 29 years), he published three articles for the Society on the use of massage in medicine. One of these, in 1817, was on the efficacy of friction massage in the treatment of palsy and apoplexy (he also practised blood-letting and dietary changes as part of the treatment). In his writings, which preceded

those of Per Henrik Ling (1840s), he also mentioned the use of devices or massage implements such as brushes and wet flannels. Some years later, in 1860, the benefits of the Movement Cure for paralysis were described and illustrated with a case history by George H. Taylor MD (Taylor, 1860). Another claim came in 1886 from William Murrell, who contended that massage was instrumental in healing infantile paralysis.

Parturition

It was the custom in many primitive civilizations to assist parturition by the use of external manipulation. This tradition dates back to the ancient Hebrews, and to Rome, Greece, the South American coast, Africa and India. In some places these methods are still in use today. Compression of the abdomen is utilized for the purpose of increasing muscular activity and to apply a mechanical force on the contents of the cavity. It can be of utmost importance in preventing or reducing haemorrhaging from a relaxed and expanding womb; it is also used to express the placenta (Crede's method) and, sometimes, to correct malpositions. The constriction of the abdomen and the uterine globe takes different forms. It can be simple pressure applied with the hands to the abdomen, and the use of aids such as bandages or belts wrapped around the abdomen is also common. Stones, and even pressure with the feet, may also be used on top of the abdomen whilst the patient lies supine. The position of the parturient varies; she may be sitting on an assistant's lap, kneeling down, squatting, suspended by her arms, resting over a horizontal pole or lying prone.

Significant assistance in parturition has also been provided by massage; for instance, among the American Indians and the natives of Mexico. Its effect is to aid with the expression of the neonate and the placenta, and also to prevent haemorrhaging. The technique most commonly used is a kneading action over the abdomen, and sometimes oils and heat are added (or even turtle fat, as among the Gros-Ventres). In ancient Arab cultures, physicians such as Rhazes advocated firm rubbing of the abdomen in childbirth. This practice is continued in some areas.

Obstetricians in Japan are said to correct mal-positions during the later months of pregnancy by the use of kneading. In Siam in the 17th century, massage in childbirth was used mostly to reduce pain. The strokes used then were light rubbing, touching, delicate pressure, tickling and friction with the fingertips. The combination of compression and vigorous shampooing, as practised later in Siam, was described by Samuel R. House MD in the journal *Archives of Medicine* (1879). Another method of massage is stripping down the abdomen. For this, the parturient is suspended by bands beneath the arms and an assistant kneels behind her and applies a heavy effleurage-type movement, or stripping, on the abdomen. This method has also been used amongst the Tartars, the Coyotero-Apaches and even in Siam, as reported by Dr Reed, a surgeon in the USA (cited by Engelmann, 1882; reproduced 1994).

Treating the wounded

The Greeks started to make use of massage in around 300 BC, coupling it with exercise as a regime for fitness. Gladiators were given regular massages to ease pains and muscle fatigue. It is said that Julius Caesar regularly had his whole body pinched and rubbed down with oils.

In the UK, massage was used by the members of the Incorporated Society of Massage to treat wounded soldiers of the Boer War. The Almeric Paget Massage Corps (later to become the Military Massage Service) was set up in 1914 to help treat the wounded of the First World War, and this service extended to some 300 hospitals in the UK. It was offered again in the Second World War.

The benefits of massage in the treatment of war injuries were highlighted in a book written by James Mennell in 1920. He was medical officer in charge of the Massage Department at the Special Military Surgery Hospital in London. Mennell worked under the guidance of Sir Robert Jones, who was director of the same hospital. In the introduction to the book, Sir Robert Jones said of massage:

As a concomitant to surgical treatment, massage may be employed to alleviate pain, reduce oedema, assist circulation and promote the nutrition of tissues.

The term he used for the practice of massage was 'Physico-therapeutics', and he defined its effect as 'the restoration of function, this also includes the use of mobilization (passive and active) to complete the treatment'.

The use of apparatus for massage

In 1864, George Taylor MD established the first American school to teach Ling's method. Whilst suffering from a broken elbow and unable to teach or to treat patients, he invented an apparatus to carry out the massage and exercises. Such assistive devices could be applied with the same proficiency as the manual techniques, and in some cases even served as useful aids to the therapist. Another graduate of Ling's Institute in Sweden had a similar idea. In 1865 in Stockholm, Jonas Gustaf Zander devised a system of machinery to carry out the same series of exercises and massage movements. One of these machines was the vibrating apparatus. It had previously been suggested that only Ling and his students could really master the art of vibration. Furthermore, gymnastics, and especially vibration movements, achieved the desired effects only when carried out at particular frequencies and intensity. The apparatus was designed to perform the same quality of movement. It was therefore an effective substitute. A choice of application meant that the whole body or certain regions only could be treated, and it was said to provide the same benefits as manual vibration. Circulation could be improved and, with this, the nutrition of the tissues. The apparatus could also improve the tone of muscles, including the involuntary muscles of the heart, stomach and intestines. Blood vessels were similarly affected, with contraction and vasodilatation of the vessels resulting in improved circulation, in particular to the extremities. Other uses for the machinery included calming the nerves, aiding a weak digestion and improving the function of respiratory organs, as well as soothing pain.

Massage today

Modern day massage owes its growth not necessarily to individual pioneers but to the great number of practitioners who are utilizing the techniques in clinics, homes, hospitals and surgeries. Through its efficacy it has secured a firm place amongst other complementary therapies. Being an art as well as a science, its progress will continue as long as practitioners and students go on to explore and research it.

INTRODUCTION TO MASSAGE THERAPY

Massage has the potential to influence emotion, biochemistry and biomechanics, usually without adding excessively to the adaptation load, and is therefore uniquely placed to be able to be applied in most situations, from minor injuries to terminal conditions.
(Chaitow L. Presentation *Journal of Bodywork and Movement Therapies* Conference London 2001)

Massage therapy can be described as the manipulation of soft tissues by a trained massage therapist for therapeutic purposes.

'Therapeutic' is synonymous with the terms healing, restorative, beneficial, remedial and curative. Any one of these terms is an appropriate description of the values of massage and can be seen to be of equal relevance to massage and other bodywork/manipulative therapies. The understanding of the reasons behind the effects of massage can, however, show a discrepancy amongst therapists. Though all equally valid, these differences will invariably influence the emphasis and subsequently the approach to the treatment. In some quarters, the benefits of massage are seen as being primarily based on the biomechanical physical principles, i.e. scientifically based. Others see massage as the medium through which an exchange of energies can take place between the therapist and the recipient and whereby, using a focused approach, a balancing of energies can be achieved. Spiritual healing and intuitive touch are similar approaches. Others place the importance on the emotional and psychological factors influencing disease and healing. The significance of each of these perspectives is not diminished even though they are not always referred to in this text and despite the fact that the emphasis here is primarily on the biomechanical, biochemical and psychosocial aspects of massage.

The therapeutic value of massage extends beyond relaxation, although this in itself is remedial and has positive consequential benefits. Most massage movements have the additional therapeutic effects of easing muscle tightness and increasing the circulation. However, some techniques are termed 'applied' because they are used for a specific effect; for instance, to improve lymphatic drainage or to assist peristalsis of the colon. Their use is determined by the condition being treated; invariably the massage is implemented not to cure a disorder but to alleviate some of its symptoms. Conversely, the massage may be contraindicated at times because of the nature of the pathology involved.

There is no set routine for a massage treatment, and no fixed number of times each stroke must be carried out. Furthermore, therapeutic or applied massage does not necessarily imply a whole body massage. Very often the treatment is carried out to one or two regions only; for example, the abdomen and the back. It may also be the case that certain movements alone are required to achieve the desired outcome; for example, to help improve the function of the visceral organs or to enhance the venous return. Consequently, massage should never be carried out 'by numbers'—a treatment does not consist of three effleurage strokes in one direction followed by three strokes in the other direction.

Massage is an art as well as a science, and every treatment, even by the novice practitioner, should combine these two aspects. In addition to knowing the all-important theoretical background, it is necessary for the practitioner to develop the skill of recognizing the most suitable techniques and how many times to carry out each one. This ability can only be achieved if the therapist manages to develop the palpatory skills needed to monitor and assess the response of the tissues to the massage. Through these palpatory skills the therapist can assess the state of the tissues (e.g. fibrotic, spasms), any discomfort which may be inflicted with a particular stroke and technique, and the response or emotional state of the patient. It is only with this continuous awareness and sensitivity that the practitioner can determine the number of strokes, pressure, speed and so forth that are appropriate on a particular region of the body and for that particular patient. The same argument is put forward to determine the duration of each treatment session or to quote the number of treatments necessary to treat a condition and over what period of time. Apart from the commercial connotations it conjures up, having a preconceived duration and number of treatments goes against the basic philosophy of the holistic approach in which each patient is seen as an individual entity, with their own healing capabilities and needs. Massage requires time, patience, empathy, pleasant surroundings, tranquillity and so forth. It is not possible to make someone relax quickly; it takes time to induce parasympathetic responses, homeostasis and healing.

FUNDAMENTALS OF MASSAGE THERAPY

The case history

Any method of massage treatment should be preceded by taking a full medical case history of the patient or client. It would be very unprofessional for the massage therapist not to follow this golden rule. A case history furnishes the therapist with all the relevant information about the patient and helps reveal any crucial condition that may be a contraindication, whilst providing a framework for the treatment. Advice to the patient can only be offered once a thorough assessment has been made; in some cases the recommendation involves referral to another practitioner or a consultant. Taking a case history does not, however, put the massage practitioner in a position to make a diagnosis. Accordingly, practitioners should not attempt to do so. The case history sheet may be divided into sections such as the ones listed here, and each part should include adequate details without being too time-consuming to complete. In addition, the case his-

tory document is confidential and nobody but the therapist should have access to it.

Section A—personal details

1. *Name and address.*
2. *Contact telephone numbers* (daytime, evening or mobile phone).
3. *Date of birth.*
4. *Marital status.*
5. *Occupation.* The patient's line of work may give rise to stress, to overuse syndromes like repetitive strain injuries or to abnormal postural patterns, all of which can lead to postural imbalances and to muscle tightness.
6. *Address of general practitioner.* Some patients may prefer to withhold details of their general practitioner, and their decision must of course be respected. These details may, however, be needed in the unlikely event of an emergency, and having them on record could prove to be a lifesaver should the massage therapist need to contact the patient's doctor.
7. *Consent to contact the patient's doctor outside an emergency situation.* Having assessed the information obtained from the case history, the observations and the treatment itself, the massage therapist may conclude that some of the findings are significant enough to be passed on to the patient's doctor. This cannot, however, be carried out without the full consent of the patient, whose authorization is therefore requested on the case history sheet.

Section B—symptoms and history

1. *Current symptoms.* A list of symptoms that may have prompted the patient to seek massage therapy is entered in this section. The symptoms are listed in order of severity and onset, and each symptom is assessed for any possible contraindications. For example, hot flushes, persistent headaches and palpitations could indicate heart problems, which require a full examination by a doctor; they certainly suggest that massage to the neck is contraindicated. Information needed for the assessment includes the duration and frequency of each symptom, any factors which

increase or reduce its severity, and the history of its onset.

2. *Recording levels of pain*. Any changes in the presenting symptoms need to be recorded. An entry can be made following the treatment or in subsequent weeks. Recording levels of pain, aching and sensitivity can be achieved by a simple grading system to which the patient can relate; e.g. pain levels on a scale of 1 to 10, with 1 depicting the lowest level and 10 the level of most severity. This and other grading systems can also be used to obtain some measure of other symptoms such as severity of headaches.

3. *History of previous and current treatments*. Details of all current and recent treatments are recorded, and should any of these raise doubts about the suitability of the massage treatment then approval should first be sought from the patient's doctor or consultant.

4. *Conditions*. An entry is made of any condition from which the patient may suffer. This information is needed to help form an overall picture of the patient's health, and to structure the treatment programme. For instance, a patient suffering from frequent colds may reflect a weak immune system, and the indicated treatment for such a case is lymphatic massage. Advice on food supplements and other treatment approaches may also be appropriate. Another case in point is a drastic unplanned or rapid drop in weight, which may indicate cancerous changes which require investigation by a doctor.

5. *Medication*. Although patients are generally willing to convey details of their medical history, some components may unintentionally be omitted. Asking about medication can therefore reveal some vital information. For instance, patients may forget to mention that they suffer from insomnia but will promptly remember when questioned about their medication. Insomnia can have underlying factors such as depression and anxiety.

6. *Additional details*. Questions on diet and modes of relaxation can be included to build up a picture of the patient's lifestyle. Whilst this is valuable information, it cannot be used to make changes to the patient's diet unless the therapist is a trained nutritionist. Similarly, advice on

relaxation methods is appropriate, but any deep anxiety states may require the help of a trained counsellor.

7. *Exercise*. For the massage therapist, the most common ailments patients present with are back pain, muscle stiffness and tension. Prescribing some simple exercises can help with the treatment of these disorders. Back pain, for instance, is often associated with a weight problem or lack of exercise. It is, however, worth bearing in mind that on some occasions the exercise itself may be a causative factor. Muscle stiffness is often related to overuse during a sporting activity.

Contraindications The question of contraindications to massage goes beyond a straightforward list, the reason being that, in theory, massage can be applied in most conditions, either to a region of the body or for relaxation. In practice, however, there are times when it is unlikely to be effective and is therefore best avoided. It may also be the case that, whilst massage is not strictly contraindicated, the presenting signs and symptoms are indicative of pathology and consequently require examination by a doctor before any massage treatment is applied. On the other hand, certain illnesses or symptoms, which can be either local (a region or tissue) or systemic, are serious enough to render massage unsuitable. Some examples of common contraindications are listed in this section. Those shown as local contraindications (Box 1.1) indicate that massage should not be carried out on the region affected by the condition. Systemic contraindications are those conditions which affect the whole body or system of the body (Box 1.2). Contraindications to massage are considered for each region of the body and for specific conditions in later chapters.

Probable contraindications There follow examples of conditions which may require investigation prior to massage.

- *Depression*. In some cases of clinical depression the sedating effect of massage can exacerbate the lethargic state of the patient. Treatment therefore should only be carried out with the doctor's approval.
- *Heart problems*. Any potential condition or pathology of the heart necessitates full investi-

---

Box 1.1   Examples of local contraindications

- Symptoms without a known cause such as:

  - Heat or redness
  - Pain
  - Indigestion

- Areas of inflammation
- Fractures
- Myositis ossificans
- Bony avulsions
- Bone disease such as Osgood–Schlatter
- Tumours or symptoms of undiagnosed cancer

  - Suspicious lumps or growths

- Peptic ulcers
- Ulcerative colitis
- Aneurysm
- Appendicitis
- Gout
- Infective arthritis
- Pneumonia
- Gastritis
- Glomerulonephritis
- Areas affected by herpes zoster (shingles)
- Intestinal obstruction
- Ascites (abdominal swelling)
- Portal hypertension
- Spina bifida
- Varicose veins
- Venous thrombosis
- Open wounds
- Acute strains
- Bacterial and fungal infections

  - Athlete's foot
  - Cellulitis
  - Ringworm
  - Impetigo
  - Abscesses

- Impaired blood supply to a tissue
- Weakness in the wall of the blood vessels as in haemophilia
- Enlarged liver or spleen associated with jaundice
- Enlarged liver of hepatitis

Box 1.2   Examples of systemic contraindications

- Toxaemia (septicaemia)
- Viral infections
- Fever
- Diarrhoea from infection
- Measles
- Tissue susceptibility to bruising as from drugs
- Symptoms of undiagnosed cancer

  - Unrelenting pain
  - General malaise
  - Temperature changes
  - Unexplained heat or inflammation
  - Unexplained weight changes

---

gation and massage should only be carried out once a medical diagnosis has been made.

- *Frequent colds.* A weakened immune system may manifest in a number of symptoms such as recurrent viral infections (colds, flu and so forth). Whilst massage helps the immune system, a weakened system can be caused by some underlying pathology that would need to be diagnosed before any massage treatment.

- *Premenstrual tension.* PMT is in fact a syndrome of symptoms, some of which can be alleviated with massage. The condition may, however, be due to hormonal imbalances and therefore requires a diagnosis if it is severe.

- *Cystitis.* This inflammatory condition, while common enough, can extend to the ureters, bladder and kidneys, and massage in these areas would be contraindicated. A full diagnosis may be required before massage is carried out.

- *Loss of weight.* A sudden or unexplained loss of weight may be indicative of cancer and therefore requires investigation

- *High blood pressure.* The aetiology of high blood pressure should always be diagnosed by a doctor before any treatment is carried out. Although massage can help reduce high blood pressure when it is stress-related, it is still given as an adjunct to other treatments. In some cases it may not be of benefit; for instance, if there is serious underlying pathology of the brain or heart.

- *Diabetes.* It is not unsafe to massage a diabetic patient, but it is important to bear in mind complications such as neuropathy, degenerative changes in the blood vessels and increased susceptibility to infection. Weakening of the connective tissues (e.g. fragility of the skin) may also be present.

- *Constipation.* This condition may be due to such pathology as twisted intestines or carcinoma, and the cause should always be established prior to any treatment.

- *Steroids*. The use of steroids may have a weakening effect on the connective tissues and, if extensive, can render massage unsafe.
- *Corticosteroids* can also impair the immune system and the subject is prone to infections. Massage should only be performed when there is no risk of contamination.
- *Jaundice*. One form of jaundice is referred to as *prehepatic jaundice*. This is when there is abnormal destruction of red blood cells or some bleeding disorder. Massage in this case is carried out with extreme care as the patient may be susceptible to bruising. *Hepatic jaundice* may be of viral aetiology, in which case massage may be contraindicated.

Cancer is a controversial yet serious enough condition to demand careful consideration. Traditionally, massage has been contraindicated in cancer patients because of the risk of metastasis through the lymph and, in some cases, the vascular systems. Caution is still necessary, albeit that nowadays massage is proposed for the terminally ill and following mastectomy. Cancers that metastasize easily through the lymphatic system and blood vessels, such as melanoma and Hodgkin's disease, are more of a question mark, and techniques for increasing circulation are therefore best omitted. Massage in the areas of lymph nodes is also avoided. As a general rule, areas in which there is active disease are best avoided so as not to increase the blood flow or metabolic rate. Other regions of the body may be massaged, particularly to promote relaxation. Consultation with, and approval of, the patient's general practitioner is always advisable.

Section C—assessment and treatment records

1. *Assessment of the case history*. Once the case history has been completed and the physical observations carried out (discussed later in this chapter), the massage therapist is able to appraise the following aspects of the treatment:

- The suitability of massage treatment for this particular patient.
- The massage treatment programme and expected results.
- Any conditions or contraindications that may call for further assessments; therefore, any immediate or possible referrals.
- Any advice that may benefit the patient.

2. *Treatment record*. This entry should include details of the treatment carried out during each visit. Examples of entries include:

- General relaxing massage; expected beneficial effects achieved and no adverse reaction to treatment.
- Applied relaxing techniques to the lumbar muscles; additional techniques applied for lordosis.
- Abdominal massage and colon drainage; patient to report on the effects of the massage over the next 24 h, to be reassessed in the next session and treatment repeated if necessary.
- Addressed overworked muscles of the right shoulder.
- Massage to improve circulation of the legs; to be reassessed in the next session and treatment repeated if necessary.

Subsequent treatments Following the initial consultation and massage treatment the patient may return for one or more subsequent visits. Some time is therefore allocated to update the case history of the patient before any treatment. It may be that the symptoms have abated but other symptoms have emerged; it could also be the case that the symptoms have increased. These details are necessary so that the massage therapist can consider the treatment programme or, indeed, new contraindications. The general entries would include:

1. Were there any symptoms following the last treatment session? Sometimes a patient may experience a headache or congestion in the sinuses following a massage treatment. The symptoms normally last a short time (perhaps an hour) and are generally caused by the body's elimination of toxins. Following heavy pressure techniques on a muscle, there may be soreness in

the area for a day or so. While care is needed so that no reaction is caused by the treatment, some techniques (e.g. deep neuromuscular work) may cause a slight inflammation of the tissues, e.g. on areas of fibrotic changes or adhesions, when the tissues are being manipulated and stretched. Any soreness is naturally best avoided, but should it occur will only last a day or so, and the patient can be advised to use a cooling pack following the treatment.

2. Have there been any changes or new developments since the last treatment? The patient may experience a reduction in some of the symptoms, which indicates that the condition is responding to the massage (as well as any other treatments). There may be an additional symptom that the patient has experienced since the last treatment. This may be a complication of the condition or may be related to a completely different condition. For instance, a patient may be responding well to their treatment for headaches but may have experienced an increase because of a bout of sinusitis. A different scenario could be, for example, that they have been free of headaches but have recently developed pain in the knees that is likely to be related to degenerative changes and a recent 5-mile walk. Where symptoms have increased following the previous treatment, it is vital that the treatment programme is reviewed and, if necessary, stopped altogether.

3. Treatment programme. The techniques to be carried out, as well as the aims of the massage treatment, are also recorded. Changes in the treatment approach may be necessary following the previous session and accordingly these are also recorded.

General assessment

Posture

The term posture refers to the kinetic position of the body when it is upright, sitting or lying. It can also be described as the structural relationship between the musculoskeletal systems and gravity. Individuals each develop their own postural patterns; these may in turn be influenced by hereditary factors, customary standing or lying positions, muscle weaknesses, abnormalities such as bony deformities, emotional states, and diseases such as asthma, emphysema and spondylitis.

Analysis and corrections of posture can only be carried out by a physician or a practitioner specializing in body mechanics. The massage therapist, unless trained in this particular field of work, cannot carry out any major adjustments to the patient's posture. Some features are, however, very apparent and are good indicators of abnormalities; they also help the therapist to assess the state of the muscles and to plan the treatment. Observation of the posture starts with the patient standing, when certain spinal deviations are noticeable. Some of the more common postural irregularities are discussed here; they can, however, only act as general guidelines because of the diversity of postural patterns. Further examination can be carried out when the patient is lying down; these observations are considered in later chapters.

Observing the patient in the standing posture The upright body fights a never-ending battle against the constant pull of gravity. Several groups of postural muscles are recruited to facilitate movement and to maintain a vertical position. Malfunction of the mechanisms involved causes the body to deviate from what is considered a normal stance. One common factor for this deviation is an imbalance in muscle function, where certain muscles are too tight whilst others are too flaccid. Bony misalignments and abnormalities are similar influences; in this case there are departures from the normal spinal curves or body alignments. Some examples are considered below.

1. *Scoliosis*. This is described as a curving of the spine to the left or right. The muscles on one side of the curve (the concave side) tend to be short and tight, while those on the elongated side (the convex side) are commonly flaccid.

2. *Lordosis*. Increased lordosis is an excessive hollowing of the lumbar spine. At times it can also be observed in the cervical spine. Lumbar lordosis is a further example of muscle imbalance;

the low back muscles are short and tight compared to those of the abdomen, which tend to be weak.

3. *Kyphosis*. Kyphosis refers to an exaggerated forward curve of the thoracic spine. The muscles of the upper back, despite being elongated, are likely to be tense from supporting the spine in a forward bending position. On the other hand, the muscles of the anterior chest wall, including the intercostals, are found to be shortened.

4. *Rotation*. Segments or blocks of the spine can be rotated around a vertical axis, sometimes in combination with one of the aforementioned deviations. The rotation shows as a prominent area to the left or right of the spine. It is not always easy to identify and could be mistaken for overdeveloped muscles.

5. *Muscle tightness*. Muscles that are contracted or shortened can be observed as prominent tissues; for instance, the levator scapulae muscles or the upper fibres of the trapezium. The muscles involved with posture, such as the back muscles, the hamstrings, quadratus group and those of the calf, are very susceptible to tightness.

6. *Atrophied muscles*. These are identified as areas where the muscle bulk is smaller compared to the opposite side of the body. For example, the infraspinatus muscle can be atrophied and observed as a flattened tissue overlying the scapula. The serratus anterior muscle, if weak or atrophied, causes 'winging' of the scapula.

7. *Hypertrophied (overdeveloped) muscles*. Muscles that appear to be bigger when compared to the opposite side are said to be hypertrophied— for example, the right leg muscles of a right-footed footballer.

8. *Genu valgum and genu varum*. In the standing posture, the abnormalities of genu valgum of the lower limbs (knock-knees) or the opposite genu varum (bow-legs) can be easily observed. These do not necessarily affect the massage treatment, but they are worth noting.

9. *Foot mechanics*. A frequent disorder of foot mechanics is dropping of the medial arch. This can be seen as a functional flattening of the foot and a medial rotation of the tibia. One or both feet may also appear to be irregular in shape and position. In this category of malfunctions the feet do not support the body structure effectively and, as a result, imbalances can arise further up the body, particularly in the pelvis and the spine. Although uncommon, it is feasible for the root cause of a headache to be incorrect foot mechanics and not a problem of the cervical or thoracic spine.

Palpatory skills

It is reasonable to assume that palpatory skills are vital to any massage therapy. Competence and dexterity are required not only for the purpose of assessing the tissues but also for their manipulation. Palpation can be carried out without the use of massage oils or cream; this is indeed an excellent method for developing sensitivity in the hands. Observation and evaluation are then continued throughout the massage treatment, even with the tissues lubricated. A sensitive and confident touch is essential to palpatory skills. Having relaxed hands is an additional requirement, and helps to enhance their sensitivity. Palpation is carried out mostly with the pads of the fingers, as these zones are very responsive; however, the whole region of the hand is very often involved in the process of 'feeling' the tissues as well as applying the pressure. This two-way action, evaluating the tissues while exerting pressure, is the very crux of massage treatment. The depth of the palpation varies with the tissues being targeted; a light touch is needed for the superficial tissues while a slightly heavier pressure is applied for some of the viscera and deeper muscles. If abnormalities are palpated, it is imperative to establish whether the deviations are in the superficial fascia, the muscles, bones or an organ. Ascertaining the tissue layer helps to assess the probable changes; for example, a nodule in a muscle, scar tissue in the superficial fascia, a thickening of a bony surface, or compacted matter in the colon. This continual adjustment of the pressure to suit the state of the tissues is essential for all massage strokes.

The methodology and interpretation of soft tissue assessment are based on the principles of long-established massage and bodywork modus operandi such as neuromuscular technique and connective tissue massage. Mutual to most of these procedures are reflex pathways, hypersensitive reflex zones, nodules, trigger points and so forth. For those practising massage, bodywork and manipulative therapies these somatic dysfunctions are vital to the assessment of musculoskeletal integrity. For this reason, the rationalization of the tissue changes, as well as the assessment procedures, are included in this section and again in later chapters. Connective tissue massage, for instance, is described later in this chapter as one of the diagnostic methods of palpatory skills. Neuromuscular technique, on the other hand, while being another method of soft tissue assessment, is introduced here and included again in the chapter on massage and bodywork techniques (Chapter 2). Information and guidance on examination and palpatory skills is therefore offered throughout the book.

Observing and palpating the skin

On observing and palpating the tissues, certain blemishes and irregularities may be found on the skin. Some of these may be of a questionable nature, such as irregular or bleeding warts, in which case massage to the affected area is avoided. It may also be necessary to draw patients' attention to these changes so that they can seek the appropriate treatment. Massage is also contraindicated if there are any contagious diseases, for instance herpes zoster (shingles). As a further precautionary measure massage is not carried out on any area where the skin is lacerated, owing to the possibility of a blood-borne infection such as AIDS. Most other types of blemishes are not contraindications, provided the massage itself does not cause any discomfort. A number of the abnormalities of the skin and superficial tissues are listed here, and any such findings should be recorded in the case history sheet and, if necessary, their progress closely monitored.

1. *Skin colour.* The colour of the skin can undergo some changes in certain conditions. Examples of colour changes include:

- Redness, which is associated with increased circulation, inflammation or an excessive intake of alcohol (red face).

- A cherry red colour, which is related to carbon monoxide poisoning (not commonly seen).
- Cyanosis (bluish colour), which is caused by a reduced haemoglobin or oxygen in the blood, and is also a sign of asthma, pulmonary disease such as tuberculosis, emphysema and whooping cough.
- Yellowing, which follows the condition of jaundice but is also related to an increase in carotenoid pigments, toxicity and renal insufficiency (uraemia).
- Brownish-yellow spots (liver spots), which can be noted in pregnancy, goitre, and in uterine or liver malignancies.

2. *Dryness.* One of the signs of hypothyroidism is dry skin, which is most common on the face but can also be widespread. In some areas the skin can also feel rough. Dry skin is also indicative of kidney problems, e.g. uraemia, and diabetes.

3. *Clamminess.* The skin may feel clammy or damp on palpation. This can be related to simple heat, anxiety or the elimination of toxins.

4. *Decreased mobility.* A common cause of reduced mobility in the superficial tissues is oedema. The tissue area is congested with fluid; it has an unyielding feel to it and will not return rapidly to normal after being prodded (decreased turgor). Changes in elasticity are discussed below.

5. *Oiliness.* Acne is commonly found in the face and back; the usual appearance is of pustules filled with pus.

6. *Lesions.* A vesicle is a small sac or blister of up to 0.5 cm in diameter. It is filled with serous fluid and may indicate herpes simplex.

7. *Rash.* A rash refers to redness in an area of skin, and can have a number of causes. For instance, a rash across the nose and cheeks is a sign of systemic lupus erythematosus.

8. *Petechiae.* These are small purplish haemorrhagic spots on the skin which appear in certain severe fevers. They may also be caused by abnormalities of blood-clotting mechanisms as can occur with some people taking drugs (for example, in the treatment of thrombosis).

9. *Ecchymosis.* A form of macula appearing in large irregularly-formed haemorrhagic areas of

the skin. The colour is blue–black and in most cases changes to greenish–brown or yellow. It is caused by haemorrhage of blood into the skin or mucus membranes.

10. *Warts and moles*. A non-healing sore, a thickening lump or an obvious change in a wart or a mole may indicate a tumour or cancer of the superficial tissues.

11. *Scales*. Flaking (exfoliation) of the epidermis occurs in psoriasis or dry skin. Red patches accompany the flaking in psoriasis which, although common in the head and elbows, can also be found on the back.

12. *Papules*. A papule is described as a tiny red elevated area of the skin of up to 0.5 cm in diameter. It is generally solid and ill-defined, and is indicative of eczema, measles, smallpox or more serious conditions like syphilis.

13. *Nodules*. (See below.)

14. *Elasticity and friction resistance*. Palpation of the skin can reveal changes that relate to the somatic dysfunction caused by stressors. Connections between the peripheral tissues, the common nerve trunks and the autonomic reflexes affect sweat gland secretions and, in turn, the water content of the epidermis. Increased epidermal hydration can lead to friction resistance or 'skin drag' when a finger is run over the skin surface, whereas profuse sweating will naturally render the skin surface very slippery. The skin elasticity is also reduced as a result of the reflex activity and, when comparing one region to another, the skin is found to be less mobile. The connection is made either by pushing the skin with one finger or by lifting it and rolling it between the fingers and thumb.

Palpation for tissue temperature

1. *Heat*. A local rise in temperature indicates underlying inflammation, mostly in the acute stage. The cause of the inflammation may be an organ malfunction, such as a kidney infection, or it may be associated with tissue damage, for instance a muscle strain or fibrosis. An increase in tissue temperature that is more systemic may be related to fever or raised blood pressure.

2. *Cold*. A local drop in temperature is associated with reduced circulation to the tissues. In most cases this is only transient, as can be observed in the hands and feet. It may, however, also be chronic, where the reduced blood supply has led to fibrotic changes in the tissues. Systemic coolness could indicate impaired circulation, mostly associated with a weak heart in old age. Cold feet and difficulty in getting warm in bed may be associated with problems of the bladder.

Somatic dysfunction

Changes in the tissues can occur when the body is subjected to stressors, and these may be chemical, mechanical or emotional (see Chapter 3). A typical stressor is an organ that is malfunctioning. As a result of these stressors the peripheral tissues undergo changes which can be observed and palpated; they include congestion, muscle spasm, adhesions and oedema (Box 1.3). Such abnormalities or dysfunctions of the peripheral tissues will themselves act as stressors and create further imbalances.

An organ that is malfunctioning can have two effects on the peripheral tissues:

1. A direct referred pain, usually felt in a dermatome, myotome or bony tissue which is supplied by the same nerve root as that of the malfunctioning organ. The pain is generally present without any palpation; for example, the

---

Box 1.3 Examples of somatic dysfunction in reflex zone areas

- Muscle spasm
- Contractures in the fascia or muscles
- Fibrotic tissue
- Reduced skin elasticity accompanied by 'skin drag'
- Sweating
- Increased or reduced skin temperature
- Nodules
- Hypersensitivity
- Adhesions
- Congestion
- Oedema
- Hypotonic states
- Atrophy
- Bony thickening

painful abdomen associated with appendicitis (Fig. 1.1).

2. Indirect tissue changes in the periphery (reflex zones). Changes in the somatic tissue are brought about by an indirect connection to the nerve supply of the malfunctioning organ, or by an impaired circulation to the tissues (see Chapter 3). As a result, the somatic connective

tissues undergo changes such as tightness, congestion and thickening, and they are generally a source of pain on palpation. This is invariably worse with movement or contraction of a muscle. A dysfunctional visceral organ will often lead to a painful stimulus, but this is not always felt in the organ itself. Through the reflex mechanisms, the malfunction creates changes in the

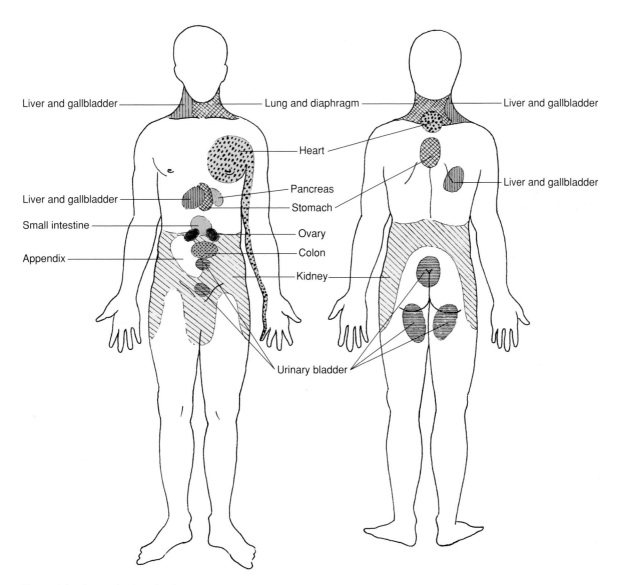

Figure 1.1   Areas of referred pain.

myotomes, leading to muscle spasms, and also in the dermatomes, causing hyperaesthesia of the overlying superficial tissues. It has been documented that this relationship was established by Sir James MacKenzie in the early 1900s (Fig. 1.2). Reflex zones are also considered in neuromuscular technique and connective tissue massage.

The areas of direct referred pain and those of tissue changes sometimes coincide. Furthermore, an area of tissue change related to one organ (for example, the stomach) can overlap another area connected to a different organ (such as the heart). It follows that, in some cases, it is difficult to con-

clude precisely which organ is mostly at fault. The case history should, however, provide sufficient information regarding the likely condition, and a specific assessment can also be made of those zone areas that are commonly connected to a particular disorder.

Nodules

A nodule is a single node or an aggregation of cells, e.g. a lymph nodule (or node), which is made up of densely packed lymphocytes.

Sometimes nodules are prominent enough to be seen as lumpy areas, for instance in the groin.

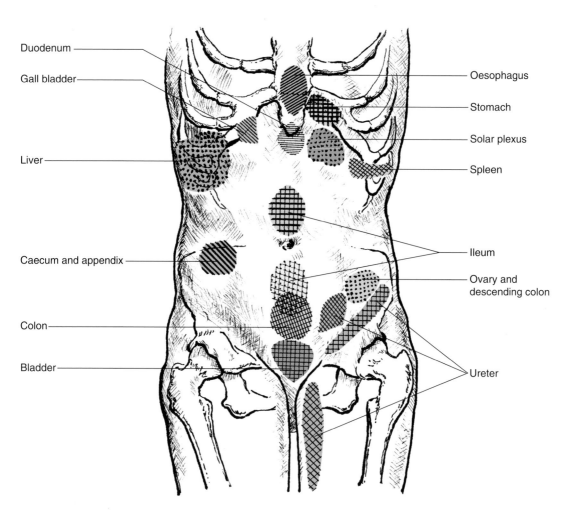

Figure 1.2 Reflex zones of the abdomen (after MacKenzie, 1923).

The term is also used to describe a 'knot' or tightness in a muscle (see Palpation of muscles) or in the superficial or deep fascia. A collection of fat cells is sometimes called a fatty nodule. Some authors refer to nodular changes in the skin, muscle, tendons and periosteum as 'trigger points'. The association is made because nodules that become chronic can refer pain to another region and are therefore known as 'trigger points'.

Nodules are hardened areas or indurations that can be observed on palpation of the superficial muscles and surrounding fascia. Their development is activated by stressors acting on the body (see Chapter 3). Somatic injury, visceral dysfunction or pathology, and infection are typical stressors which cause somatic sensory impulses to the central nervous system. A reflex vasospasm occurs in the corresponding somatic tissue (Travell and Simons, 1983). In addition, there is increased tissue tension and hypertonicity of muscles. These tissue changes are in themselves stressors and will cause further reflex activity and chemical imbalances. The outcome is the formation of nodules or trigger points with chronic ischaemia, chemical imbalances and pain sensations.

These hypersensitive zones take the form of a collection of fat cells in a roughly laid layer of connective tissue, together with fibrin and some elastic fibres. Some nodules are described as 'fatty nodules', as they contain mostly fat globules and are softer when palpated; these are generally found in 'endomorphs' (persons with stocky type structure). Hypersensitive zones can, in most cases, be reduced by the pressure of massage, which is increased in gentle stages.

Neuromuscular technique

The most significant development in the assessment methodology of soft tissues is perhaps neuromuscular technique (NMT). It has a fascinating history which is well presented in Leon Chaitow's book *Modern Neuromuscular Techniques* (Chaitow, 1996a). NMT was introduced and developed in Europe by Stanley Lief and Boris Chaitow, and has proved to be a very effective diagnostic tool in the assessment and treatment of soft tissue lesions (somatic dysfunctions), e.g. congestions of local connective tissues, adhesions, nodules, hypersensitive zones and changes in muscle tone. NMT is increasingly being used in conjunction with other soft tissue manipulative methods as well as massage. It is therefore one of the fundamental methods with which the massage therapist may wish to be familiar and, accordingly, for this reason it is incorporated with the massage techniques.

In its simplest form NMT is applied with the thumb, which is moved over the tissues to be assessed (Fig. 1.3). The fingers are spread and they support the weight of the hand. While the fingers remain stationary and using minimal lubrication the thumb is moved towards the fingertips. The short stroke applied with the thumb covers an area of about 5–8 cm (2–3 inches) and is completed in 4–5 seconds. Pressure with the thumb is variable, adjusting to the feel and resistance of the tissues being addressed. For the purpose of assessment pressure is minimal, at least initially, and may be increased for deeper palpation. Any force is exerted through the straight arm and the practitioner's own body weight is used to add force behind the movement. To facilitate the palpation and assessment of the tissues it is vital that the thumb, fingers and, indeed, the whole hand are relaxed and not held in a 'tense' posture. Contact is made with the very tip, or with the lateral or medial aspect of the tip of the thumb. Using such a small area of the thumb allows for a more specific and precise 'reading' of

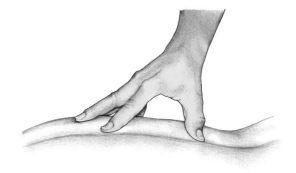

Figure 1.3   Position of the thumb and fingers for the neuromuscular technique.

the tissues. For a more general assessment the whole pad of the thumb may be employed; very likely this would be the initial choice of the novice practitioner. With a little practice the various tissue structures can be targeted more specifically as the contact with the thumb becomes more precise.

Palpation of the subcutaneous fascia

Beneath the skin there is the subcutaneous fascia and the first layer of deep fascia. The easiest tissue to palpate is the subcutaneous fascia, with its content of fat and fluid. The deeper fascia is indistinguishable, as it is sandwiched between the subcutaneous fascia and the uppermost muscle layer. The subcutaneous fascia is the site for a number of changes that can give rise to symptoms or to tenderness on palpation. Disorders may include:

1. Excessive fat, which is easily detectable.
2. Fatty nodules (a small area of fat encapsulated in soft tissue)—these can undergo structural changes and become a tumour or lipoma.
3. Tumours.
4. Hardening of the fascia.
5. Flaccid tissue associated with old age or a weak constitution.
6. Cellulite.
7. Ischaemia and congestion of tissues caused by a reduced blood supply; for example, oedematous tissue.
8. Adhesions, which are fibrous infiltrations into the tissues. They are caused by the laying down of collagen fibres in a very similar way to the process of fibrosis.

Hypersensitivity

Palpation of the tissues can elicit tenderness or pain, which may arise from dysfunction of either a local structure or a distant organ. Pain caused by a local malfunction tends to increase considerably on palpation of the tissues, even with minimal pressure, whereas pain that is referred tends

to increase only in proportion to the pressure applied. The hypersensitivity in the superficial tissues can therefore have a number of causative factors:

1. Hypersensitivity on palpation may be because of irritation or inflammation of a nerve. As a result, the sensory nerve endings in the peripheral tissue become hypersensitive; for example, paraesthesia from a trapped nerve in the spine.
2. It may also be a referred pain from malfunction of a distant organ, such as a kidney infection.
3. Another causative factor that is both local and partly systemic is a viral infection, such as that of herpes zoster (shingles).
4. Local and superficial irritation of the tissues may be caused by a chemical irritant or an allergen.

Connective tissue massage (CTM)

Connective tissue massage has its place somewhere between the 'more traditional' massage and the 'bodywork' techniques. Although it is termed as 'massage' it is carried out mostly without any lubrication and therefore could easily be classified under soft tissue techniques. The concepts of CTM, however, apply to both massage and bodywork techniques; indeed, several other methods are based on the same principle. The concept of connective tissue massage was based on the principles of reflex processes that were pioneered by Sir James MacKenzie (MacKenzie, 1923). The development of CTM was carried out by Elizabeth Dicke, a German physiotherapist who developed the *Meine Bindegewebsmassage* (Dicke, 1953; 1956) and founded her school in Uberlingen, West Germany, and later on by Maria Ebner in the UK and the USA. Alongside the development of the *Meine Bindegewebsmassage* were those carried out by Head (an English neurologist), who also showed changes in well-defined areas of the body surface, referred to as 'Head's Zones' and which related to malfunction of specific organs. Whereas Head pointed out changes in the skin, MacKenzie

(MacKenzie, 1923 as cited in Tappan, 1988) concentrated on changes in the muscle tone and hypersensitivity in areas sharing the same root supply with pathologically affected organs.

The hypothesis for CTM and other treatment approaches such as NMT (Chaitow, 1996a) is based on the connection between the somatic tissues and organs, glands, etc. through the viscerosomatic and other nerve pathways (described in Chapter 3). Maria Ebner, in her book *Connective Tissue Massage* (1962) describes the connections as:

The close interrelation between the somatic, autonomic and endocrine systems makes it impossible for pathological changes to take place in any one structure without causing adaptive changes in other structures.

Diseased or stressed organs, as well as dysfunction of the musculoskeletal system, are therefore seen as causing somatic changes in the fascia layers and muscles through viscerosomatic activity. Changes can be observed and palpated on the back, abdomen and in other regions of the body. Ebner's reflex zones offer a good example of changes in the somatic tissues of the back and their corresponding organs (Fig. 1.4). Some techniques assess and treat one or two regions, others are applied more systematically. CTM is often applied primarily to the tissues of the back even though the method is equally suitable for other areas. Sir James MacKenzie concluded that a strong relationship exists between the walls of the abdomen and the internal abdominal organs (MacKenzie, 1909 as mentioned in Chaitow, 1996a). The tissue changes include tightness in the superficial fascia layers, hypersensitive zones, trigger points, muscle wasting or hypertonicity (Box 1.3). Assessment and treatment of the somatic dysfunction can help normalize the related organs, viscera and other tissues.

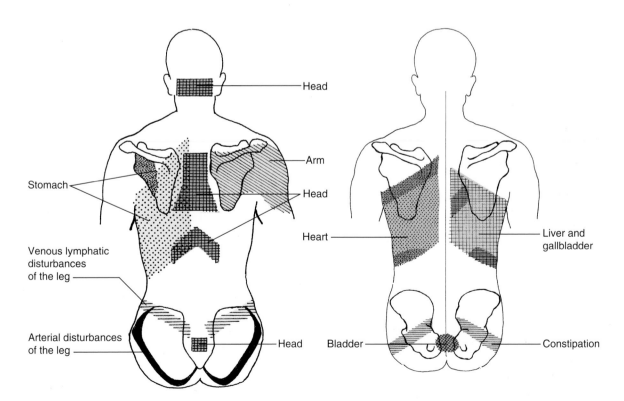

Figure 1.4   Reflex zones on the back (after Ebner, 1962).

CTM incorporates soft tissue manipulation and 'rolling' of the fascia layers (Fig. 1.5). The mechanical stimulation of the connective tissues is seen as a stimulus that is strong enough to elicit a nervous reflex. Stimulation of the somato-visceral and visceral cutaneous reflex pathways helps to harmonize the activity of autonomic nervous system (sympathetic and parasympathetic stimulation). This in turn helps to normalize endocrine responses and balance the circulation and reflex activity between organs, systems and tissues. The theory and methods of CTM are distinct and well established. It is therefore not the intention here to instruct the reader in the full and extensive practice of CTM but to illustrate the viscerosomatic connections in the assessment of somatic dysfunction.

Pain

Pain may be elicited on palpation of the superficial tissues, and the discomfort can be of variable intensity, sharpness, etc. It may be due to several factors.

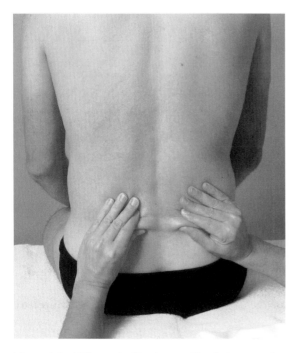

Figure 1.5 Lifting and rolling layers of fascia in connective tissue massage.

1. Cellulite tissue contains hard fibrotic fibres, and excessive compression of these fibres can irritate the pain receptors in the subcutaneous fascia and underlying structures.

2. Oedema causes an increase of pressure within the interstitial tissues, and an excessive build-up of fluid stimulates the nerve receptors and elicits pain. Palpation or heavy massage on an oedematous area can have a similar effect.

3. Stressors or trauma can create fibrotic changes in the superficial layers (fascia or muscles), and pain can be elicited if these hard tissues are pressed against the underlying structures during palpation or massage.

4. Nodules (see also Palpation of muscles). These are small areas of hardened tissue found mostly in the superficial fibres or fascia of the muscles. They are initially tender to palpation, but are generally yielding and become less painful as the massage progresses.

5. Lymph nodes that are overactive or chronically congested give rise to pain on palpation. Common sites are in the intercostal, groin, axillary and breast tissues.

Palpation of muscles and associated fascia

1. *Heat*. Heat within the muscle tissue can be related to overuse or to a strain of the fibres. If either condition is chronic it may cause the onset of fibrosis. In this process, the continued strain on the muscle fibres or the associated fascia leads to inflammation and the laying down of fibrotic tissue.

2. *Aches and soreness*. Aches and soreness on palpation are indicative of increased metabolites in an overworked muscle. The condition is invariably exacerbated by congestion and ischaemia.

3. *Muscle spasm and tenderness*. These are synonymous with muscle tightness and muscle stiffness, and pertain to localized contractions of the muscle bundles, mostly acute. Sustained or chronic muscular activity can lead to hypomobility in the associated joints. Increased muscle tone is due to a number of causes, ranging from postural imbalances to strains and reflex responses from stressors such as organ or tissue malfunctions. This reaction is associated with the fight-

or-flight response and the general adaptation syndrome. Sustained muscle spasm leads to ischaemia, toxins and pain in the muscle.

- Tender and unyielding muscles can be indicative of emotional states such as anxiety.
- Mechanical disorders may give rise to tenderness and tightness in the muscles; e.g. misalignments of the spine can bring about muscle contraction in an attempt to correct the misalignment, and the tenderness may result from irritation of the nerves associated with the misalignment.
- Palpation of a strained muscle, particularly in the lumbar area, will invariably elicit pain.
- Malfunction of an organ can refer pain to the superficial tissues and cause muscle contractions; e.g. appendicitis causes tenderness and tightness in the abdominal muscles.

4. *Muscle contracture.* A muscle and its surrounding fascia can become contracted from a chronic spasm of the same muscle. If a muscle spasm, from whatever cause, is prolonged to more than a few weeks it changes to a chronic state with the laying down of fibrotic fibres. On palpation the muscle feels very tight and decreased in length. The thickening and shortening occurs mostly in the fascia, that is, the epimysium (covering the muscle), the perimysium (covering the muscle bundles) or the endomysium (covering the muscle cells). An overall shortening of the muscle fibres and fascia occurs and this is not easily reversible, if at all. Paralysis creates a similar state.

5. *Fibrotic changes.* Fibrotic states occur in muscles which are subject to repetitive strain or microtrauma. Collagen fibres are laid down along the muscle fibres and the fascia layers during the repair mechanism and as a protective measure. A case in point is postural imbalances, which cause some muscles to be overworked, e.g. the paravertebral muscles. On palpation the segment of muscle involved feels 'ropey' and does not yield much when stretched across its fibres. Contracture of a muscle is often accompanied by some degree of fibrotic change.

6. *Nodules* (*hypersensitive zones*). See pages 16 and 17.

Trigger points

Nodules that become chronic can themselves develop into trigger points. These act as stressors to the body and can spontaneously cause irritation, pain or sensation in another region referred to as the 'target area'. Trigger points and their target areas share the same nerve pathway and are additionally connected via the autonomic nervous system (see Chapter 3). Trigger points can be 'active' and therefore cause reflex activity without being palpated. The reflex effects and malfunctions that are experienced in a region distant from the trigger point include the following:

- Hypersensitivity to pressure.
- Spasm, weakness or trembling of voluntary muscles.
- Hypertonicity or hypotonus of involuntary muscles affecting mostly the blood vessels, the internal organs and glands. Manifestations of these changes in the involuntary muscles are seen, for instance, as altered levels of gland secretions in the eye, mouth and digestive tract and as disturbances in the process of elimination. Such disorders can themselves lead to other dysfunctions in the peripheral tissues.

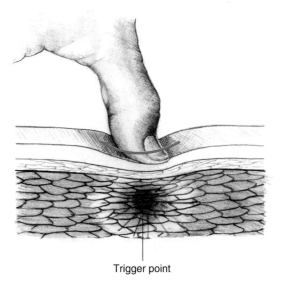

Trigger point

Figure 1.6 Assessment of hypersensitive nodular changes and trigger points.

A trigger point can be assessed and located using either one or more fingertips or the thumb. The technique with the thumb is that of NMT so that the tip or pad is used to palpate the tissues (Fig. 1.6). Short strokes are applied with the thumb to assess the tissues for nodular changes and trigger points. Sometimes trigger points are dormant and will only cause a sensation, mostly of pain, when pressure is applied or when the tissues in which they are located are manipulated. Trigger points are most commonly found in 'shortened' muscles, but they can also be located in any tissue (the treatment for trigger points is described in Chapter 2). Examples of trigger points include:

- Trigger point: splenius capitis, below the mastoid process. Target area: pain in the lateral parietal area of the head (Fig. 1.7).
- Trigger point: inferior aspect of the iliac crest, in the medial origin of the gluteus medius muscle.Target area: pain in the region of the glutei muscles.

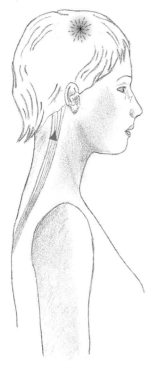

Figure 1.7 Trigger point in the upper end of the splenius capitis muscle, below the mastoid process. The target pain is in the lateral parietal area of the head.

In some situations, scar tissue may function as a trigger point. If it is undetected and untreated it may give rise to reflex symptoms in other regions. These changes can be located in connective tissue or indeed in organs, and can therefore be associated with conditions that are either chronic or not responding to treatment. The scar tissue area is palpated for adhesions and for hypersensitive zones that are exacerbated when the skin is stretched.

Palpation of the skeletal tissue

1. *Tenderness*. Tenderness may be elicited on palpation of a bony surface, and could be caused by relatively minor causes such as bruising of the bone or a hairline fracture. Both are mostly related to trauma. Causes of a more serious nature, such as osteoporosis, are less common but worth bearing in mind.

2. *Abnormality*. Observation or palpation may reveal an abnormal bone line or surface. The abnormality may be associated with hypertrophy of the bone following a fracture or with arthritic changes.

Palpation of joints

1. *Tenderness*. Simple palpation or articulation of a joint can indicate some common conditions. For instance, pain that is elicited on passive articulation of the hip can reveal arthritic changes.

2. *Heat*. Heat in a joint is easily palpated and indicates inflammation, mostly related to conditions such as rheumatoid arthritis. Trauma may also create heat within the joint.

3. *Vertebral column*. A gentle pressure can be applied to the side of the spinous processes of the spine. If this manoeuvre brings about pain, it could indicate some disorder with the mechanics of the vertebral column (see Chapter 5).

Prudence and ethics

Patients' expectations

Some patients may not have a full appreciation of their ailment, and consequently expect the therapist to carry out a diagnosis and treatment. Furthermore, they may be unaware of the fact that massage, although beneficial, does not offer an 'instant cure' for all conditions, and that the massage therapist is not the person to make a diagnosis. This situation requires the practitioner to clarify the role of massage to the patient. It also highlights the necessity for the massage practitioner to be well prepared, with knowledge on assessment, indications, contraindications, acute and chronic conditions and the practice of referral.

Referrals

On rare occasions the therapist may conclude that the patient would benefit from an examination by a doctor or a specialist consultant. Any such advice is passed on with consideration to the patient's own sensitivity, and with the understanding that the patient may choose to do otherwise. If the patient is in agreement the therapist can prepare a report of the presenting symptoms, observations and any treatments given to date, and forward this to the patient's doctor or consultant.

Care of the patient during the treatment

It is vital that the patient is in a comfortable position, whether lying down on the treatment table or sitting in a chair. Cushions can be used to support the back, the knees and the feet. When the patient is lying prone, a cushion or folded towel is placed underneath the abdomen; this prevents unnecessary hollowing of the back and is of particular importance if the patient has a lordotic lumbar spine. Towels can be used to cover those regions of the body that are not being massaged; this in itself is a requisite of ethical correctness. The covers are also needed to preserve body heat and thereby prevent involuntary muscle contractions.

The patient–therapist relationship

An essential dynamic of massage therapy, as in any other therapy, centres on the relationship between the patient and the therapist. In the ideal situation this rapport is built on a professional foundation, and does not verge on the extremes of being either too businesslike or too familiar. However, finding and maintaining the appropriate degree of closeness is a challenge for the therapist and may require constant adjustment.

Without any doubt it is vital for the therapist to show empathy with patients; this implies understanding their feelings as well as offering comfort and consolation. While patients will undoubtedly appreciate this compassion, they may also feel safe and comfortable enough to want to share certain personal feelings with the massage therapist. It is fundamental, however, that the therapist is in control of the situation and is explicit about which emotional issues he or she can, or wants to, deal with. Some emotional issues can be overwhelming to an untrained therapist. Such a situation is best avoided and, to this end, a patient may be encouraged to seek help from a professional counsellor. Furthermore, any attempt to handle delicate emotional matters, unless fully trained, is a disservice by the massage therapist. An example of a difficult and sensitive situation is transference, when a person transfers emotions from the past to the present. Undoubtedly this is a negative action, albeit an unconscious one, and feelings and expectations a person may have had in previous relationships are negatively transferred to present interactions with people. Clients may unwittingly transfer emotions such as anger, love or power onto the therapist because, in their mind, the practitioner represents someone from the past. This may be done subtly or in a more overt way, but in any case the therapist becomes the recipient of these undeserved feelings. The situation can lead to problems not only for the therapist but also for the patient, who is unable to deal with these emotions; hence the need for professional counselling.

Safeguards for the massage therapist

It is perhaps superfluous to advise the massage therapist to safeguard him or herself against the danger of contracting an infectious disease from the patient. It is none the less sufficiently important to warrant a reminder. The importance of obtaining and updating information about certain diseases cannot be stressed enough. One example is hepatitis A, B, C, D and E. Each type of this condition is infective and the person is likely to be a carrier. Massage in this situation, if carried out at all, must be administered with extreme care and preferably with the patient dressed or in their underclothes. Any towels used during the massage are disinfected and the hands washed thoroughly before and after the treatment. Hepatitis that is related to drug or alcohol abuse is not usually infective and massage should not require any precautions. However, approval of the patient's doctor is always advisable prior to any treatment. Viral infections that affect the skin are also contagious and must be avoided. Herpes simplex types I and II can affect the genitalia, while herpes simplex type I affects mostly the regions above the waist. Herpes zoster is another infectious viral condition affecting spinal or cranial nerves and causing chickenpox. Massage is therefore best avoided during the acute stages of these conditions.

2

The massage techniques

THE ELEMENTS OF MASSAGE TECHNIQUES

Introduction

In its modern history, the terminology which describes the massage movements is derived from the English and French languages. Terms such as *effleurage, petrissage, massage à friction* and *tapotement* are merged with words like rubbing, shaking and vibration. Whilst the theory remains more or less constant, variations and additions to these basic techniques have been developed to facilitate easy application, deep pressure and specific treatment. A further expansion has been the inclusion of certain aspects of 'bodywork', such as neuromuscular movements and treatment of trigger points, into the massage work. As a result of this progress a great number of names for the massage techniques have emerged and, to minimize the confusion, the massage movements in this book have been classified into the seven categories that are listed here. It is important to emphasize at this point that the classification of massage movements varies from one therapy approach to another. For example, what is referred to as petrissage in physiotherapy may be listed as kneading in massage teaching. The category of massage techniques depicted in this book is therefore only one interpretation. A description of the basic methods is also presented in this chapter. Further techniques, together with details of their effects and application, are included in subsequent chapters.

Massage techniques fall under one of the following main headings (see also Table 2.1):

1. Effleurage or stroking techniques
2. Compression movements
3. Lymphatic massage movements
4. Percussive strokes
5. Friction techniques
6. Vibration and shaking movements

7. Bodywork techniques.

The postures in massage

Postural awareness

It is a common mistake to assume that an adequate massage requires the therapist to apply hard, strong and heavy strokes, or that powerful

Table 2.1 Category of massage techniques

Stroking movements	
• Light stroking effleurage	
• Deep stroking effleurage	
• Examples	Palm effleurage
	Forearm effleurage
	Thumb effleurage
	Effleurage *du poing* (fist effleurage)
	Fingertip effleurage

Lymph massage movements	
• Effleurage	Very light and slow stroking
• Intermittent pressure	Gentle on-and-off pressure combined with a stretch

Compression movements	
• Kneading	Compression with the thenar/hypothenar eminences or the palm of the hand
	Compression combined with a rolling and stretching action
• Petrissage	Stretching, lifting and twisting movement using both hands
	Circular compression movements using the pads of fingers

Percussion movements	
• Hacking	Fingers open and straight fingers
	Fingers together and curled
• Pounding	Palmar side of the fisted hand
• Cupping	Cupped hand
• Flicking	A flicking action with the fingers

Friction methods	
• Cross-fibre friction	
• Circular friction	
• Parallel friction—along line of fibres	

Vibration techniques	
• Vertical oscillation	

Bodywork techniques	
• Neuromuscular movement	
• Trigger point pressure	
• Muscle energy technique	Post-isometric relaxation
• Passive stretching	
• Soft tissue manipulation	
• Joint mobilization	

hands and considerable body strength are necessary. The most significant requisite for an effective massage is a good technique, which is applied with the minimum of effort. In the majority of massage movements the therapist's stance is an essential aspect of the technique. The position of the therapist in relation to the treatment table and the patient influences the efficacy and flow of the stroke and, consequently, the therapist's posture has to be assumed before the hands are placed on the recipient's body. Moreover, appraisal of the body's stance has to be maintained throughout the movement. Postural awareness is therefore a combination of body position, body weight and direction of pressure. These components can be adapted to suit the therapist's own structure, the height and width of the treatment table, and the therapist's own preferred massage methods.

The therapist's body weight is used to apply pressure to the massage movement. To this end, adjustments in the posture are made before each movement so that a comfortable and practical stance is taken. This position should enable the therapist to shift the body weight backwards and forwards, or from side to side. It should also allow for a coordinated action between the body and the hands during the massage movement. A good posture is therefore one in which the therapist feels well grounded, whilst having the freedom to move (Box 2.1).

Box 2.1 Benefits of a correct posture for the practitioner

- The direction, pressure and rhythm of the movement are easily controlled
- Each technique is carried out with very little energy expenditure
- Mechanical stress on the therapist's own body is avoided
- The hands are relaxed, applying little or no pressure
- The breathing pattern is deep and effortless
- Relaxation extends to the whole body and subsequently to the recipient
- The therapist's own 'chakra' or energy source is focused
- The therapist is 'well grounded' throughout the treatment

Several body postures are described in this section and are depicted again with the massage movements in later chapters. Readers can use the postures as illustrated, or make any necessary adjustments to suit their own preferences. Comfort and ease of movement are very significant if mechanical stress on the body is to be avoided and, to this end, one or two postures are described with the practitioner leaning against the treatment table. This arrangement is safe and appropriate, provided it is carried out with the right intention and does not infringe upon any professional or ethical codes. On a similar note, there may be a need (albeit only occasionally) for the practitioner to sit on the edge of the treatment table. This is also professionally acceptable as long as adherence to ethical codes is maintained.

Lunging posture

This posture facilitates long massage strokes, for instance along the length of the patient's lower limb, without any forward bending of the trunk. It can be described as a mid-upright position, with the legs set apart as in the 'lunging' pose of fencing. The front foot is in line with the treatment table whilst the back foot is rotated laterally. Another adjustment is for the practitioner to be in a position slightly away from the treatment table or leaning against it, depending on the massage movement being applied. As the front knee is flexed, the body moves forward and the weight is shifted to the front foot. As the knee extends and straightens, the body moves backward and the weight is shifted to the back foot. During the forward movement the back leg remains locked straight; as the body moves backward it can flex at the knee or remain in the same position. The back is more or less upright throughout the movement. In this posture, the pressure is applied through the arms and onto the hands. The arms are either straight or slightly flexed at the elbow (Fig. 2.1).

Lunging posture with the elbow flexed

This posture is similar to the previous lunging posture, but only one hand is used to apply the

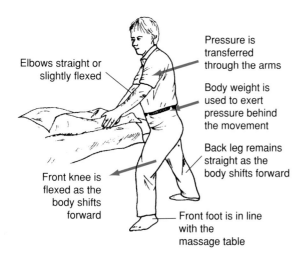

Figure 2.1 Lunging posture—the arms are held away from the body and both hands apply the stroke.

massage stroke and the elbow is held in a different position. The posture can be utilized to increase the body weight behind the massage movement and on certain regions of the body. For the purpose of adding pressure, the more lateral elbow is placed on the abdomen or pelvis whilst the wrist remains straight without any abduction or adduction. As the body moves forward, pressure is applied through the forearm onto the hand. It is then reduced when the body moves back and the weight is shifted to the back

foot. This position is taken up for the deep effleurage movement to the back when the patient is lying on one side (Fig. 2.2).

T'ai chi posture

The stance in this posture is similar to that of a t'ai chi pose or a plié in ballet. For ease of movement, the therapist stands at a slight distance away from the treatment table whilst parallel to it. With the back held upright, the body weight is shifted from one leg to the other, moving from side to side. For a number of massage movements the posture is used in a stationary position or with only a slight shift to the side. A gentle rotation of the trunk adds pressure through the arm, for instance in a criss-cross effleurage to the patient's back. This manoeuvre is, however, marginal, and is performed with the back still in the upright position. Rotating the trunk can similarly exert a gentle pulling action with the arm, and this is used to exert pressure from the front of the massage movement (Fig. 2.3).

Upright posture

In this posture, the practitioner stands with the back straight and the feet together or slightly apart. The body is parallel to the treatment table and invariably rests against it. Whilst maintain-

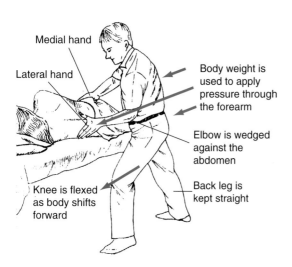

Figure 2.2 Variation of the lunging posture—the elbow is flexed and the massage applied with one hand.

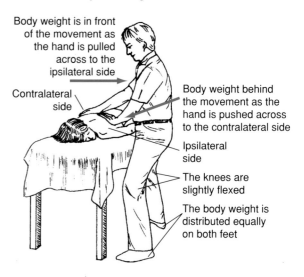

Figure 2.3 T'ai chi posture—the back is straight and the knees slightly flexed.

ing a straight back, the therapist can lean forward slightly by tilting the pelvis and without tensing the back muscles. This adjustment is often necessary when massaging the contralateral side of the patient. It also helps to add weight behind the movement. Massage to the patient's contralateral scapula is a typical stroke when this posture is used. It is also engaged with the practitioner facing in the direction of the patient's head rather than across the body. For some techniques the practitioner takes up this upright posture whilst standing at the foot end or the head end of the treatment table (Fig. 2.4).

To-and-fro posture

For the to-and-fro posture, the therapist stands away from the treatment table with the feet placed one behind the other. The position of the feet is determined by how much weight is necessary for the massage movement, and by what is a comfortable position for the therapist. Having the feet farther apart allows for more body weight to be transferred through the arms. Body movement in this posture is forwards and backwards (to-and-fro). Forward movement is performed as the body weight is shifted onto the

front foot. At the same time, the heel of the back foot is raised slightly to elevate the body and alter its centre of gravity. As a result the body tilts forward, which exerts pressure through one or both arms. Raising the heel adds more body weight to the movement. To accomplish this transference of weight, the arms are held in a straight position or flexed slightly at the elbow. Although the back is more or less straight, some forward bending is inevitable; this should, however, be kept to a minimum. Pressure through the arms is released as the body shifts backward, and the heel of the back foot is lowered to the floor. The to-and-fro posture is used to apply strokes from the head end of the massage treatment couch (Fig. 2.5), or to the contralateral side of the body (Fig. 2.6).

Leaning posture

Before leaning forward, the therapist takes up a position at a slight distance from the treatment table. The legs are parallel to each other and the feet wide apart; this stance provides a safe grounding and a stable base. As the body leans forward, pressure is transferred through the arms onto the hands. By standing at a slight distance away from the treatment table, the therapist can lean forward without too much

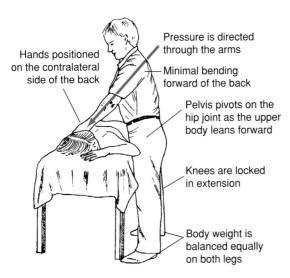

Hands positioned on the contralateral side of the back

Pressure is directed through the arms

Minimal bending forward of the back

Pelvis pivots on the hip joint as the upper body leans forward

Knees are locked in extension

Body weight is balanced equally on both legs

Figure 2.4 Upright posture—the knees are locked in extension, and there is minimal forward bending of the trunk.

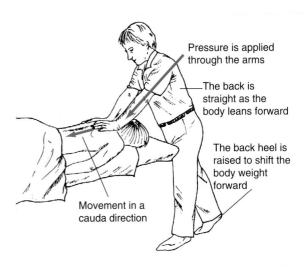

Pressure is applied through the arms

The back is straight as the body leans forward

The back heel is raised to shift the body weight forward

Movement in a cauda direction

Figure 2.5 To-and-fro posture—applied from the head end of the treatment table.

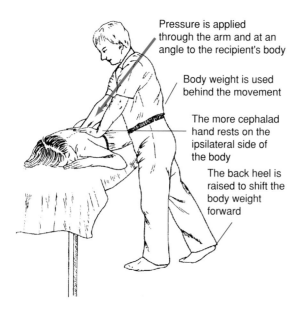

Pressure is applied through the arm and at an angle to the recipient's body

Body weight is used behind the movement

The more cephalad hand rests on the ipsilateral side of the body

The back heel is raised to shift the body weight forward

Figure 2.6 To-and-fro posture—the back heel is raised to shift the body weight forward.

bending of the back. The greater the distance, the more body weight is applied behind the movement and through the arms. Once the massage stroke is completed, the body shifts backward towards the upright position. The leaning posture is mostly used for applying massage movements from the head end of the treatment table (Fig. 2.7); it can also be used as an alternative to the to-and-fro posture.

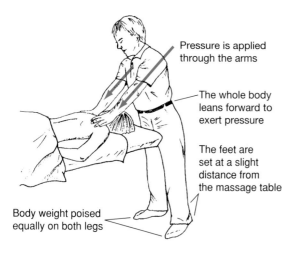

Pressure is applied through the arms

The whole body leans forward to exert pressure

The feet are set at a slight distance from the massage table

Body weight poised equally on both legs

Figure 2.7 Leaning posture—the whole body leans forward to apply pressure through the arms.

Sitting on the edge of the treatment table

Some massage techniques are easier to carry out while sitting on the edge of the treatment table. In this posture, however, the body weight is not so easily applied. The arrangement is very useful none the less, as it precludes excessive bending and twisting of the trunk. Sitting on the edge of the treatment table is counterbalanced by having one foot on the floor; this is also advisable for ethical reasons. For most massage movements in this position, one hand is used to apply the stroke whilst the other one stabilizes the recipient's body. This sitting posture is utilized, for example, when the patient is lying on one side (Fig. 2.8).

Additional components of the techniques

The use of body weight and pressure

A component of the massage movement is the angle at which the pressure is applied, and this is determined by the therapist's posture, as already discussed, and the direction of the body movements. The body weight is therefore used to apply pressure from different angles:

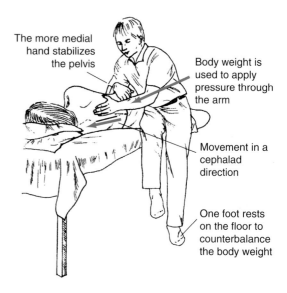

The more medial hand stabilizes the pelvis

Body weight is used to apply pressure through the arm

Movement in a cephalad direction

One foot rests on the floor to counterbalance the body weight

Figure 2.8 Some massage movements are best applied while sitting on the outer edge of the treatment table.

1. Body weight may be applied behind the movement, and pressure is exerted by applying the body weight more or less in line with the direction of the stroke (see Fig. 2.1).

2. Pressure may be applied at an angle to the recipient's body. In some movements, especially those on the back, the pressure is applied at an angle to the body surface. This is in addition to the force exerted by the body weight behind the movement (see Fig. 2.6).

3. Body weight is applied from in front of the movement. In one or two instances, the body weight is used to pull the hands towards the therapist's own body. This implies that any pressure applied to the tissues is being exerted by a pull rather than a push, and therefore from in front of the movement (see Fig. 2.3).

The correct use of the hands

The manner in which the hands are used is as relevant to the massage technique as the body posture. Any tension in the therapist's hands may reflect anxiety, which can easily be transferred to the recipient and eradicate any attempt to induce relaxation. Pressure for the massage stroke is predominantly exerted by the weight of the body and not with the hands, and muscle contractions of the hands are therefore minimized. Palpation and assessment of the tissues is likewise most effective when the hands are relaxed. In a similar manner, any changes in the tissues that may occur as a reaction to the massage technique are also easily detected when the hands are relaxed.

Particular attention is needed when using the thumbs. Extending the distal interphalangeal joint when applying pressure with the thumb exerts a great deal of stress on the joint itself and can lead to pain and degeneration. It is therefore advisable always to keep the thumb straight or in a slightly flexed position (see Fig. 2.10).

In some situations, especially during back massage, effleurage with the forearm is very effective and a good alternative to other effleurage techniques that are carried out with the palm of the hands, fists or thumbs. The health and condition of the therapist's own hands and, indeed, the whole body is of equal importance as the treatment being administered. It is also worth remembering that a massage treatment with heavy pressure, no matter how forceful, should not replace the patient's responsibility for exercises, change of lifestyle and so forth. The position or movements of the hand and wrist during a massage technique are described as flexion, extension, abduction and adduction. Although these are self-explanatory terms it is worth bearing in mind the directions of the deviation.

Pressure

At this stage it is appropriate to introduce the concept of the 'invitation' rule. In all soft tissue work the muscles, and indeed the recipient, cannot be forced to relax. Increasing the pressure therefore does not lead to deeper relaxation; it may in fact cause further spasms. Tranquillity is therefore best achieved by 'encouraging' the muscles, and the individual, to let go of tension. In turn, this is accomplished when the hands are relaxed and sensitive to responses from the tissues. Put another way, the therapist must not 'barge in' through the muscular wall but must wait to be 'invited' in as the tissues relax and yield to the pressure. By feeling the way through the tissues the sensitivity in the therapist's hands is allowed to develop, and invariably the therapist can reach a degree of skill where excessive pressure is always avoided. Furthermore, causing pain is almost anticipated and the pressure or the technique is adjusted before the tissues, or the recipient, have time to protest. This approach constitutes an essential factor in the palpatory skills and the art of soft tissue work. As well as being relaxed, the hands are used without any excessive abduction or adduction at the wrist. In addition, the thumb is never held in extension but in a horizontal position or in slight flexion. The pressure of the massage strokes is also discussed later on with the effects of massage and the perception of pain (see Chapter 3).

The rhythm of the massage stroke

When all the scientific theory on massage movements has been studied and absorbed, what remains is the art of the techniques. Part of this involves the rhythm of the movements, not because they necessarily have to be performed in an artistic fashion but because the rhythm increases their effectiveness. In addition to all the mechanical and reflex effects of massage, relaxation remains one of its most potent outcomes. As noted elsewhere, the fact that the recipient is able to relax and remove anxiety is sufficient to set the body in a self-healing mode. A correct rhythm, therefore, is important for each movement. The slow and continuous stroking of light effleurage is the best example of massage for relaxation, and the rocking technique (see Chapter 4, pp. 161–2) is another example in which the appropriate rhythm is an essential aspect of the treatment. The speed of the movement, however, is not as important as its regularity. This is particularly so when certain massage movements such as petrissage and kneading are being carried out, both of which can be relaxing as well as imparting other benefits. Another point that is worth bearing in mind is that the rhythm of the movements sets up the pace of the overall massage treatment, and there is a considerable difference between a treatment that is unhurried and reflective and one that is speeded up and superficial. It is also important to mention that establishing a good rhythm to the overall treatment helps the practitioner to focus and tune in to the recipient, which means that the treatment is more about healing the patient than the tissues. Furthermore, when the therapist is relaxed and working to a rhythm, the treatment can be expanded to include other aspects, i.e. the energy and subconscious levels. By visualizing the body as healthy, the therapist can also use intuition to feel and manipulate the tissues.

TERMINOLOGY

The study of anatomy and the practice of massage necessitate the use of terms which describe the location of organs, the direction of movements and the position of the hands in relation to the regional anatomy. The following is a list of terms that are used frequently in this book.

- *Anterior*. The front of the body, in front of, before. For example, the abdomen is on the anterior side; the stomach is anterior to the spine. An illustration or observation showing the front of the body or of a region is referred to as the anterior view. A massage movement towards the front of the body is said to be in an anterior direction, or anteriorly.
- *Caudad* or *caudal*. Caudad is from the Latin *cauda*, meaning 'tail', and *ad*, meaning 'towards'; opposite to cephalad. A similar word is caudal, from the Latin *caudalis*, meaning 'pertaining to the tail'. The term refers to the location of a body organ or region which is situated nearer to the 'tail' (coccyx) than a particular reference point; for example, the abdomen is caudad to the chest. This is in some ways synonymous with the term 'inferior'. Caudad or caudal is also used to indicate a direction that is towards the posterior aspect of the body, and can be used for a movement or to indicate that an organ lies deeper inside the abdomen or below another organ (therefore more posteriorly). In this book, the term is employed to describe the direction of a massage movement when it is carried out towards the pelvis or the feet. Another application is to specify which hand is needed for a particular stroke; for example, 'the caudad hand (the one nearest to the patient's feet) applies the effleurage whilst the cephalad hand (the one nearest to the patient's head) stabilizes the limb' (see Fig. 2.5).
- *Centrifugal*. From the Greek *kentron*, meaning 'centre', and the Latin *fugere*, meaning 'to flee'. Describes a movement moving away from the centre and towards the periphery.
- *Centripetal*. From the Greek *kentron*, meaning 'centre', and the Latin *petere*, meaning 'to seek'. Describes a movement towards the centre of the body from the periphery.
- *Cephalad* or *cephalic*. Cephalad from the Greek word *kephale*, meaning 'head'; opposite to caudad. A similar word is cephalic, from the Latin *cephalicus*, meaning 'cranial' or 'pertaining to the head'. The term is also synonymous with 'superior', and indicates the position of an organ or region that is closer to the head than a particular reference point; for example, the

chest is cephalad to the abdomen. In this text, the term is used to describe the direction of a massage movement when it is carried out towards the head (see Fig. 2.8). It also used to demonstrate which hand is needed for a particular manoeuvre, as described above in the paragraph on Caudad or caudal.

- *Contralateral*. From the Latin *latus*, meaning 'side'. This indicates the location of a region that is on the opposite side of the midline from the point of reference; for instance, the right side of the spine may be affected by a nerve impulse originating in the contralateral (left) side. In massage, the term is used to indicate the opposite side of the body to where the massage therapist stands (see Fig. 2.4).
- *Coronal plane*. See frontal plane.
- *Distal*. From the Latin *distare*, meaning 'to be distant'. Indicates the farthest point away from the centre of the body or from the trunk. The term is mostly used to describe the position of the part of a limb that is farther away from the trunk than the point of reference; for example, the wrist is distal to the elbow.
- *Frontal plane*. A plane which divides the body into the anterior and posterior portions, at right angles to the midsagittal plane.
- *Hypothenar eminence*. The prominent fleshy part of the palm, just below the little finger.
- *Inferior*. The location of a body part or organ which is beneath or deeper to the more superficial point of reference; for instance, the ribs are inferior to the pectoralis muscle group. The term is also used to describe the position of an organ, tissue or bony landmark that is further towards the feet than its point of reference; for example, the inferior border of the iliac crest is further towards the feet than the superior border. This bearing primarily applies when the subject is in the standing posture (anatomical position), but it is equally relevant when lying down. In this context it is synonymous with the term caudad.
- *Ipsilateral*. From the Latin *ipse*, meaning 'the same', and *latus*, meaning 'side'. Indicates the same side of the body as the point of reference; for instance, a reflex action such as that of the patellar reflex is created by tapping the patellar tendon just below the knee, which causes contraction of the thigh muscles on the ipsilateral side. In massage it is used to describe a movement carried out on the same side of the body as where the therapist stands (see Fig. 2.6).

- *Lateral*. Towards the outside of the body; for instance, the lateral aspect of the femur is in the region of the iliotibial band. In this text the term is also used when describing a massage movement (see Medial, below).
- *Midsagittal plane*. An imaginary line passing through the body, dividing it into symmetrical halves (right and left).
- *Medial*. Towards the central axis of the body; for example, the medial aspect of the femur is in the region of the adductor muscles. The term is also used when describing a massage movement, and in this case the medial hand is the one which is positioned nearest to the midline or to the spine of the patient. The 'lateral' hand is the one which is positioned closer to the lateral border of the body. For instance, when a deep effleurage is applied to the back the medial hand carries out the stroke and it is reinforced with the more lateral hand (see Fig. 5.5).
- *Paravertebral* or *postvertebral*. Alongside or near the vertebral column. These terms are frequently used to indicate the muscles of the back that are close to the spine.
- *Passive movements*. These are actions or movements of joints which are carried out by the therapist without any assistance from the subject; for example, the hamstring muscles are stretched passively when the subject is lying supine and the lower limb is raised and flexed at the hip joint by the practitioner.
- *Periphery*. The outer part or outer surface of the body. The peripheral tissues are therefore those of the skin and subcutaneous fascia and their integrated soft tissue structures.
- *Posterior*. The back area of the body; for instance, the spine is located on the posterior region of the body.
- *Prone*. When the subject is lying face down.
- *Proximal*. Describes the position of that part of a limb which is nearer to the trunk than the point of reference; for example, the elbow is proximal to the wrist.

- *Somatic.* As a general term it is often used to differentiate between the innermost (visceral) regions of the body such as the thoracic and abdominal cavities, and those areas that are more superficial and make up the structures of the body wall, e.g. the skin, muscles, tendons, ligaments and skeletal structures.
- *Superior.* The position of a body region or organ that is situated above or higher than the point of reference; for example, the scapula is superior to the ribs. The term is also used to describe the position of an organ, tissue or bony landmark which is farther towards the head than its point of reference, e.g. the superior border of the iliac crest is farther up than the inferior border. This bearing primarily applies when the subject is standing (anatomical position) but it is equally relevant when they are lying down. In this context it is synonymous with the term cephalad.
- *Supine.* Opposite to prone; the body is lying down, facing upwards.
- *Systemic.* Pertaining to the whole body rather than to one part.
- *Thenar eminence.* From the Greek *thenar*, meaning 'palm'. This term refers to the fleshy part of the hand at the base of the thumb, where the abductor and flexor muscles of the thumb itself are located.
- *Thoracic.* Pertaining to the upper back or thoracic spine.
- *Transverse plane.* A plane which transverses the body horizontally at any level.

AN INTRODUCTION TO THE MASSAGE AND BODYWORK TECHNIQUES

In this section the methods and basic procedures of massage and bodywork techniques are explained and illustrated. The aim of these basic descriptions is to introduce the range of techniques so that the reader is already familiar with them when they are referred to in the next two chapters. More detailed representations, together with guidance on posture and application, are given in Chapters 5–10.

Effleurage or stroking techniques

Effleurage comes from the French word *effleurer*, meaning 'to touch lightly'. Also referred to as 'stroking', it is indisputably the most natural and instinctive of all massage techniques. As a basic movement, effleurage is used at the beginning of all massage routines and has a number of applications, but perhaps the most important is the initial contact it provides with the patient. This in itself is a crucial aspect of the therapist–patient relationship; a positive outcome of the massage treatment often depends on how the patient perceives this touch. As in other movements, the effleurage stroke can be adapted for a particular region of the body or for a particular effect. Variations include a change in the pressure, rhythm, method of application and direction of the stroke.

The effects of effleurage are reflex as well as mechanical, although these frequently overlap (see Chapter 3). A reflex response does not call for a particular direction of movement. In contrast, a mechanical effect is applied in a specific direction; for example, massage to empty the large colon is carried out with the flow of its contents. The general effects of effleurage are as follows:

1. *Mechanical effects.* The mechanical effect of effleurage is direct. It moves the blood along the blood vessels and, in a similar direct manner, it pushes the contents of hollow organs such as those of the digestive system. Most effleurage movements for the circulation are directed towards the heart and therefore along the venous return. Sometimes the effect sought is an increase in local circulation and therefore a more circular movement may be applied. At other times effleurage along the arterial flow is applied, e.g. along the arms towards the hands, to improve blood flow to the extremities. Arterial flow is naturally under the influence of the pumping action of the heart and, indeed, the blood circulation is generally constant. If the general circulation is impaired, however, perhaps due to bed confinement, even the arterial blood flow can benefit from effleurage.

2. *Relaxation.* Light stroking effleurage strokes, in any direction, are of great value when relaxation is the aim of the treatment.

3. *Reduction of pain*. This is a very significant effect of the effleurage massage, involving both mechanical and reflex mechanisms. The increased venous blood flow helps to remove inflammatory agents, which are a common source of pain. Oedema is also reduced by the massage movement. A build-up of fluid increases the pressure within the tissues and causes stimulation of the nociceptors (pain receptors), and draining of the oedema with effleurage and lymphatic massage strokes helps to alleviate the pressure and the pain. Furthermore, massage has the effect of blocking the pain impulses travelling to the spinal cord and of stimulating the release of endorphins (natural painkillers).

4. *Reflex effects*. A reflex effect of effleurage involves the sensory receptors of the superficial tissues. These nerve endings are stimulated by the massage movements and this has an indirect beneficial effect on other regions of the body. The connection is via a reflex pathway involving the autonomic nervous system. Effleurage on certain regions has an additional reflex effect; it enhances contractions of the involuntary muscles of the gut wall (peristalsis).

5. *Reduction of somatic dysfunction or referred pain*. As with all massage movements, effleurage can also be applied to areas of somatic dysfunction or referred pain. The effect is to reduce the sensitivity and other disturbances in the tissues and, in so doing, improve the function of related structures or organs (see Chapter 3).

There are no significant contraindications to effleurage other than those pertaining to the skin (see Chapter 1).

Pressure of effleurage—light stroking

Light effleurage is comparable to the gentle stroking of a pet. As an assessment stroke, it helps to evaluate the superficial tissues for heat, tenderness, elasticity, oedema and muscle tone. It also serves as a comfortable approach to 'making contact' with patients and considering their levels of stress. Palpating the skin for such minute and subtle changes necessitates that the hands be relaxed, as tension lowers their sensitivity. The pressure

applied is neither very light nor heavy enough to make the hands sink into the tissues (Fig. 2.9). Light effleurage is extremely effective in inducing relaxation. The process involves receptors in the superficial tissues which, when stimulated by touch, produce a relaxation response via the parasympathetic nervous system. The local and systemic circulation is also improved with light effleurage, which has a direct and mechanical effect on the venous return, increasing its flow. Reflexively, it has a toning effect on the involuntary muscles of the arterial walls (see Chapter 3).

Pressure of effleurage—deep stroking

Deep stroking techniques are often preferred to the light effleurage movements. By and large, the subject considers the heaviness of the movement to be just as relaxing, if not more so, as a lighter weight. Reflexively, the deep pressure has an inhibitory effect on the muscles and their proprioceptors, i.e. nerves, muscle spindles and Golgi tendon organ (Leone and Kukulka, 1988). The motor impulses arriving from the spinal cord at the neuromuscular end-plates (nerve junctions) are also inhibited by the deep pressure and, as a result, the contractions are weaker and the muscles relax (see Chapter 3). The heavy pressure is transmitted to the deeper tissues, and venous circulation and lymphatic drainage in these deeper

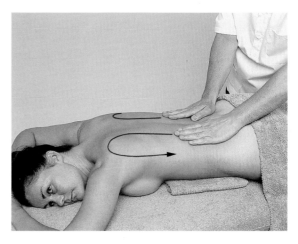

Figure 2.9 General effleurage movement applied with both hands simultaneously.

structures are thereby improved (Brobeck, 1979). As the veins are drained, more space is created for the arterial blood flow. Muscle tissue will also benefit from the increased blood flow, which supplies it with oxygen and plasma fluid. Enhancing the venous return facilitates the removal of lactic acid and other by-products of muscle activity, and this helps to relax the muscles and simultaneously to prepare them for strenuous physical sports. Deep stroking movements have a stretching effect on the superficial fascia and also reduce nodular formations (hardened areas) and congestion. As in all other movements, deep stroking massage should only be carried out to the tolerance levels of the recipient. An initial slight tenderness is often experienced in the superficial tissues; this generally reduces gradually during the treatment. If the pain is exacerbated with the deep stroking, the movement should be discontinued on that region.

Deep effleurage can be carried out using the hand as in the light stroking movements. A 'fisted' hand is a second tool that can be used for the same effect (see Effleurage *du poing*—Chapter 5). Effleurage with the forearm can also be used, particularly when heavy pressure is required to increase the local circulation. The forearm can be very effectively substituted for the hands when carrying out effleurage stroking (see Chapter 5). Whilst this method can be used to avoid a strain on the hands it does not provide the same precise contact with the tissues that the fingers and palms can offer; sensory receptors in the palmar surface of the hands far outnumber the ones on the forearms. For the assessment of tissue dysfunction, therefore, the hands are better tools. Forearm effleurage is best applied to increase the circulation and for the relaxation of muscles. Theoretically, it can be applied on most regions of the body. It is advisable, however, that the head, chest and abdomen are avoided at all times and the technique restricted to the back, legs and arms.

Thumb effleurage

Thumb effleurage is another form of deep stroking massage (Fig. 2.10). As it is applied with

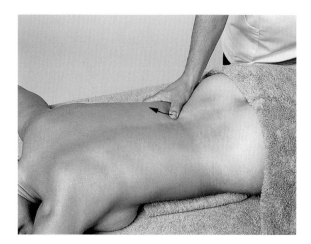

Figure 2.10 Deep effleurage with the thumb is carried out on the lumbar muscles on the ipsilateral side of the spine.

only one or two digits it makes it possible for the pressure to be concentrated on small areas of muscle tissue, and it is also of particular use where the muscles lie flat to the bone (such as the infraspinatus of the scapula). The alternating thumb strokes of this effleurage are very short and are repeated several times on the one area. It is continued until the tissues begin to yield and soften, and the 'knotted' feel of the fibres is reduced. The hands can then be moved to another section of the same muscle and the effleurage resumed. Thumb effleurage has the following applications and effects:

1. *Reduction of pain*. It can be applied in conditions such as lumbago where there is general achiness and muscle tightness in the lumbar region.

2. *Reduction of fatigue*. As it increases the local circulation through the muscles, it counteracts the effects of fatigue.

3. *Reduction of oedema*. Thumb effleurage is also used to reduce oedema and adhesions (fibrous congestion); these can be present, for instance, in the soft tissues surrounding an arthritic joint.

4. *Heat*. The pressure of the thumb effleurage increases the temperature of the fascia matrix in the deep tissue layers. Heating the fascia facilitates stretching of the collagen fibres in fibrotic tissue.

Compression movements

Compression movements are also referred to as soft tissue manipulations. This is a somewhat inappropriate use of the term, because all massage movements can be considered to manipulate the tissues. A distinction does, however, exist, as some compression movements, especially kneading, are at times carried out without any lubrication to the tissues. Furthermore, a degree of manipulation is also involved. Both kneading and petrissage, the primary compression movements, displace and contort the tissues either by lifting or by pressing them against the underlying structures. The direction of the stretch can therefore be applied in different directions. Some authors classify petrissage as a primary soft tissue technique, with subgroups of kneading, rolling, lifting and shaking. Disparity therefore lies in the terminology used by different authors and practitioners, although the treatment of the soft tissues entails very similar manipulations. For instance, shaking is described in conjunction with vibration movements in this text, whilst rolling and lifting come under soft tissue manipulation. 'Compression movements', as a classification of soft tissue manipulation, is perhaps an old term but it is credited to one James B. Mennell, who was medical officer at the Physio-Therapeutic Department at St Thomas' Hospital in London (see History of massage, Chapter 1). Mennell was amongst the pioneers in the use of massage and exercise therapy in hospitals, most probably even preceding the role of physiotherapists. In his work *Massage: Its Principles and Practice* (1920) he classifies the 'petrissage' movements under the heading of compression techniques. Although slightly dated, this terminology is still applicable as it describes the technique well. A compression movement that is carried out with the palm and fingers of the flat hand, for example, is classified as petrissage in some books (Fig. 2.11).

Compression movement—kneading

Kneading generates a pressure which is transmitted to the underlying structures; it can there-

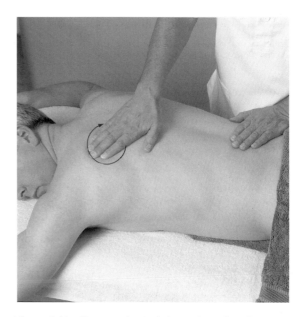

Figure 2.11 Compression technique, also referred to as petrissage, is applied in small circular movements with the palms and fingers.

fore affect the deep as well as the superficial tissues. There are several kneading methods; some are described in this section whilst others are included in later chapters.

The effects and applications of kneading include:

1. *Stretching and release of adhesions*. The essential effect of kneading is that it stretches muscular tissue and its surrounding fascia. This has the additional outcome of reversing any shortening within these tissues and releasing any adhesions.

2. *Reduction of oedema*. The pump-like action of kneading is likely to aid the flow of lymph and reduce oedema. Draining the interstitial fluid will also remove waste products from the tissues.

3. *Increased circulation*. The local circulation is improved through a reflex effect, which causes vasodilatation of the superficial arterioles. Transportation of nutrients to the tissues is therefore increased because of the enhanced blood perfusion, and the venous flow of the blood is also enhanced by the mechanical action of the movement.

4. *Reduction of pain and fatigue*. The improved circulation helps to reduce pain and fatigue in

the muscles. An accumulation of metabolites, including carbon dioxide and fluid (catabolized lactic acid), is created by the repeated or sustained muscle contractions. The arterial blood vessels are also occluded. As a result, the muscles are susceptible to acidic congestion, ischaemia, pain and fatigue. Clearing away these by-products counteracts fatigue and prepares the muscles for strenuous physical activity such as exercise.

Kneading with the fingers and thumb

On some muscles, such as those of the calf, the kneading movement is carried out using only one hand. In this case, the thumb is placed on the lateral side of the calf and the fingers on the medial side (Fig. 2.12). Pressure is exerted simultaneously on each side of the calf, and the tissues are compressed and rolled over the underlying structures using a semi-circular action. The grip is then released so that the tissues resume their normal resting state. When the movement has been repeated a few times the hands are moved to another section and the technique carried out again. This procedure is continued over the whole region of the calf.

Kneading with the thenar/hypothenar eminences

This method of kneading is used on muscles that are large enough to be pressed firmly and stretched transversely. They include the paravertebral muscles (close to the spine), the upper fibres of the trapezius and the gluteal muscles. No circular movement is involved in this method of kneading. The tissues are first pulled by the fingers towards the thenar/hypothenar eminences, and a slight pressure is applied during this manoeuvre, sufficient to pull the tissues. The thenar/hypothenar eminences are next employed to apply compression and to roll the tissues forward over the underlying structures; this manoeuvre also stretches the fibres transversely. Whilst some counterpressure is applied with the fingers, the emphasis is on the pressure with the thenar/hypothenar eminences (Fig. 2.13). The tissues are therefore convoluted forward rather than simply squeezed. If there is sufficient yield in the tissues, they can also be rolled over the fingertips. The compression is released as the heel of hand approximates the fingers. When the tissues have returned to their normal resting state, the hand is repositioned and the technique repeated on the same area.

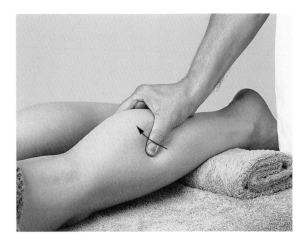

Figure 2.12 Kneading is carried out using only one hand. A circular pumping action is simultaneously applied with the fingers and thumb.

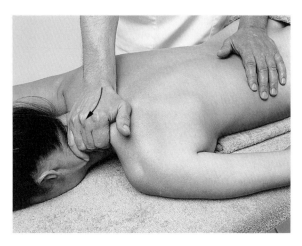

Figure 2.13 Kneading with the thenar/hypothenar eminences rolling the tissues towards the fingers.

Kneading with the fingers

An on-and-off compression technique can be applied with the fingers, which are placed flat to the skin surface. The hands are positioned on top of each other and exert an equal pressure with the extended fingers. Simultaneously with the compression, the tissues are stretched in a circular direction. Minimal sliding of the hands takes place during this manoeuvre. Both the pressure and the tissues are then released for the procedure to be resumed. The technique is indicated on muscles that are tense without being chronically tight or fibrotic. It is therefore applied with other techniques such as the light effleurage movement. This movement is similar to the compression method described earlier (Fig. 2.11) but is carried out with one hand on top of the other.

Compression movement—petrissage

In some books petrissage is also referred to as wringing, kneading, rolling, picking-up and shaking. As mentioned earlier, identical movements are grouped under different headings (in this and other books), e.g. as kneading and soft tissue manipulation techniques.

Although petrissage is a compression movement, it differs from kneading in that the tissues are lifted off the underlying structures instead of being rolled over them. Compression is applied between the fingers of one hand and the thumb of the other, and the tissues are also simultaneously lifted and twisted slightly in a clockwise or anticlockwise direction (Fig. 2.14). The pressure is then released and the position of the hands reversed. In this manner the movement is carried out by alternating the grip position of the hands. Once the left fingers and the right thumb have compressed the tissues, they are swapped with the right fingers and left thumb for the next compression. The technique is most suitable for the larger muscles such as those of the lower limbs, lower back, glutei region and arms.

The effects of petrissage include:

1. *Increased circulation*. Petrissage increases the circulation through the dermis and the subcutaneous (superficial areolar) fascia. This effect is

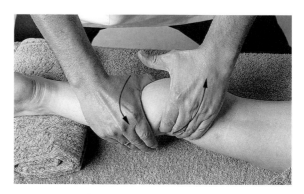

Figure 2.14 Petrissage—the fingers of one hand compress the tissues against the opposite thumb.

significant, as the superficial blood vessels (unlike the deeper ones) are not surrounded by fascia layers. Consequently, they cannot be compressed against a fascia wall to assist their blood flow and are therefore susceptible to collapse and to varicosity. Petrissage also compresses the deeper blood vessels against the lower fascia planes, and the flow of blood in the venous as well as the arterial vessels is therefore improved.

2. *Pain reduction*. Like kneading, the movement of petrissage relaxes tight muscles by increasing their circulation and stretching the fibres. The improved circulation has the additional effect of reducing pain and fatigue in the muscles.

3. *Improved lymphatic drainage*. Petrissage improves the lymph drainage of the muscular and superficial tissue. When muscles contract, they cause the lymph vessels to be compressed against the deep fascia planes; this has the effect of pumping the lymph forward. The squeezing action of petrissage provides a similar compression for the lymph vessels.

4. *Fat emulsification*. When performed vigorously, petrissage is likely to have the effect of emulsifying the fat in the superficial connective tissue cells. In this emulsified state the fat globules have a better chance of entering the lymphatic system and also of being metabolized.

5. *Stretching and release of adhesions*. Synonymous with the action of kneading, the twisting component of petrissage helps to break up any adhesions between the muscle bundles

and muscle layers. It stretches the deep fascia layers, the investing layers between muscles and other tissues, plus the epimysium, perimysium and endomysium. It also helps to break up the fibrous collagen capsules of cellulite.

Lymphatic massage movements

A considerable number of lymph drainage techniques have been developed for the remedy of oedema, to the extent that the treatment is often detached from massage and practised as a separate therapy altogether. However, massage still has a significant role to play in the treatment of oedema, as most movements have some influence on the flow of lymph. Two massage techniques that are specifically applied for lymph drainage are described in this section; they are also included in subsequent massage routines in later chapters.

Lymph massage—effleurage

Lymph effleurage is distinguishable from similar strokes in that it is very light and extremely slow. Hardly any pressure is required for this stroke; the weight of the hand alone exerts sufficient pressure to move the lymph through the superficial vessels. The direction of the stroke is always towards the next proximal group of nodes, and the stroke is performed at a very slow speed to match that of the lymph flow. Very little lubrication is applied for this movement, and the hands are very relaxed as they move over the tissues. Contact is made with the whole area of the hand, including the fingertips and the thenar and hypothenar eminences (Fig. 2.15).

The benefit of lymph effleurage extends also to the muscular tissue, although a heavier effleurage is needed to drain the muscles than that used for the superficial tissues. The reason behind this move is that a greater build-up of pressure is required within the deeper vessels for their walls to contract by reflex action (see Chapter 3). As a general rule, the direction of the lymph effleurage stroke for treating muscles follows that of the venous return. However, in the case of long muscles the stroke is carried out

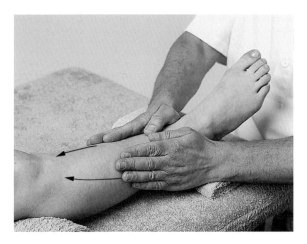

Figure 2.15 Lymph effleurage to the anterior lower leg traces the lymph channels towards the popliteal nodes.

from the periphery of the muscle towards its centre, and this is considered to be a more accurate direction of its lymph drainage.

The therapist can either be standing or sitting to carry out the lymph effleurage movement. To keep the hands relaxed and to maintain the slow rhythm of the effleurage movement, it is suggested that a sitting posture is adopted whenever possible. As already discussed, the direction of lymph effleurage follows that of the lymph vessels. For instance, lymph massage on the posterior aspect of the thigh is carried out in two directions. One stroke is from the midline towards the medial aspect, and this traces the channels towards the inguinal nodes; a second pathway is from the same midline towards the lateral aspect, and these vessels also drain into the inguinal nodes but follow a different route. On the anterior aspect, the lymph vessels travel from the lateral towards the medial region, and the lymph effleurage is carried out in the same direction.

Lymph massage—intermittent pressure

This movement is different from the usual massage techniques in that it is applied using an intermittent pump-like pressure. Only the fingers and the palm of the hand are used; the thenar and hypothenar eminences do not make contact with the tissues. A small degree of pressure is applied for less than a second and removed completely for the same period. This on-and-off cycle is repeated continuously for a short time. With each compression, the tissues are stretched in two directions; the first is in line with the fingers, and therefore in the same direction as they are pointing; the second is in a clockwise or anticlockwise direction, towards the next proximal group of nodes. For instance, the practitioner stands on the left side of the supine patient and places the hands on the anterior/medial region of the left thigh. The direction of the stretch is clockwise, i.e. towards the inguinal nodes (Fig. 2.16).

Using the same guidelines, the intermittent pressure technique can be adapted for other regions of the body. On the calf, for instance, the movement is applied using only one hand (Fig. 6.26). In this case, the position of the hand resembles that for the compression kneading technique on the same area. The two methods must not be confused, however; the lymph massage is carried out very lightly and without any sliding of the fingers, whereas kneading is applied with a heavy pressure and a degree of sliding over the tissues.

During the intermittent pressure technique, it is essential for the hands to maintain good contact with the tissues to facilitate the stretch. Lubricants are therefore avoided or restricted to very tiny amounts. In contrast to the lymph effleurage movement, the intermittent pressure

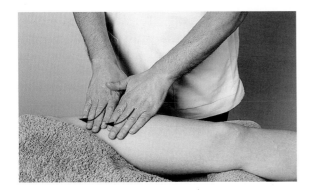

Figure 2.16 Intermittent pressure technique on the anterior region of the thigh.

technique is best carried out whilst the therapist is standing.

The on-and-off pressure of this movement has a dual effect. A pump-like action is created, which assists in the movement of fluid through the vessels. In addition, the tissues and the lymph vessels are stretched in two directions, longitudinally and transversely. As a result of this action there is a reflex contraction of the muscular wall of the vessels, which also pushes the lymph forwards (see Chapter 3).

Percussive strokes

The common term used for the percussive-type strokes is *tapotement*, a French word meaning 'light tapping'. Other phrases and techniques include hacking, pounding and flicking. These percussive-type strokes have a hyperaemic effect (an increase in the local circulation) on the skin. They also stimulate the nerve endings, which results in tiny muscular contractions and an overall increased tone. As a general rule, most recipients find the percussive strokes very invigorating whilst others find them relaxing.

As already noted, the percussive-type striking is of a mild traumatic nature and the body responds by contracting the muscles. Another interpretation is that the pressure is registered by the mechanoreceptors in the fascia and the Golgi tendon organ in muscles. A reflex action ensues, which results in tiny contractions of the involuntary and voluntary muscles. Skeletal muscles are said to benefit from this reaction, which helps to increase their tone. However, this toning effect on the skeletal muscle is somewhat hypothetical, and the more likely effect of the percussive-type strokes is on the involuntary muscles of the blood vessels (see Chapter 3). The initial response in the superficial and deep blood vessels is contraction of the involuntary muscular wall; this is followed by nerve fatigue and therefore vasodilatation, as demonstrated by the ensuing hyperaemia.

It is possible that percussive strokes that are continued for a long time may fatigue the nerve receptors and become counterproductive. In addition, muscles that are already weak can

Box 2.2 Contraindications to percussive-type strokes

- Bony areas
- On the head
- On the neck
- On the back of knee
- On the spine
- Tissue or area which is inflamed
- Varicose veins
- On the kidney area
- Any muscle that is strained or abnormally contracted
- Areas of hypersensitivity
- Any paralysed muscle

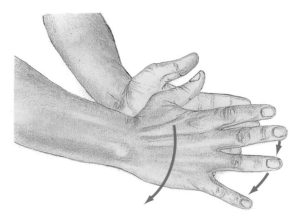

Figure 2.17A Hacking—the little finger strikes the tissue as the other digits cascade onto it.

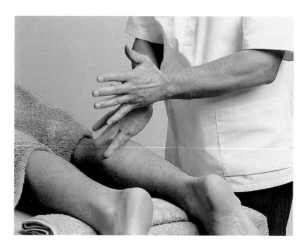

Figure 2.17B A flicking action of the wrist is used to peform the hacking movement.

only contract for short periods at a time and should not therefore be subjected to long treatment, in the same manner as a novice runner cannot be expected to run a marathon. On healthy tissue, percussive strokes are safely used to maintain or improve the existing tonicity. They can however be contraindicated in some regions (Box 2.2).

There are four types of percussive strokes:

1. *Hacking*—little finger strike with open and straight fingers or curled fingers
2. *Pounding*—flat fist, palmar aspect
3. *Cupping*—cupped hand
4. *Flicking*—a flicking action with the fingers (misleadingly referred to as slapping).

Hacking—little finger strike

When hacking with straight fingers, the fingers are spread open and held in this position for most of the time. Only the little finger strikes the tissues; the ulnar border of the hand does not make any contact or exert any pressure. As the little finger comes down and hits the tissue, the other fingers cascade onto it; they are then spread apart again as the hand is raised. The hand is brought down with a flicking action of the wrist, and rapidly raised again by the same flicking manoeuvre. An alternating striking takes place with the hands; as one hand is raised the second one is brought down. This alternating action is repeated several times (Figs 2.17A and B).

A heavier hacking movement is carried out with the fingers flexed and closed together. Only the little finger strikes the tissues as the hand is brought down; the ulnar border of the hand does not make contact or apply any pressure. The hand is then raised again with a similar flicking movement of the wrist. An alternating striking action is used; one hand is raised as the second is brought down (Figs 2.18A and B).

Pounding

The percussive movement of pounding is performed with the hand in a fist and with the

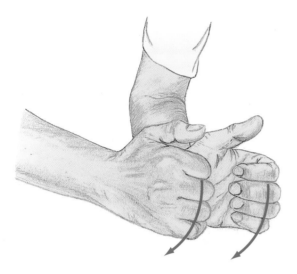

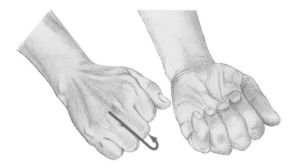

Figure 2.19A Pounding—one hand is supinated to show the flexed fingers for the pounding movement.

Figure 2.18A Hacking—a heavy hacking movement is applied with the fingers curled and closed together.

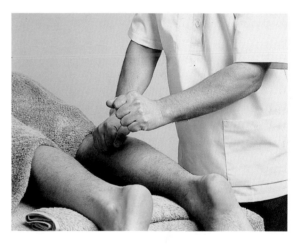

Figure 2.19B Pounding is carried out with the palmar side of the fist striking the tissues.

Cupping

Cupping is performed with the fingers slightly flexed and squeezed together. The hand is put into a cup shape, as if holding a small round object in the palm without closing the hand. This shape is maintained as the hand is lowered, making a hollow sound as it strikes the tissues, and raised again rapidly. There is no flicking action of the wrist; the bending takes place at the elbow and the forearm is lowered as the hand is brought down (Figs 2.20A and B).

Flicking

Flicking is carried out with the fingers together and more or less straight; the wrist is locked or

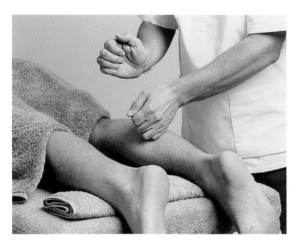

Figure 2.18B Hacking—the alternating hacking movements are applied by the same flicking action of the wrists.

palmar side striking the tissues. If a lightweight pounding is required, the hand is brought down with a slight flicking action of the wrist. For a heavier pounding, the wrist is locked and the bending takes place at the elbow; the whole forearm is therefore lowered as the hand strikes the tissues. An alternating action is used, as already described. Pounding is applied to large muscles, such as the belly of the gastrocnemius and the quadriceps group of the thigh (Figs 2.19A and B).

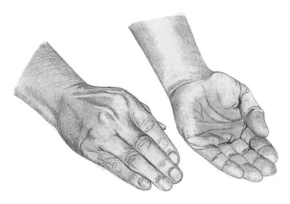

Figure 2.20A Cupping—one hand is supinated to show the fingers slightly flexed and squeezed together into a 'cupped' position.

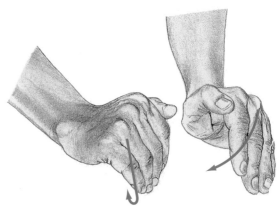

Figure 2.21A Flicking—all the fingers are close together and straight to *strike* the tissues. The movement is applied by flexing the metacarpophalangeal joints.

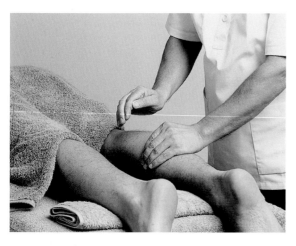

Figure 2.20B Cupping—the hand strikes the tissues, making a hollow sound.

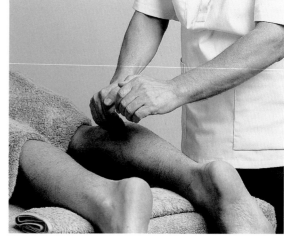

Figure 2.21B Flicking—the *flicking* action is performed by a slight flexion of the interphalangeal joints.

with very little flexion. A light striking action is first carried out with the palmar side of the fingers as they rapidly flex at the metacarpophalangeal joints. This is combined by a gentle flicking action of the tissues, mostly with the fingertips; at this stage there is a slight flexion of the interphalangeal joints. The fingers are straightened out once more for the striking to be resumed. In a similar fashion to the other percussive strokes, flicking is repeated several times and with alternate hands (Figs 2.21A and B).

Friction techniques

Friction movements are carried out on both the superficial and deep tissues. Using the fingertips or the thumb, and in most cases only one hand, the more superficial tissues are moved over the underlying structures. The technique is performed with very little sliding of the digits and, to this end, minimal lubrication is used. Friction movements can be applied in a number of directions. As their effect is, to a large extent, local to the tissues being addressed they do not have to follow the venous return or lymphatic drainage specifically. They may be circular, transverse (across the fibres) or in a straight line along the fibres, although the latter two methods tend to be preferred. Although not always applicable, a rhythm can be incorporated into the movement by coordinating the action of the body and that of the hands. Pressure is exerted by the body weight, leaning forward to apply the pressure and easing backward to reduce it. Heavy friction pressure can lead to fatigue of the involuntary muscles, such as those of the arterioles, but this temporary situation has to be tolerated to carry out the treatment effectively. Local hyperaemia is in fact one of the main effects and, in some cases, the primary goal of friction.

Friction movements have the following effects and applications:

1. *Local hyperaemia*. Local circulation and temperature are both increased with the friction movements. The effect is achieved in the superficial and deeper tissues, depending on the depth of pressure which is used for the technique. Friction massage has the effect of releasing a substance resembling histamine which is liberated by the cells of the skin (Jacobs, 1960). The effect of this histamine-type substance is dilatation of the capillaries by its direct influence, and arteriole dilatation by an axon reflex mechanism.

2. *Dispersion of pathological deposits*. Friction movements disperse pathological deposits (calcifications), in particular around joints (for example, in gouty or rheumatic areas). These types of pathological changes may be tender on palpation, in which case the friction movements are applied with very little pressure. If the tenderness elicited is very severe, the movement is omitted altogether.

3. *Stretching and release of adhesions*. Friction movements can release adhesions between tissue layers such as skin, fascia, muscle, tendon, aponeurosis, periosteum, bursae and ligaments. The heat produced by the repeated action of the

movements encourages fibrotic tissue to yield and stretch.

4. *Reduction of oedema*. This technique helps to reduce chronic oedema. The consistency of progressive oedema is likely to change towards a more solid state, which is therefore more difficult to disperse; friction movements can be used for this effect.

5. *Gastrointestinal effects*. Friction movements can also be applied to treat the colon, provided the techniques are comfortable for the patient. The involuntary muscles of the digestive tract are stimulated by this movement but, if the treatment is drawn out, the same muscles are susceptible to fatigue.

6. *Neurological effects*. In some special cases, friction movements are used to treat the main nerves such as the sciatic branch. The fingertips are placed to the side of the nerve, and small circular frictions are then carried out along the course of the nerve. Because of the close proximity of the fingers to the nerve, this method is used very rarely and only with the approval of the patient's doctor. Friction movements cannot affect the nerve axon or its neurolemma (sheath) directly; these get their nutrition from the cell, which is located a distance away in the spinal cord. The nerve sheath, however, has its own blood supply, the comes nervi communicans, and improving the circulation to this area indirectly improves the blood supply to the nerve. There are also lymph spaces in and around the sheath that can fill up with debris, e.g. from pathology. Removing this build-up frees the axon and its neurolemma. However, treatment of nerves with friction movements does carry some very specific precautions and contraindications (Box 2.3).

7. *Persistent neuralgia*. One of the causes of this condition is minute adhesions, which pull or press upon the nerve. Reducing the adhesions by friction massage can therefore alleviate the neuralgia.

8. *Pain reduction*. Stimulation of the receptors in the skin and fascia layers is seen as activating the pain gate mechanism, i.e. creating sufficient stimuli along C fibres to block the perception of pain.

Box 2.3 Precautions when applying friction movements over nerves

- Friction movements are not applied if the nerve is inflamed
- No treatment is given on a nerve if the axon or the cell is diseased or injured
- Friction technique is carried out very gently and the pressure increased with the utmost care
- The technique is immediately stopped if it exacerbates the nerve pain
- Friction massage is avoided on any region which reacts to the treatment with a protective muscular contraction
- Referral to a doctor may be necessary if the aetiology of these reactions has not been diagnosed

Transverse friction movement

Fingertip pressure of small amplitude is one method used for friction massage. The fingers are spread out and short strokes are applied, forward and backward, with the fingertips. Pressure is regulated throughout the treatment, commencing gently and progressively increasing. Fingertip friction is performed, for example, across the fibres of the intercostal muscles (Fig. 2.22).

Circular friction movement

In this method of friction, the fingers are closed together or slightly apart. Pressure is applied with the fingertips and maintained as the fingers describe a series of small circles. The tissues are rolled over the underlying structures and in this respect the circular friction technique has a slight resemblance to a kneading stroke. The main difference is that the pressure is maintained throughout the friction movement, whereas it is intermittent in the kneading stroke. One region very suitable for circular friction movement is the infraspinatus area of the scapula (Fig. 2.23).

Thumb friction

On some regions, the thumb can be substituted for the fingertips. Forward and backward strokes are applied in the same manner as in the fingertip friction movement.

The paravertebral muscles provide one area that is suitable for thumb friction. In this region the friction can be applied across or along the fibres. However, using the thumb for these muscles can prove rather tiring and, in most cases, the fingertips make a better choice. On the other hand, the common insertion of the extensor muscles in the elbow is easily treated with thumb friction across the fibres (Fig. 2.24).

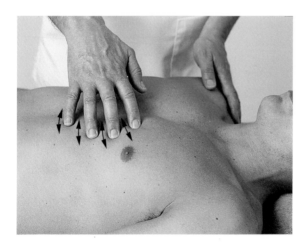

Figure 2.22 Transverse friction massage over the intercostal muscles.

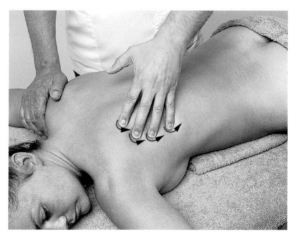

Figure 2.23 Circular friction on the scapula. The fingers apply pressure and move the tissues over the underlying structures.

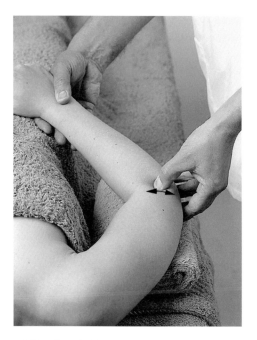

Figure 2.24 Thumb friction across the fibres of the extensor muscles at the elbow.

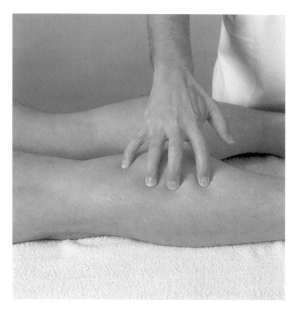

Figure 2.25 Vibration movements are applied over the calf muscles.

Vibration and shaking movements

For the vibration movement, the fingers are mostly held in a splayed out position; however, they can also be used closed together. The pads or the fingertips are used to grip the skin and superficial tissues gently. An on-and-off pressure is applied with the whole hand in this position, and without breaking the fingertip contact with skin. Pressure is of low amplitude and applied very rapidly to create fine vibration movements (Fig. 2.25). This technique is different from percussive strokes in that it does not cause a reflex contraction of the skeletal muscles (although it does affect the involuntary muscles).

Shaking is a similar, but coarser, operation to vibration. One hand is used, and rests on the muscle or tissue in a similar fashion to the effleurage stroke with the fingers close together. However, when carried out on areas such as the abdomen, the movement is applied with the fingers splayed out. The shaking action is performed from side to side and without any sliding of the hand, creating a vibration that travels into the superficial and deep tissues. It also influences the visceral organs. Apart from being administered as a massage stroke, and therefore worth adding to the massage routine, vibration is very efficiently achieved with a contemporary electrical device. On some regions the shaking is unavoidably combined with a vibration movement; the abdomen is a good example. Vibration movements that are carried out continuously for about 2–3 min are seen as having an inhibitory effect, which is most likely to be because of the adaption of the mechanoreceptors. When the vibratory movement is applied with an on–off pressure and therefore in short bursts, the effect is said to be stimulating.

Vibration and shaking movements have the following effects and applications:

1. *Increased lymphatic flow.* A beneficial application of the vibration technique is for dislodging and loosening the lymph. In disease, usually when there is lymph stasis, the consistency of the fluid changes so that it resembles treacle or liquid glue. It can harden further, to the consistency of dough, and this renders it more difficult to shift. The vibrations have the effect of reversing this

state and, as it becomes more liquefied, the lymph can flow into and along the lymph vessels. The lymph is also encouraged to move through the fascia planes from one compartment (for example, that containing an organ) to the next.

2. *Reduction of oedema.* Injuries to the soft tissues, such as sports injuries, produce oedema. This too can change and become viscous if it is untreated and longstanding. Vibration is applied to reverse this situation. The oedema which precedes the onset of cellulite may be fluid enough to drain with other massage techniques although, as the condition progresses, the viscosity of the interstitial lymph can change to a more gluey state. Vibration movements are beneficial for reversing this, along with other massage movements. However, this condition is an example of when mechanical devices can be more effective than 'hands on' efforts.

3. *Contraction of involuntary muscles.* The vibration technique is used on the abdomen to secure a reflex contraction of the involuntary muscles of the viscera. It is crucial that the abdominal muscles are relaxed when vibration massage is carried out, and that a reflex protective reaction does not occur. The technique may be difficult to perform if the abdomen is bloated with wind or the patient is obese.

4. *Stimulation of thoracic organs.* Organs under the cover of the rib cage are stimulated by the vibration effect transmitted through the chest wall.

5. *Neurological effects.* Vibration can also be applied to nerves, in a similar fashion to friction. The effect is to reduce surrounding adhesions and to improve lymph drainage within the nerve sheath.

6. *Muscle tone.* Fast vibration movements can also stimulate muscle tone when carried out for short intermittent periods. Continuous vibration movement can have the opposite effect, i.e. to reduce muscle tension.

7. *Stretching and release of adhesions.* Whilst other massage movements such as friction and thumb effleurage are likely to be more effective, adhesions can be reduced and scar tissue stretched by vibration movements. Joint mobility is also improved, as restriction is often associated with adhesions and scar tissue.

8. *Peripheral arterial circulation.* Vibratory movements have an effect on the involuntary muscles of the arterioles. Movements that are carried out on the superficial tissues at a low rate of about 80 times per min create an initial response of vasoconstriction. This is soon followed by relaxation of the arterioles and vasodilatation. Lowering the resistance in the peripheral arteries helps to lower the blood pressure. When carried out at a higher rate the vasospasm is prolonged and so blood pressure is raised.

Precautions for vibration techniques are shown in Box 2.4.

Bodywork techniques

Bodywork is a general term used to describe a number of soft tissue manipulation techniques. These fall somewhere between the stroking-type movements such as those used in Swedish massage and the more specific joint manipulations of other modalities such as osteopathy and chiropractic work. Some bodywork techniques are based on the emotional–mind–body aspects, while others deal primarily with the biomechanical function of the body. The physiological mechanisms of bodywork involve the nervous pathways in visceral, muscular and somatic tissues. Major components therefore are the sensory nerves, motor nerves, reflex pathways, Golgi tendon organs and muscle spindles. Other factors include the fasciae (superficial, deep, subcutaneous) as well as the muscles and tendons.

Box 2.4 Precautions when applying vibration movements

- Vibration movements are discontinued if they elicit any pain, particularly when they are applied on nerves
- Acute conditions are contraindicated to the vibration movements
- The technique is omitted in the presence of inflammation

Bodywork groups together a number of treatment procedures such as neuromuscular technique, muscle energy technique, Rolfing and myofascial release. Heading the endorsements and advancements in this field of work have been authors and researchers such as Leon Chaitow, Karel Lewit, Janet Travel, David Simons and Ida Rolf. Each therapy incorporates its own physiological hypothesis and practical approach. Overall, however, the bodywork methods share some common concepts and certain similarities in techniques. Furthermore, various elements of these procedures have been integrated into other therapies, massage being one example. In some respects the extensive use and similarity of the techniques makes the line between massage and bodywork an ambiguous one, and indeed massage is sometimes synonymous with bodywork. However, the advancements made in some of the bodywork therapies are very extensive, extremely commendable and have become a sphere of specialism for bodywork therapists. With this in mind, and therefore without any claims to these domains, a few bodywork movements are included in this book for the reason that they serve to enhance the effect and scope of the massage treatment. It is also considered appropriate for the massage therapist to use techniques other than massage when treating somatic tissue dysfunctions.

Common targets for bodywork techniques include soft tissue dysfunctions such as contracted fascia, muscle tightness, flaccidity, fibrotic tissue, nodules and trigger points. These tissue changes are very common, and are therefore significant to the massage therapist. Nodules, for instance, are hard areas that occur in shortened and tight muscles as well as in the fascia. The nodules are generally tender, but respond to massage, friction or pressure, although the response is less if they are chronic. Treatment of these soft tissue changes has a normalizing effect on the musculoskeletal structure and, in many cases, on the associated organs.

Neuromuscular technique (NMT)

The neuromuscular technique (NMT; Chaitow, 1987 and 1996a) has the dual and synchronized effect of assessment and treatment of the superficial somatic tissues and muscles. Irregularities are palpated with the thumb or the fingers as they slide over the tissue or muscle, and the same stroking movement has the additional effect of treating these structures by reducing nodules, tightness, sensitivity, etc. This technique is used to address the following tissues and related malfunctions:

1. *Changes in the superficial and deep fascia.*

   - Congestion in the fascia layers can result from a reduced blood supply and an impaired drainage of the blood and lymph. The circulation is improved by the mechanical effect of NMT, and it is further enhanced by a reflex response to the movement, which relaxes the involuntary muscles of the blood vessels and thereby causes vasodilatation.
   - Nodules. If the circulation within the fascia layers is impaired it causes an instability in the acid–base balance, and this is a precursor to the formation of nodules. In addition to enhancing the circulation, NMT exerts sufficient pressure to reduce the rigidity of the nodules and the hypersensitivity which accompanies them. The pressure applied with the thumbs on the local tissues initially creates vasospasm in the superficial blood vessels. As the stroke is completed and the pressure released there is reflex vasodilatation which helps to reduce the ischaemic state of the trigger point.
   - Fibrous infiltration (adhesions) can develop between tissue layers and consequently prevent them from sliding over each other, thereby restricting movement between muscle groups. Adhesions can also form within a muscle and, as a result, the muscle loses elasticity and may become painful when it is contracted. In the chronic stage these fibrous infiltrations can replace some of the active fibres of the muscle. Adhesions are reduced with the NMT and other massage movements.

2. *Changes in muscle tone.*

   - Chronic muscle contractions can be brought about by a number of factors, including postural imbalances, psychogenic factors and organ malfunction. Sustained contractions in the muscle are reduced by the pressure of the technique, which inhibit the motor impulses to the muscular endplate. The technique also inhibits the sensory impulses from the muscle spindle to a degree, leading to relaxation of the extrafusal fibres (see Chapter 3). Furthermore, it stretches the fibres of the musculotendon junction, which overloads the Golgi tendon organ and thereby inhibits contraction of the same muscle.

- Flaccidity in a muscle can be a consequence of severe contraction or tightness in its antagonist. This tension is reduced with the NMT and, in turn, the muscle tone of the antagonist is improved.

3. *Impairment of nerve pathways.* Adhesions and contracted muscles can entrap nerves, blocking the nerve supply to the tissues. Muscles are also subjected to this impairment, and will malfunction as a result. Hypersensitivity is also common. By reducing adhesions and congestion in the tissues, the NMT has the effect of releasing entrapped nerves and restoring their function.
4. *Limitation of joint mobility.* The full mobility of a joint is dependent on the flexibility of all the muscles associated with it. Any tightness or malfunctioning in these muscles can therefore have a limiting effect on its movement. Conversely, improving the resilience of the tissues surrounding a joint by using the NMT improves its mobility.
5. *Malfunctioning organs.* Changes in the superficial tissues, i.e. the fascia and muscles, can be a reflex response to organ malfunction. Conversely, treatment of the superficial tissues with this technique and other massage movements has a normalizing effect on organs and glands.

Method of application of the neuromuscular technique

The NMT can be applied using several methods, including the fisted hand and the elbow, as depicted in later chapters. The basic stroke is carried out with one thumb and this is the most straightforward manner of palpating and assessing the tissues (Fig. 1.3). It is often more practical, however, to apply the technique with both thumbs when using it on certain regions of the body (for instance, on the muscles and fascia of the upper back; Fig. 2.26), as this allows for easier control of the body posture and the pressure of the technique.

Each stroke is carried out over an area of about 5–8 cm (2–3 inch) in one direction. To allow for the tissues to be palpated, assessed and treated, the speed of the stroke is very slow, lasting about 4–6 seconds to complete. Contact is made with the lateral border of the ball of each thumb or with the very tip; the smaller the contact area the more precise is the information picked up by the sensory nerve ending on the thumb.

When used together, the thumbs are positioned one behind the other. They palpate the tissues and assess them for any changes such as nodular areas. These are then treated by an increase in the pressure and a repetition of the same stroke. The intensity is immediately reduced if an area of 'give' is encountered; similarly, the pressure is eased once the nodules themselves yield to the pressure. The strokes are repeated several times, and once the treatment is completed on one region the hands are posi-

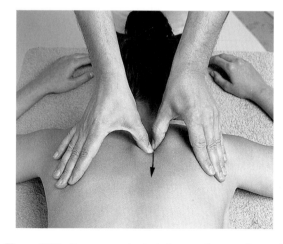

Figure 2.26 Neuromuscular technique on the muscles and fascia of the upper back.

tioned on another area and the procedure resumed.

Pressure of neuromuscular technique

As already indicated, the pressure of NMT is adjusted according to the state of the tissues and the degree of sensitivity in the area. The pressure does not exceed the subject's pain threshold. If the threshold is exceeded a reflex muscle and tissue contraction is likely to occur which would intensify the sensitivity. In addition, the contraction may affect the circulation of the muscles and superficial blood vessels, causing ischaemia.

Excessive pressure can also cause some trauma and inflammation in the tissues. This would be counterproductive as the outcome of inflammation is infiltration by collagen fibres as part of the repair mechanism and therefore, to some degree, of scarring and adhesions.

When treatment is carried out on certain tissue states (for example, on fibrotic or hypertonic areas), the tendency is to increase the pressure. An increase in pressure may be necessary to reduce fibrotic tissue, bearing in mind that these changes are often very difficult or impossible to reverse. Inflammation of the tissues is very likely to ensue and it is therefore important to treat this area with a cooling pack following the treatment. In most cases the inflammation is a result of microtrauma and will resolve quickly. However, it is also good practice to advise the subject to apply cooling packs at home should the tenderness or the heat of inflammation persist. Some gentle passive stretching can be applied following treatment with NMT as it helps to realign tissue fibres. Further stretching can be carried out by the subject a day or two after treatment to maintain the flexibility of the tissues and reduce adhesions.

Trigger points

A trigger point (Travell and Simons, 1983, p. 12) is located by assessing a tissue area that is likely to house a hypersensitive nodule. Trigger points may be found in fascial or muscular tissue, ligaments or tendons, scar tissue, or deep within a joint capsule or the periosteum of bone (see Chapter 1). Palpation of such a reflex zone will refer a sensation to a distant region, either increased sensitivity or purely a sensation. Common trigger points are often active; one such example is the upper area of the splenius capitis muscle (Fig. 1.7). The patterns and location of trigger points are distributed in all body regions. Examples of frequently found trigger areas are in the sternocleidomastoid, levator scapulae, lower fibres of the latissimus dorsi, infraspinatus, trapezius and rhomboid muscles.

Once a reflex zone is established as a trigger point, it is treated in the manner described here. The procedure is also included in Chapter 5.

1. Pressure is applied on the reflex area using the pad of a finger or a thumb and, whilst gentle, the pressure is sufficiently deep to activate the trigger point and so refer the sensation to a distant region. The pressure applied on a trigger point area must not exceed the subject's pain threshold. Protective muscular tension is very likely to occur if the pressure is excessive, especially if the subject experiences a pain sensation.

2. Pressure into the tissue is held for a few seconds and then released for a few seconds; it is then resumed once more, and this procedure is continued either until the sensation in the distant region reduces or for approximately 1–2 min.

3. The tissue housing the trigger point, e.g. muscle, tendon, fascia or ligament, is passively stretched for a minute or thereabouts. During this stretch or just prior to it the tissues are rapidly cooled. A cooling spray or an ice cube can be used; these will restrict the cooling to the specific muscle, tendon or ligament. Using a very cold wet towel is another option, but this chills a wider area.

4. The process of applying the on-and-off pressure can be repeated if necessary, and the tissues stretched once more.

Soft tissue manipulation

The term 'soft tissue manipulation' is frequently used in bodywork and manipulative therapies. It is applied to shift and modify the soft tissues (such as fascia layers and muscles) so that they are stretched longitudinally or transversely, compressed, or lifted off the underlying structures.

Most of the time, soft tissue manipulations are carried out without any lubrication to allow for a good grip, and therefore with minimal sliding of the hands. These methods can be employed on most regions of the body as palpatory skills during assessment of the tissues' resilience. They can also be used to reduce adhesions, fibrotic states, muscle tightness and so forth. Invariably, soft tissue manipulations are applied in combination with other bodywork techniques such as neuromuscular strokes and treatment of trigger points. Some of the massage strokes, even though applied with a lubricant, are soft tissue manipulations, e.g. petrissage. Strictly speaking, however, manipulations of the soft tissues are ideally carried out without any lubrication. This method of treatment is in itself a useful method of improving the palpatory skills as the hands can be trained to 'feel' the tissues rather than slide over them. For this reason the massage therapist will do well to practise soft tissue manipulations and, indeed, to combine them with the massage treatment. Soft tissue manipulations can be easily adapted for most regions of the body, and applications of these methods are depicted in later chapters.

A simple manipulation is carried out with the fingers and thumb of each hand, which gently grip the tissues and lift them off the underlying structures. In this method, all the digits are extended and rest flat to the skin surface to prevent any 'pinching' of the skin as the tissues are lifted. The technique can be applied with one hand (already described as a kneading movement) or with both hands simultaneously. What is termed as 'skin rolling' is another example of soft tissue manipulation that can be applied to the superficial layers of the back. Soft tissue manipulations can equally benefit large muscle groups. When working on the calf muscles for example, the gastrocnemius and the soleus muscles are lifted off the deeper muscle layers and the tibia and fibula. This applies a transverse stretch to the fibres of the muscles and also reduces adhesions between fascia layers (Fig. 2.27).

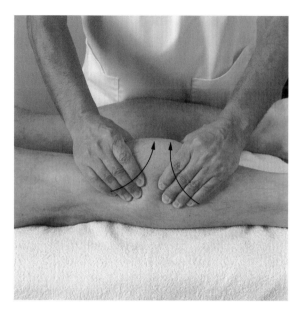

Figure 2.27 Soft tissue manipulation of the calf muscles.

A longitudinal stretch can be applied to the soft tissues of the back. While standing on one side of the treatment table, the operator places both forearms on the contralateral side of the back. Initially these are positioned next to each other in the middle thoracic region. Some pressure is applied so that the forearms grip the tissues and take up some of the slack. While this pressure is maintained the tissues are stretched further as the cephalad forearm is taken further into that direction and the caudad one is pushed further towards the pelvis (Chapter 5, Fig. 5.2). Pressure can be adjusted as the body weight is used to exert the necessary force. This has to be sufficient to stretch not only the superficial tissues but also the muscle layers. The position of stretch is held for a few seconds before the tissues are released and the whole procedure repeated. Variations of the position of the forearms can be used, and the technique can also be applied on the ipsilateral side of the back.

Passive stretching

Returning to the archetypal discipline of Swedish massage movements, or physical therapeutics as they were known in the early days, the tissues and joints are passively manipulated following the massage strokes. The premise for this practice was that passive mobilization of joints and tissues helps to secure their newly adjusted flexibility and provides a base for further improvement, for example with exercise. Nerve pathways and reflexes are additionally stimulated and restored with these manipulations. This principle is still valid and therefore some basic passive stretching and mobilizations can be carried out as part of the massage treatment. It is important to add, however, that complicated pain conditions affecting the spinal column or any joint of the extremities are best left to the expertise of other practitioners, such as osteopaths, chiropractors and physiotherapists. General stretches and mobilizations can be applied, albeit not necessarily in every massage treatment; during a relaxing full body massage, for example, bodywork techniques can take up too much time and may be too disruptive to the process of relaxation. These techniques are of great value for many conditions, and consequently are discussed in the chapters on the applications of massage.

Passive stretching involves extending the muscle to its full resting length, or as near to it as possible. It is easily applied to the limbs, where a long lever system can be used. This technique, however, must not be limited to these regions, as other areas such as the back and neck derive great benefit from it. Once the muscle has been gently taken to its full length, it is held in that position for about 5 seconds and is then returned to its shortest resting position. The procedure may be resumed once more if necessary.

One method of passively stretching the quadriceps is carried out with the patient lying prone. The massage therapist holds the lower leg with one hand and stabilizes the pelvis by applying some gentle pressure. Flexion of the knee exerts a passive stretch to the quadriceps and this can be gently increased as the foot is taken towards the pelvis (Fig. 2.28).

Joint mobilization

Mobilization of joints is more involved, because of the number of structures that may be malfunctioning. The joint to be moved is taken through its full range of movement. Limitation of movement is caused by malfunction in any one of the structures: the bone surfaces, capsule, bursae or associated muscles. For the massage therapist, the aim of carrying out a passive movement is not to diagnose or treat any pathological dysfunction but to increase the mobility of the joint. The technique itself is restricted mostly to the joints of the extremities and is only applied in some of the conditions being treated with massage.

Mobilization of the hip joint is carried out with the patient supine. Essentially, the limb is first held in a secure position, in most cases using both hands. The massage therapist holds the patient's knee with both hands and moves both the hip and the knee joints into flexion. It may be easier to hold the knee with one hand and use the second hand under the foot to offer more support (Fig. 2.29). The femur is then moved in the various directions of flexion, internal and external rotation, abduction and adduction. Both clockwise and anticlockwise movements are suitable. It is worth noting that pain in the hip joint itself

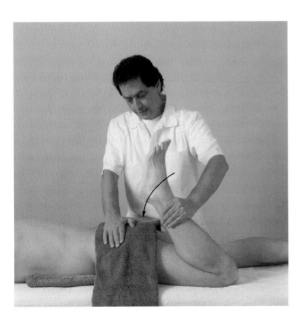

Figure 2.28 Passive stretching of the quadriceps muscles.

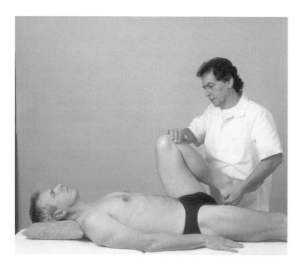

Figure 2.29 Joint mobilization of the hip.

may be indicative of arthritic changes. While this condition would indeed benefit from passive articulation, hip joint mobilization may be uncomfortable and would therefore be contraindicated. Approval from the patient's manipulative therapist or doctor may be needed before further treatment.

Muscle energy technique

Muscle energy technique (MET) is another of the bodywork methods that are employed to help normalize skeletal muscles and somatic tissue dysfunctions. As with other bodywork treatment, the theory and applications of the methods are very comprehensive, as illustrated in Leon Chaitow's book *Muscle Energy Techniques* (1996b), and necessitate the appropriate training. A basic approach, however, such as the post-isometric relaxation (PIR) can be easily integrated into the massage therapy and effectively applied for enhancing relaxation of muscles. The term MET covers a number of procedures, which include PIR, isolytic contraction, reciprocal inhibition, resistive duction, isokinetic contraction or progressive-resisted exercise, and integrated neuromuscular inhibition technique. Of these, PIR is perhaps the most frequently used and the simplest method to incorporate in a massage treat-

ment. MET can help achieve the following changes:

1. Reduce muscle tension.
2. Stretch shortened muscles. A passive stretch can be applied to a shortened muscle following relaxation.
3. Treatment of trigger points. Trigger points are treated by stretching of the muscles where they are located. This is normally carried out following treatment of the trigger points with NMT or ischaemic compression with 'on-and-off' pressure.
4. Improve muscle tone. Shortened muscles prevent their antagonists from maintaining full tonus. A short agonist muscle therefore results in a weak antagonist. Conversely, when a postural muscle that is in a 'contracted' and shortened state is treated with PIR and lengthened, the tonus of its antagonist is improved. This in turn can be further toned up with exercise.
5. Improving the muscle tone can also be achieved by applying one of the methods of contraction:
   - Isometric contraction, where the muscle is working against a resistance but remains static so that it does not lengthen or shorten.
   - Isotonic concentric contraction, where the muscle is working against resistance but is also shortening at the same time so that the origin and insertion are in approximation.
   - Isotonic eccentric contraction where the muscle is working against resistance but is also lengthening so that the origin and insertion are moving further apart.
   - Isokinetic contraction or progressive-resisted exercise. This is akin to an 'isotonic concentric contraction', but it is called isokinetic as the joint is being mobilized at the same time. The patient is asked to start with a weak contraction of a muscle against a resistance offered by the operator. Without any rests or breaks the patient rapidly increases this to a full strength while the operator is taking the associated joint through its movement. This manoeuvre should be very rapid and takes about 4 seconds for each contraction. It is worth noting,

however, that in some cases the patient may not be able to conduct such a change in effort. The technique is most suitable for smaller joints such as those of the upper and lower extremities. The same toning effect can also be achieved by using an 'isotonic eccentric' contraction.

6. Improve joint mobility by normalizing associated muscle groups.
7. Nerve impulses travelling to and from muscles are normalized.
8. Fibrotic tissue can be broken down (to a degree) and stretched (using isolytic technique).

Any one method, or a combination of methods, can be used to achieve the desired effect. As already noted, the most frequently used technique in massage is that of PIR. Justification for its use lies in that the technique helps to reduce muscle tension, even that associated with emotional anxiety, and therefore enhances the effect of the massage. It can also be used to ease tightness and temporary shortening of a muscle or muscle group, and this is a valuable supplement to the massage treatment.

Post-isometric relaxation

PIR is very similar to, and is likely to have its origins in, proprioceptive neuromuscular facilitation, a system applied in rehabilitation programmes. Other terms which describe this method include 'hold–relax'; 'contract–relax' and 'myokinesis'. As already discussed, PIR is particularly useful for relaxing and stretching muscles. To increase relaxation of a muscle the patient is asked to carry out an isometric (static) contraction. After a few seconds the patient releases the contraction and allows the muscle to relax. The concept is that the muscle achieves a greater relaxation following the isometric contraction, and this can be of benefit in two ways. It may be a means of relaxing tense muscles, especially if the tension is associated with emotional anxiety. It may also be used to stretch the muscle passively during the relaxation phase. When treating areas of considerable emotional tension like the neck region, the contraction–relaxation phase

is carried out but the passive stretching following the relaxation is omitted. The reasoning behind this approach is that the patient may be too tense to tolerate any passive stretching. In any case, the contraction followed by the letting go, if repeated several times, may be sufficiently effective to induce relaxation.

In this section the technique is demonstrated and described for the hamstrings and gluteal muscles (Fig. 2.30); other regions are covered in later chapters.

Procedure

- The patient lies supine with one knee and hip flexed; in this manner the upper fibres of the hamstrings and the gluteus muscles are slightly stretched. When PIR is performed, with the aim of stretching, the muscle or muscle group is first put into a position of maximum stretch.
- The practitioner stands next to the patient and uses one or both hands to exert some pressure on the flexed knee.
- The patient is first asked to apply an isometric contraction by pushing the knee against the operator's hand, whilst the operator applies an equal pressure so that the gluteal and hamstring muscles are contracted but in a static position. The patient need use only about 20% of their strength, but this can vary depending

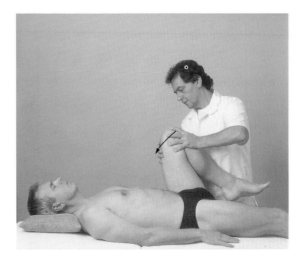

Figure 2.30 Post-isometric relaxation carried out on the gluteal and the hamstring muscles.

on the degree of muscle contraction and the person's own response.

- This contraction is held for about 6–10 seconds.
- Following this static contraction the patient is then asked to release the force, as the operator similarly eases the pressure.
- As the patient lets go, the muscles relax into a greater state of relaxation than they were before the contraction.
- During this relaxation phase, the muscles can be passively stretched as the operator pushes the knee to increase the hip flexion.

Physiology of post-isometric relaxation

The physiology of the technique is that a passive stretch of a muscle (at maximum stretch) also stretches the Golgi tendon receptor organ. Golgi tendon receptors are situated in series with the fibres and so are stimulated by both active and passive contractions of the muscles (see also Chapter 3). When the muscle is maintained at full stretch and worked isometrically the Golgi tendon receptor senses the increased muscle tension. As the Golgi tendon receptor is loaded and stretched, it reflexively inhibits the extrafusal fibres of the muscle, albeit temporarily. The reflex arc causes the neuromuscular end-plate and the muscle membrane to be hyperpolarized, leading to muscle relaxation. The muscle is stretched during the 'refractory period', i.e. when the muscle is being polarized after working. During repolarization there are no motor impulses and therefore no contraction taking place. According to Karel Lewit (Lewit, 1991), during the relaxing phase and stretch, the stretch reflex involving the muscle spindle is avoided (the stretch has to be gentle). Normally the muscle spindle responds to stretching passively or actively, but as long as the stretch is gentle firing of the muscles spindle is avoided.

3

The effects of massage

INTRODUCTION

Substantiation for the efficacy of massage is often sought by massage therapists and, increasingly nowadays, by the authorizing bodies, health providers and the medical profession. Several papers and books covered the subject during the Victorian age (Brunton and Tunnicliff, 1894–1895) and throughout the 20th century. Overall, however, research into the subject has been rather scarce until more recent times.

In the past, most research focused on the physiological effects of massage, e.g. on the blood circulation, lymphatic flow and muscle function. Some of the more recent studies have placed a greater emphasis on the relaxation aspects of massage. Despite the fact that many of the 'old' studies were somewhat inconclusive as to the positive effects of massage, a great proportion of the historical information still holds some value today. At the very least it provides some evidence of the relationship between the manipulation of tissues and some of the body systems. Accordingly, references to some of the old literature are made in this and other chapters. Supplementary and more up-to-date data is taken from recent studies and clinical trials. While these are still not always conclusive in their findings, they are now much more clearly designed and controlled, and provide some statistical confirmation needed to meet the current demand for 'evidence-based' therapies.

In addition to the relaxation and emotional support that it offers, massage therapy is of benefit because of the influence it has on a number of bodily processes. These consequences or effects of massage are considered to be mechanical, neural, chemical and physiological (Yates, 1989), or simply mechanical and reflex (Mennell, 1920). All of these hypotheses are significant, and indeed interrelate with each other and with underlying psychotherapeutic factors.

The biomechanical effect refers to the direct influence massage has on the soft tissues being manipulated. Crediting a massage movement with an effect that is solely biomechanical is, however, difficult because even the simple action of contacting the patient's skin sets up a neural reflex loop. A psychotherapeutic–energy interaction is also likely to take place between the patient and the therapist as a result of this contact. However, for the purpose of classification, it is acceptable to tabulate some techniques as being predominantly biomechanical and having a direct physical effect. Stretching and loosening of muscles is one example. Improving the flow of fluid through the blood and lymph vessels as well as the onward movement of the intestinal contents represent other biomechanical actions.

A reflex effect of massage occurs indirectly. Neural mechanisms are influenced by manual intervention and action on the tissues, and massage is one such intervention. The process is centred on the interrelationships of the peripheral (cutaneous) and central nervous systems, their reflex patterns and multiple pathways. The autonomic nervous system and neuroendocrine control are also involved (Greenman, 1989).

The psychotherapeutic or psychosocial effect of massage is very relevant to the outcome of the treatment. As a result of the relaxation provided by massage therapy, the recipient's sensitivity to anxiety and stress is likely to be reduced. This in itself may be the only change needed for healing to take place. A placebo effect may also be in place, where a strong belief that massage can be helpful has a powerful influence on the recipient's self-healing mechanisms. Equally feasible is that, with relaxation, the subject becomes more receptive to the other therapeutic effects of massage, for example on hormones and immunity. It is noteworthy that the systems which appear to respond most to massage (namely the integumentary, the cardiovascular, autonomic nervous and the neuroimmune systems) are also the ones which respond very well to relaxation techniques such as guided imagery (Menard, 2002).

Biochemical changes, such as a reduction of stress hormone levels, have been shown to occur with massage (Field, 1998). These may take place through any one, or a combination, of the biomechanical, reflex and psychotherapeutic effects. The immune system is also helped with massage. Findings indicate that massage can produce specific effects, such as an increase in the eradicating properties or activity (cytotoxicity) of natural killer cells (Ironson et al., 1996) through the pathway of perception and adaptation involving the higher centres and the limbic system.

The outcome of a treatment is frequently influenced by 'non-measurable' factors such as the mind–body–soul connection, subtle healing energies, and the interaction between the patient and therapist. As massage is very much a 'touch' therapy, an appropriate approach and contact by the therapist are also vital to the treatment. Other components include the frequency of the treatment, the rhythm, the protocol and the environment.

The effects of massage on the various tissues and systems of the body are considered in this chapter. As already stated, the pathways can be primarily biomechanical, biochemical, psychotherapeutic or reflex. More often, however, they are likely to involve more than one of these factors.

The information presented here is by no means comprehensive but it provides some fundamental theoretical background and the rationale for the clinical application of massage on the systems of the body. It is also used to support the application of massage in some common pathological conditions, as discussed in Chapter 4.

Neural mechanisms

Introduction

While it is not the intention of this book to cover physiology in great detail, familiarization with some aspects of the nervous system is vital to the comprehension of the effects of massage. By way of facilitating this task for the reader, aspects of the nervous system pertaining mostly to the physiology of massage are revised in some detail in this section.

Stressors

The malfunctions and changes that are often observed and palpated in the tissues during the assessment stage of the massage treatment have already been discussed in Chapter 1. Closely linked with these tissue states are stressors, which act as their precursors. The body is subjected to a number of stressors (Box 3.1), which cause reflex and involuntary responses involving the sensory nerves, the autonomic nervous system and the motor nerves. These stress factors can vary in their severity and frequency. They may be mild, severe, episodic or chronic. As a general rule, they fall under four headings: chemical, physical, emotional and congenital.

Neural connections with the peripheral tissues

The connection between soft tissue manipulation and organ function is closely related to the neural supply of dermatomes and myotomes. These segmental distributions occur as part of the embryonal development, and represent the innervation of the peripheral tissues by the spinal nerves. In many cases, branches of the spinal nerves innervate other body tissues and organs; for example, muscles, superficial tissues and visceral organs often share common spinal nerves. As a consequence of this association, malfunction of an organ may be reflected in those dermatomes and myotomes that share the same spinal nerve as the organ in question (Schliack, 1978), and the connection manifests itself and can be observed as changes in the peripheral tissues (also referred to as reflex zones; Ebner, 1962; 1968; 1978). These irregularities can also occur as a result of other stressors besides organ malfunction. The tissue changes in reflex zones can therefore develop after some weeks of visceral pathology or dysfunction, and also after a few days of somatic

---

Box 3.1   Stressors

Chemical stressors
- Toxins which can result from acute or chronic infection
- Bacteria can also give off toxic chemicals, and can enter the body through a cut, a burn, the nose or through the skin
- Visceral disease gives off toxins, which act as irritants. These can cause or intensify somatic changes in those areas that are supplied by the same spinal segment. A similar connection can occur via an adjacent spinal segment, for example appendicitis leading to pain in the abdominal region
- Organic poisons such as acids, sugars, alcohol and tobacco
- Simple chemicals such as drugs, additives and colourings
- Metabolic imbalances such as allergic reactions and endocrine factors. These lead to disturbances in gland secretions (hormonal, digestive, etc.), which have an effect on the autonomic nervous system
- Nutritional imbalance, for example deprivation of ascorbic acid creating a deficiency in the connective tissue

Physical stressors
- Trauma: an accident or repetitive strain of the muscles
- Unaccustomed or excessive exercise
- Micro-trauma: postural strains or repetitive actions
- Vascular accident: a stroke leading to obstruction of the blood supply to the tissue cells
- Oedema
- Excessive heat or cold temperatures, for example changes in atmospheric pressure and draughts
- Nerve compression: spinal misalignments or nerve entrapment by muscles
- Spinal lesions (chronic or acute) and structural imbalances
- Arthritic changes
- Faulty muscular activity: spasms, spasticity, contractures
- Changes in visceral positioning, for example visceroptosis

Emotional stressors
- Anxiety, fear, anger, etc.

Inherited and congenital factors
- Haemophilia
- Spina bifida

dysfunction (in superficial tissues, muscles, nerves and so forth).

The relationship between the peripheral tissues and visceral organs has been described by many physicians and authors. Pathology of the viscera is a primary contributory factor to peripheral tissue changes, and this was first pointed out by Head (1989). A few years later, myotome involvement and pain sensibility from pathology were described by Sir James MacKenzie. He described the reflex process as 'a vital process which is concerned in the reception of a stimulus by one organ or tissue and its conduction to another organ which, on receiving a stimulus, produces the effect' (1923). One common example of this is the muscle tension and pain in the abdomen associated with appendicitis, where inflammation of the abdominal organ causes tension in the abdominal muscle wall, together with a referred pain. The theory of pathological conditions and their connection with subcutaneous changes was also presented by Elizabeth Dicke (1953, 1956). It was further postulated that a reflex connection or pathway runs in the reverse direction, from the periphery to the central structures. Observations were made of connective tissue malfunction causing disturbances in an organ that shares a common spinal nerve. One study looked at the cutaneous tissues, which are located in dermatomes supplied by the same spinal nerves as the heart. Malfunctions in these peripheral tissues led to symptoms within the heart, and the disturbances disappeared once the peripheral connective tissues were treated (Hartmann, 1929). Another study on animals showed that stimulation of the sensory afferent nerves by massage creates local vasodilatation. This is brought about first, by inhibition of the vasoconstrictor fibres in the tissues by the massage and, second, by excitation of the vasodilator fibres in the local area (Bayliss, as quoted in Jacobs, 1960).

Manipulation of the soft tissues, and in particular Ebner's connective tissue massage, may therefore induce reflex and beneficial effects in the associated organ or organs. The process involves a number of reflex effects:

- Reflex mechanisms can reduce sympathetic activity and promote vasodilatation.

- Local and systemic circulation, including that of the parasympathetic ganglia, is increased.
- The improved circulation helps to promote the healing process, reduce muscle spasm and improve the extensibility of connective tissue.
- There is also a general balancing of the autonomic nervous system. Research on the effects of massage on the autonomic nervous system shows variable results (discussed later in this chapter).

Neural pathways

The reflex pathways involved in massage can be clarified further by reviewing some aspects of the nervous system. Three types of neurons make up the nervous system:

1. Afferent (sensory) neurons transmit information from the tissues and organs of the body to the central nervous system (CNS).

2. Efferent (motor) neurons transmit information out from the CNS to effector cells (muscles or glands), which receive and react to the impulse. The axons of afferent and efferent neurons join to form the spinal nerves, which emerge between the vertebrae.

3. Interneurons are found only within the CNS, and form connections between the afferent and efferent neurons. In some cases, however, an impulse is transmitted between afferent and efferent neurons without passing through an interneuron. One example is the patellar tendon or 'knee-jerk' reflex, where tapping of the patellar tendon stimulates the muscle stretch receptors and results in immediate muscle contraction. Interneurons also act as switches that can turn on an impulse or switch it off and inhibit its transmission.

The nervous system is divided into two parts: the CNS comprises the brain and spinal cord, and the peripheral nervous system consists of nerves outside the CNS. The peripheral nervous system transmits signals between the CNS and all other parts of the body, and consists of 12 pairs of cranial and 31 pairs of spinal nerves. All spinal nerves and most cranial ones contain axons of afferent and efferent neurons, and can therefore be classified as belonging to the afferent (sensory) or efferent (motor) divisions of the peripheral nervous system. Some cranial nerves contain only afferent fibres (for example, the optic nerves from the eye).

The efferent aspect of the peripheral nervous system is divided into somatic and autonomic parts. The somatic system is made up of nerve fibres (motor neurons) leaving the spinal cord to innervate skeletal muscle cells. The autonomic nervous system innervates cardiac and smooth muscle, the glands and the gastrointestinal tract neurons. The latter group of the gastrointestinal tract neurons make up a specialized nerve network (enteric nervous system) in the wall of the gastrointestinal tract, which regulates its glands and smooth muscles. The afferent division of the peripheral nervous system conveys information from receptors to the CNS. One end of the afferent neuron (the central axon) joins the spinal cord and the other portion (the peripheral end) terminates in the tissue or organ.

Receptors

Receptors are the first to be touched by the massage therapist when contact is made with the skin, superficial fascia and muscles.

Furthermore, receptors are the starting point of many relay pathways, involving afferent and efferent impulses, that are instigated by the massage.

In view of their relevance in massage it is appropriate that a revision is made of some characteristics and properties of receptors and their pathways.

- Somatic receptors are found in the peripheral tissues or outer wall of the body, which encompasses the skin, the superficial fascia, tendons and the joints. The skin alone is said to contain between 7 and 135 sensory receptors per square centimetre. Sensory neurons conduct information from the receptors to the spinal cord.
- Receptors are situated at the peripheral ends of afferent (sensory) neurons, and their function is to respond to changes both in the outside world and within the body's own internal environment. The peripheral fibres or endings of the sensory neuron (like those in the skin or subcutaneous tissues) can make up the receptor. An adjacent cell can also perform the same function, transmitting the impulses to the peripheral endings of the neuron.
- Sensory receptors respond to changes in their environment by initiating neural activity within the afferent neuron; these initial neural activities are referred to as graded potentials, which are translated into action potentials. The stimulus or energy that activates a sensory receptor can take many forms, such as touch, pressure, temperature, light, sound waves, chemical molecules, etc. Most receptors respond specifically to one form of stimulus; however, virtually all can be activated by several different forms of energy if the intensity is sufficiently high. Pain receptors, for example, are stimulated by pressure, temperature and toxins.
- After entering the spinal cord some of the impulses are conducted along ascending pathways within the cord and thus to the different regions of the brain (brainstem, thalamus, cerebrum and cortex).
- Many of the sensory impulses, having synapsed with interneurons along the pathway, are conducted to the cerebral cortex. When they reach this region of the brain the sensory stimuli will produce conscious sensations. Other impulses terminate in the spinal cord or the brainstem and these do not typically produce conscious sensations.
- Some of the ascending pathways (spinal tracts) carry information about one type of stimulus only; for instance, a stimulus from mechanoreceptors, and these tracts are called specific pathways. Other tracts are non-specific ascending pathways and carry stimuli from different receptors.
- Stimulation of a sensory receptor can lead to a reflex mechanism whereby motor efferent impulses travel down the cord to synapse with lower motor neurons. One typical outcome is increased tension in the same tissues from which the sensory impulses originated. This is not always the case, however. Sensory impulses do not always lead to motor impulses emerging

from the anterior horn of the spine. In some cases the response is a 'negative feedback', which will inhibit motor impulses.

- Adaptation. Adaptation is a decrease in the frequency of action potentials in an afferent neuron despite maintenance of the stimulus at constant strength. Some receptors adapt completely so that, in spite of a constantly maintained stimulus, the generation of action potentials stops. A typical example of adaptation is the awareness of the touch pressure exerted by a ring when it is first put on a finger. This is then followed by a gradual decrease in the sensation of pressure. Some receptors, such as those responding to touch, pressure and smell, adapt rapidly. Others are slowly adapting receptors and amongst these are the nociceptors and the proprioreceptors.
- A sensation describes the conscious awareness of a stimulus; for example, pressure being applied to the tissues. In addition to feeling a direct stimulus, sensation can also be understood or perceived; for example, the sensation of pain can be perceived as coming from an infection or injury.

Classification of receptors

One classification of receptors is based on the type of stimuli they detect, as catalogued here. Those used most in massage are the mechanoreceptors and the nociceptors.

1. *Photoreceptors* detect light on the retina of the eye.
2. *Chemoreceptors* detect taste, smell and chemicals in the body fluids.
3. *Temperature receptors (thermoreceptors)* detect changes in temperature.

- These are found as free nerve endings and are dispersed randomly throughout the skin.
- Those in the skin are classified according to their responses to cold and heat.
  Type-1(warm receptors):
  – Free nerve endings
  – Respond to temperatures between 30°C and 40°C
  – Increase their discharge rate upon warming.

Type-2 (cold receptors):
– Structure unknown
– Stimulated by temperatures between 20°C and 35°C
– Increase their discharge rate upon cooling.

4. *Mechanoreceptors* detect mechanical changes within the receptor itself or in nearby structures.

- These type of receptors are stimulated by touch, pressure, vibration, proprioception, hearing, equilibrium and blood pressure.
- Mechanoreceptors also respond differently to stimuli and are therefore of two types:
  – Type a: Quickly adapting. In response to sustained pressure these receptors will quickly adapt to the stimulus and respond with a burst of action potentials. When activated, these receptors generally give rise to the sensations of touch, movement, vibration and tickling.
  – Type b: Slowly adapting. In response to sustained pressure these receptors will slowly adapt to the stimulus and respond with a sustained discharge throughout the duration of the stimulus. These receptors generally give rise to the sensation of pressure.

5. *Pain receptors*

- Most pain receptors are nociceptors. They are located at the end of small unmyelinated or lightly myelinated afferent neurons.
- They are sensitive to any stimulus which can cause tissue damage.
- Pain receptors respond to different stimuli such as:
  – intense mechanical pressure
  – mechanical and thermal stimulation
  – irritant chemicals as well as to mechanical and thermal stimulation. Chemicals such as histamine, bradykinin and prostaglandins are released from damaged tissue and depolarize nearby nociceptor nerve endings, initiating action potentials in the afferent nerve fibre.
  – excessive stretching, swelling or expansion of a structure
  – muscle spasm or prolonged muscular contractions
  – ischaemia to a tissue or organ.

When stimuli from other receptors, such as those for touch, pressure, heat and cold, reach a certain threshold, they will also stimulate the pain receptors.

- Pain receptors differ from other receptors because:
  - emotions such as fear, anxiety, etc. are experienced along with the physical sensation
  - a painful stimulus can evoke a reflex escape or withdrawal response
  - a painful stimulus can evoke physical changes similar to those elicited by fear, anxiety and aggression; these are mediated by the sympathetic nervous system and include increased heart rate and blood pressure, greater secretion of adrenaline, and increased blood glucose concentration.

Skin receptors—general grouping

The most superficial receptors are found in the dermis and epidermis of the skin, and also in the connective tissue (subcutaneous layer) just under the skin (Fig. 3.1). These receptors are mostly nociceptors, thermoceptors or mechanoreceptors. However, one further classification of these receptors is based on the myelin covering of the axons, which are referred to as:

a. *Free nerve endings*

- These have little or no myelin covering and can be described as the branching ends of dendrites of certain sensory neurons.
- They are dispersed randomly throughout the structures.
- They are sensitive to stimuli that give rise to pain and temperature, and are therefore mostly nociceptors and thermoceptors.
- They can also act as mechanoreceptors and respond to objects that are in continuous contact with the skin, such as clothing.
- Their impulses travel to the brain via the lateral spinothalamic tract in the spinal cord.

b. *Thick myelinated axons*

- End in receptors that can be quite complex.
- All are sensitive to skin displacement, i.e. indentation or touch pressure.
- Examples include:
  - Pacinian corpuscles
  - Meissner's corpuscles
  - Ruffini corpuscles
  - Merkel discs.

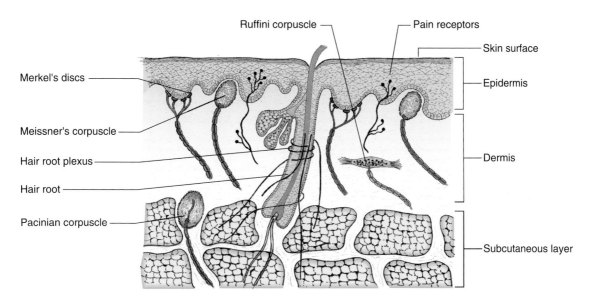

Figure 3.1   Sensory receptors in the dermis and epidermis of the skin.

Tactile (touch) sensations

Stimulation of the receptors found in the skin and subcutaneous layers gives rise to tactile sensations. While tactile sensations can be divided into those of touch, pressure and vibration they all originate from the same category of receptors, namely the mechanoreceptors. They are all sensitive to deformation of the tissues as previously discussed but can be further differentiated by the type of stimulus they convey. The sensation of touch conveyed by these tactile receptors can be:

• Light touch sensation that can be perceived as a vague feeling.
• Discriminative touch that is more specific and conveys an exact area of contact.

The tactile receptors for touch are mostly:

a. *Hair root plexuses.* These are dendrites that are wrapped around the base of hair follicles. They are sensitive to movements on the surface of the skin. Like free nerve endings, they are not surrounded by supportive or protective layers.

b. *Free (naked) nerve endings.* These are widespread in the skin and most other tissues. Although their primary function is as pain receptors they also sense continuous touch, as when something is worn next to the skin.

c. *Tactile or Merkel's discs.* These are mostly located in areas of hairless skin. They also follow the same distribution as the corpuscles of touch, and function in a similar way, i.e. relay discriminative touch.

d. *Corpuscles of touch* or *Meissner's corpuscles.* As these receptors contain a mass of dendrites they are ideally suited for discriminative touch. They are found in great number in areas of hairless skin such as the palms of the hands, the soles of the feet and the fingertips. In addition, they can be located in the eyelids, tip of the tongue, lips, nipples, clitoris and tip of penis.

e. *Type II cutaneous mechanoreceptors* or *end organs of Ruffini.* The sites for these receptors are deep in the dermis and the deeper tissues of the body. Their primary function is to detect heavy and continuous touch sensations.

Pressure sensation

Some of the tactile receptors are located in deeper tissues of the body and these are used to transmit sensations of pressure. Pressure is very similar to touch but can be heavier or sustained. Sensations of pressure are felt primarily on larger areas than those sensations perceived as touch.

The receptors for pressure are:

a. *Free nerve endings.*
b. *Type II cutaneous mechanoreceptors.*
c. *Lamellated corpuscles* or *Pacinian corpuscles.*

These are located deep within the skin, deep to mucous membranes, in serous membranes, surrounding joints and tendons, in the perimysium of muscles, in the mammary glands, in the external genitalia of both sexes and in certain viscera.

Sensations of vibration

Tactile receptors are also used to transmit sensations of vibration. A vibration impulse can be described as the repetitive signal of touch.

The receptors for vibration are:

a. *Lamellated corpuscles* or *Pacinian corpuscles.* Located in the dermis of the skin and the subcutaneous tissue, Pacinian corpuscles are the primary receptors of vibration (Intyre, 1975). They detect vibrations of high frequency (albeit that some authors put this as low as 50 and as high as 500 Hz). They adapt quickly, which means that they reduce their firing rate soon after the vibration is applied. To keep these corpuscles activated the vibratory movements need to be carried out intermittently, i.e. as short bursts.

b. *Corpuscles of touch* or *Meissner's corpuscles.* These can respond to a low frequency vibration and may be found in the ligaments, tendons and periosteum.

Reflexes

A reflex is an involuntary response to a stimulus (defined as a detectable shift in the environment such as a change in temperature or pressure). A familiar example is pulling one's hand away from a hot object. Reflexes also form part of the body's own homeostatic mechanism. This process can be observed when there is a fall in the body's external temperature, resulting in the involuntary contractions of the skeletal muscles (shivering) and of the smooth muscles surrounding the blood vessels in an attempt to maintain the body temperature.

A reflex pathway or arc (Fig. 3.2) is set up when the receptors are stimulated. Impulses from the receptors travel along afferent neurons to the integrating centre in the brain or spinal cord, and information from the integrating centre is sent along efferent (motor) neurons to the effector tissue. Almost all cells in the body can be effectors, but the most specialized and easily affected are those of muscles and glands. The outcome of a reflex action is contraction or relaxation of the muscle tissue. In some cases the efferent information from the integrating centre is conveyed in the vascular system rather than a nerve fibre, and here the messenger is a hormone. Glandular secretions are therefore affected by muscle contraction or by hormonal stimulation. Reflexes are modified by higher centres; for example, emotional tension increases the patellar reflex and exacerbates muscle tension generally.

The following examples of reflexes illustrate their application in massage.

1. The cutaneovisceral pathway or somatic reflex

Manipulation of the cutaneous soft tissues stimulates the sensory receptors in the dermis and subcutaneous fascia. As a result, afferent impulses travel to the posterior horn of the spinal cord. Here they synapse with anterior horn cells and emerge as motor impulses, which travel to the sympathetic ganglia of the autonomic nervous system. The motor impulses continue along the postganglionic fibres and end in the target tissue, namely the involuntary muscles of a visceral organ or gland. One of the beneficial effects of massage is that it can stimulate these visceral structures via this reflex pathway.

2. Viscerocutaneous reflex

Stimulation of the receptors within a gland or organ leads to changes in the peripheral cutaneous tissues. Activation of the organ's receptors can result, for example, from pressure,

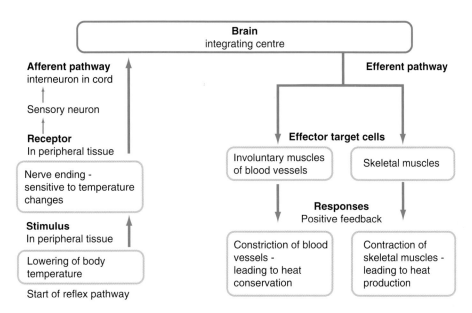

Figure 3.2 Reflex pathway showing the afferent and efferent nerves.

inflammation or bacterial toxins. The changes occurring in the periphery may be vasoconstriction of the superficial blood vessels, hyperaesthesia and pain.

3. The visceromotor reflex

A visceromotor reflex involves the contractions (tenseness) of muscle tissue, either unstriated or skeletal. It results from a stimulus, usually a painful one, originating in a visceral organ. Muscle tightness can therefore be related to a visceromotor reflex in addition to having more direct causative factors.

4. Abdominal reflex

The lightest touch to the abdominal skin results in an instant and visible contraction of the abdominal muscle wall. This involuntary reaction demonstrates the sensitivity of the abdomen and the gentle approach needed when massaging this region.

5. The abdominocardiac reflex

This is a change in the heart rate, usually a slowing down, resulting from mechanical stimulation of the abdominal viscera. Massage movements on the abdomen achieve some degree of visceral manipulation, and can therefore be seen as affecting the heart.

STRESS RESPONSES

Stress

Stress can be described as the body's reaction to stressors (see Box 3.1), which can disturb the body's physiological equilibrium (homeostasis). The biological concept of stress was developed by the Canadian physician Hans Selye (1984), who used the term 'stress' to indicate the outcome or effect which the stressors have upon the body. Another phrase associated with Selye is the 'general adaptation syndrome'. This can be described as an organism's non-specific response to stress (Taber, 1977). The process is said to occur in three stages: the alarm stage, the resistance stage and the exhaustive stage.

1. The alarm stage The first stage is the alarm (fight-or-flight) phase. During this period, the body recognizes the stressor and responds by producing the necessary hormones to deal with it. These hormones include cortisol and catecholamines.

Cortisol (hydrocortisone) is an adrenal cortical hormone. Its physiological effects are closely related to cortisone, which regulates the metabolism of fats, carbohydrates, sodium, potassium and proteins. Saliva cortisol and urine levels are used as stress indicators.

Catecholamines (norepinephrine, epinephrine and dopamine) are a class of neurotransmitters (chemical agents) which can affect mood. Norepinephrine and epinephrine are produced in response to stress; dopamine is related to motor function and mental disorders such as Parkinson's disease. Epinephrine and norepinephrine have a significant influence on the nervous and cardiovascular systems, the metabolic rate, temperature and smooth muscles. Urine levels of catecholamines are also used as stress indicators.

Other changes can be observed and monitored as indicators of stress. These include an increase in heart rate, elevation of blood sugar, dilatation of pupils, a slowing of digestion, sleep disturbance and muscle tension. In the fight-or-flight stage the body's response to the stress situation includes an increase in blood pressure and heart rate, increased oxygen consumption and increased muscle tone (Jenkins and Rogers, 1997; Murphy, 1996).

2. Resistance stage The second stage of the general adaptive syndrome is the resistance, or adaptive, stage. In this phase, the body attempts to restore its physiological equilibrium and to reverse the negative effects of the stressor. In situations in which the stressor exerts a mild and brief influence, the acute stress symptoms will diminish or disappear. On the other hand, if the impact of the stressor is strong and prolonged, the body's capability to adapt is weakened.

3. Exhaustive stage In the third stage, the body suffers from exhaustion and can no longer respond to stress. This weakening makes it susceptible to the onset of diseases, including emotional disturbances, cardiovascular disorders, renal problems and certain types of asthma.

Inner and behavioural emotions

The psychogenic effects of massage involve the emotions, as experienced or expressed by the individual. Two aspects of emotions have been distinguished: inner emotions and emotional behaviour (Vander et al., 1990). Inner emotions are within the person, and are the feelings such as fear, love, anger, joy, anxiety, hope, etc. These feelings are consciously experienced through the cerebral cortex and the various regions of the limbic system.

Emotional behaviour refers to the actions that result from the inner emotions or accompany them, and includes crying, laughing, sweating, aggressive behaviour, etc. These actions occur due to the integrated activity of the autonomic nervous system and the somatic system (which involves the efferent motor nerves). The autonomic activity is primarily under the control of the hypothalamus but it can also be influenced by the brainstem and spinal cord. Neural mechanisms for the motor efferent activity are provided by the cerebral cortex.

Massage has a very significant effect on the emotional state of the person and, in turn, on the emotional behaviour. The cumulative effect of relaxation, originating in the muscles and extending to the whole person, is to create a change in the patient's emotional state. One primary transformation is that inner feelings of tension and anxiety are replaced by calmness and tranquillity. As a result of these positive adjustments, other inner emotions such as depression and anger may also abate. In turn, the emotional behavioural responses will become less severe or may disappear totally. The outcome is a decrease in heart rate, lowering of blood pressure, improved breathing, enhanced circulation, improved digestion and so forth. Muscles will also register this change, and their relaxation becomes deeper and more permanent.

The limbic system

Emotions are also closely associated with the limbic system in the brain. The limbic system is made up of certain structures of the cerebrum and the diencephalon (hypothalamus, thalamus and pineal gland). It has an important function in the responses to emotions as well as autonomic reactions, subconscious motor and sensory drives, sexual behaviour, biological rhythms, and motivation, including feelings of pleasure and punishment.

The thalamus is a major relay centre; nuclei in the thalamus serve as relay stations for all sensory information, except smell, to the cerebrum. In addition, the thalamus plays a part in the association of feelings (pleasantness or unpleasantness) with sensory impulses. Behavioural actions involved with expressing emotions such as rage or fear are also influenced by this portion of the brain, as well as by the hypothalamus.

Despite it being only a small part of the brain, the hypothalamus is considered to be the control centre of the autonomic system. It exerts strong controlling properties and thus helps regulate an impressive number of mechanisms essential to maintaining homeostasis. For example, the hypothalamus acts as a very important relay station and output pathway between the cerebral cortex and the lower autonomic centres. Stimulation of various areas of the hypothalamus can increase or decrease arterial blood pressure, rate of heart beat, movements in the digestive tract, and several other visceral functions. The hypothalamus therefore serves as an important link between the brain (cerebrum) and the body (physiological mechanisms). Furthermore, it provides a connection between the nervous and endocrine systems. Through its close anatomical and physiological association with the pituitary gland, the hypothalamus produces several 'releasing hormones', which in turn regulate the secretion of specific hormones from the anterior pituitary. For example, corticotropin-releasing hormone (CRH) is produced by the hypothalamus in response to stress and it stimulates the pituitary gland to synthesize adrenocorticotrophic hormone (ACTH). In addition to its influence on the endocrine system the hypothalamus helps the body to combat stress by stimulating the sympathetic nervous system (Fig. 3.3).

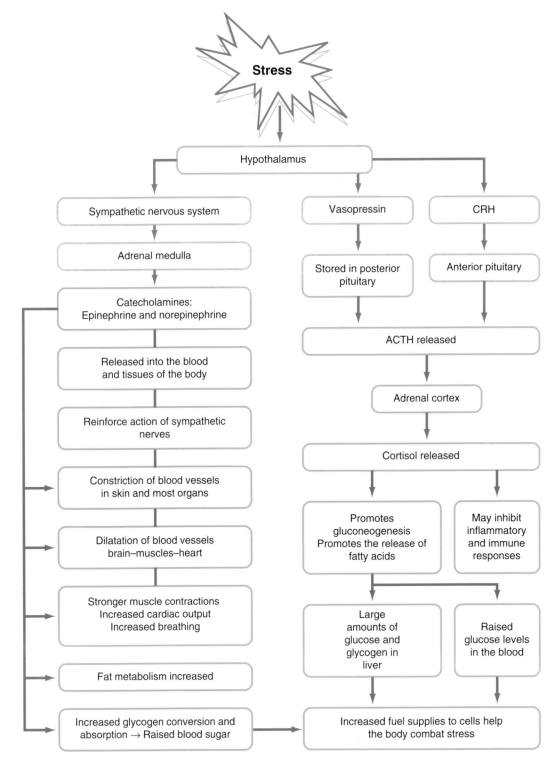

Figure 3.3 Example of the sympathetic and hormonal response to stress.

The autonomic nervous system

Most organs in the body are innervated by both sympathetic and parasympathetic fibres. Each organ, however, tends to be dominated primarily by one or the other system rather than served equally by both. The two systems function together smoothly to coordinate the numerous complex activities continuously taking place within the body.

During stress situations the sympathetic system is associated with mobilizing energy within the body for the individual's fight-or-flight response. When stimulated, it increases blood pressure, speeds the rate and force of the heart beat, increases blood sugar concentration, and reroutes the blood flow so that skeletal muscles receive the amounts of blood necessary to support their maximum effort.

Conversely, the parasympathetic system helps to conserve and restore energy and, when stimulated, decreases blood pressure, decreases the rate of the heart beat, and stimulates the digestive system to process food. This system predominates when the individual is in a 'relaxed state' and is therefore one of the desired outcomes of the relaxation provided by massage.

The adrenal medulla

Appropriately referred to as the emergency gland of the body, the adrenal medulla prepares the body physiologically to cope with threatening situations. While belonging essentially to the endocrine system, the adrenal gland (or more precisely the adrenal medulla) is also considered to be part of the sympathetic nervous system. In response to stress the hypothalamus exerts a stimulating influence on the sympathetic system. Some of the preganglionic sympathetic fibres innervate the adrenal medulla and stimulate it to secrete two catecholamines, epinephrine and norepinephrine, directly into the blood. These hormones are then carried to all the tissues of the body, where they reinforce the action of sympathetic nerves. Some of the sympathetic nerves in the body also release norepinephrine, but its influence is much less than that produced by the medulla.

Epinephrine and norepinephrine

Epinephrine and norepinephrine play an important role in the fight-or-flight reaction to stress, and prepare the body through their effect on the brain, the heart, smooth and skeletal muscles, the bronchioles, blood sugar levels and so forth.

The effects of epinephrine and norepinephrine include:

- Constriction of blood vessels to the skin and most internal organs.
- Dilatation of blood vessels to the brain, muscles and heart.
- Increased strength of contraction of skeletal muscles.
- Increased rate and strength of heart muscles.
- Increased alertness caused by a lowering of the thresholds in the reticular activating system of the brain.
- Increased breathing as the airways enlarge.
- Increased levels of both glucose and fatty acid levels in the blood rise. This provides the much needed fuel for extra energy. Epinephrine and norepinephrine raise fatty acid levels in the blood by mobilizing fat stores from adipose tissue. They raise the blood sugar level by increasing the amount of glucose absorbed from the intestine, thereby stimulating glycogenolysis. They also promote the conversion of muscle glycogen to lactic acid.

The adrenal cortex

Stimulation of the hypothalamus by one of the stress factors triggers its production of CRH which is then transported to the anterior pituitary. Under this influence the pituitary produces ACTH which is then transported to the adrenal cortex. This part of the adrenal gland is used to manufacture the stress hormone cortisol. ACTH is also stimulated by hormones other than CRH. These include vasopressin and epinephrine, both of which are increased in stress. Vasopressin is the antidiuretic hormone (ADH) which is manufactured in the hypothalamus but stored in the posterior pituitary. Another hormone that influences the production of ACTH and therefore of cortisol is the monokine interleukin-1, which is made by monocytes and macrophages (Vander et al., 1990).

Cortisol

Cortisol (also called hydrocortisone) accounts for about 95% of the glucocorticoid secretions by the adrenal cortex. Other glucocorticoids produced by the cortex are corticosterone and cortisone. Cortisol plays an important role in the provision of adequate fuel supplies to the cells when the body is under stress. This is achieved through the actions listed below. As a result of these actions large amounts of glucose and glycogen are formed in the liver, and blood glucose levels are raised.

The functions of cortisol include:

- Glucocorticoids, and in particular cortisol, promote gluconeogenesis, i.e. the production of glycogen from non-carbohydrate sources such as proteins and fats. It occurs in the liver. Increased plasma cortisol levels therefore stimulate protein catabolism.
- Cortisol plays an important function in gluconeogenesis as it helps to provide the nutrients by stimulating the transport of amino acids into liver cells. It also inhibits amino acid transport into other types of cells.
- It inhibits glucose uptake and oxidation by many body cells but not by the brain.
- Another function of cortisol is that it promotes the mobilization of fat from adipose tissue and therefore helps to release fatty acids into the blood.
- It helps to sustain vasoconstriction in response to norepinephrine and other stimuli.
- It may inhibit inflammation and specific immune responses.

Effects on the autonomic nervous system

The most frequently experienced effect of massage is the general feeling of wellbeing, which manifests from autonomic activity. The relaxation achieved with massage has an indirect effect on the autonomic nervous system and, in particular, on the parasympathetic division.

Deep relaxation is said to increase parasympathetic stimulation, and it appears that the more relaxed the subject becomes during and after the massage the greater the stimulation. As already stated, one primary centre in this complex circuit is the hypothalamus, which largely controls the autonomic nervous system and integrates it with the endocrine system.

Some research findings have demonstrated the reflex connection between massage and the sympathetic/parasympathetic branches of the autonomic nervous system. In response to the touch of massage, changes have been observed and measured in heart rate, arterial blood pressure, peripheral skin temperature, respiratory rate, skin response to galvanic current, pupil diameter and body temperature. Positive tactile contact has been associated with stimulation of the immune system (Montagu, 1986). These are some indicators of autonomic function; other results, however, have been varied and in some cases contradictory.

A study was conducted on the effects of connective tissue massage on the autonomic nervous system. Connective tissue massage was administered to middle-aged and elderly adults, and the variables monitored were skin temperature, galvanic skin response, mean arterial blood pressure and heart rate. The study showed no significant changes during or after the massage (Reed and Held, 1988). Although this is contrary to expectations, it may be due to a number of factors. For example, the effects are likely to be more significant in individuals with pathological disturbances rather than in the healthy subjects who took part in the research. Any tension or anxiety, as may be experienced in a controlled environment, can influence the outcome. It may also take longer for a subject to relax than the 15-min sessions performed in the experiment. On the other hand, a reflex response to cutaneous tissue manipulation, as proposed by the connective tissue massage theory, would indeed have an instant result.

In one report it was found that petrissage caused an immediate and transient increase in blood pressure, followed by a decrease (Edgecombe and Bain, 1899). This is in line with the concept that massage causes an initial increase in muscle tone of the blood vessels followed by fatigue and relaxation (Mennell, 1920). Other observations showed no change in blood pressure during or after massage treatments (Cuthbertson, 1933). One study showed an immediate parasympathetic response, which was indicated by a decrease in diastolic and systolic blood pressure, and there were also delayed responses some time after the treatment, but these varied from subject to subject (Barr and Taslitz, 1970).

Further research reported that an obvious increase in sweating was observed throughout the massage periods (Barr and Taslitz, 1970). Because sympathetic branches (sympathetic postganglionic neurons releasing acetylcholine) from the autonomic nervous system are the only supply to the sweat glands, this response is therefore sympathetic. The temperature control centre in the hypothalamus can also stimulate the sweat glands to reduce body temperature. As massage tends to induce a parasympathetic response, the interpretation of sweating because of massage contradicts other research findings (Reed and Held, 1988), and, indeed, clinical observations. Under normal circumstances, increased sweating in the patient does not occur during massage unless the recipient is stressed or has a raised body temperature.

The effects of sensory stimulation on the pre-operative patient were recorded in another study (Tovar and Cassmere, 1989). It was reported that touching the surgical patient with techniques such as stroking the back of the hand stimulates skin receptors, which in turn produce a relaxation response from the parasympathetic nervous system. A decrease in both blood pressure and heart rate was observed, and an increase in skin temperature was also in evidence, even in ventilated patients. This indicates an increase in peripheral blood flow and, therefore, a parasympathetic response. Vasodilatation and an increase in skin temperature may be the results of hormonal influence. Massage has been said to stimulate the mast cells to release a histamine-like substance, which acts on the autonomic nervous system. Histamine is normally present in the body and causes vasodilatation during tissue damage. A study on the effects of connective tissue massage showed marked hyperaemia and a feeling of heat, which lasted for 6 h or more after the treatment. These effects can be attributed to a parasympathetic effect. However, the sweat glands were also stimulated, and this indicates a sympathetic response (Ebner, 1962; 1968; 1978).

The vagus nerves emerge from the medulla, pass downward through the neck and branch to innervate many structures within the thorax and abdomen. Sensory neurons from many structures such as the throat, heart and abdominal viscera relay information to the medulla and pons; vagal motor neurons innervate almost all of the thoracic and abdominal organs. The vagus nerve has the most branches throughout the body and contains 75% of all parasympathetic nerve fibres in the cranial and sacral outflow (Solomon et al., 1990). Through its connection with the autonomic nervous system, the vagus nerve is said to be closely related to heart rate variability, the rate of respiration, to emotional responses and to digestive secretions. It has been suggested that massage can stimulate the vagus nerve and this occurs via the peripheral afferent pathways (Uvnas-Moberg et al., 1987). Stimulation of the pressure receptors by massage is seen as promoting activity of the vagus nerve (parasympathetic action), leading subsequently to a lowering of the stress hormones and a quietening down of the fight-or-flight state (Field, 2002). Increased vagal tone and parasympathetic activation can also increase digestive secretions (especially insulin) and improve the function of the gastrointestinal tract (Uvnas-Moberg et al., 1987). Studies have also shown changes in EEG (electroencephalogram) readings, indicating heightened alertness following massage therapy (Field et al., 1996a).

Reducing stress

Several relaxation protocols, including massage, have been found to be very effective in bringing about a reversal of the acute stress reaction (the fight-or-flight stage). The *relaxation response* to the reduced level of stress initiates a number of physiological changes, including reductions in blood pressure and heart rate, decreased oxygen consumption and reduced muscle tone (Benson, 1976; Jacobs, 1996).

In one study, carried out on preterm infants at the Hammersmith Hospital in London, the effects of massage on the levels of cortisol and catecholamines were determined. Neonatal procedures are designed to improve the quality of life for preterm infants; however, stress can still affect the infants despite interventions such as sheepskin bedding, mattresses filled with polystyrene balls, and soft music. This may be because of their underlying illness or painful disorders. Anxiety or fear may also have an effect, particularly if the infant is undergoing operations. A strong biochemical response to stress is the increased concentrations of catecholamines and cortisol. However, some researchers suggest that an increase in urine catecholamines in adults is indicative of stress, whereas raised urine catecholamines in the preterm infant signify a normal development of brain function. In the study, blood samples were obtained to determine the levels of cortisol and catecholamines before and after the massage. Cortisol concentrations were decreased consistently after the massage; the catecholamine levels in this study, however, remained constant or increased (Acolet et al., 1993). Other studies have indicated that massage has the effect of increasing serotonin levels and thereby promoting restorative sleeping patterns (Field et al., 1996a).

Experiments carried out on child and adolescent psychiatric patients revealed a decrease in anxiety, and positive changes in behaviour following a period of daily massage treatments. Stress level indicators were observed and monitored, including heart rate, saliva cortisol, urine levels of cortisol and catecholamines (norepinephrine, epinephrine and dopamine), and sleeping patterns. A reduction in the levels of these indicators was observed, as well as deeper sleeping sessions and improved cooperative behaviour (Field et al., 1992).

IMMUNE FUNCTION

Defence mechanisms offered by the body can either take the form of generalized barriers and reactions or they can be organized as direct and specific mechanisms. The general methods of defence are designed to prevent the entrance of foreign invaders into the body and to destroy those that have managed to penetrate it. This form of protection includes barriers such as the skin, acid secretions in the stomach, and inflammatory responses.

The more specific defences involve immunity, which is a state of being immune to or protected from a disease, especially an infectious disease. The protection by immunity can occur either by having been exposed to the antigenic substances peculiar to the disease while infected or by having been immunized with a vaccine which has the capability of stimulating production of specific antibodies. Immunity can also be described as the response of the body and its tissues to a variety of foreign antigens. The immune responses are therefore the production of cells and antibodies specifically tailored to attack particular antigens that gain entrance to the body, and in some cases even to the individual's own cells (autoimmunity). One immune response is that provided by antibodies. Specific B lymphocytes are activated when exposed to specific antigens so that they differentiate and secrete particular antibodies that chemically attack the antigens. A second immune response is referred to as 'cell-mediated immunity'. In this type of protection, specific T lymphocytes are activated when exposed to specific antigens. As a result, they multiply and differentiate, producing cells that attack the antigen.

T cells originate from stem cells in the bone marrow, and from here they move on to the lymph nodes via the thymus gland. The thymus gland exerts its influence on the differentiation of these T lymphocytes so that they become capable of immunological response. There are three main types of T cells. One group is the cytotoxic T cells, sometimes called killer T cells (natural killer; NK cells). These can recognize cells with foreign antigens on their surfaces and destroy them by producing materials, mostly proteins, which are toxic to the invading target cell. The second main group is the helper T cells. These assist other types of T cells, as well as B cells, in responding to antigens. The third group is the suppressor T cells that can inhibit the activity of helper T cells and cytotoxic T cells. At the front line of defence in the immune system, therefore, are the NK cells, and their cytotoxicity (activity) and part of their work is to attack cancer cells and viruses.

Immune cells are susceptible to damage and obliteration by other invading cells and viruses. They can also be attacked from within the body; for instance, NK and other immune cells can be destroyed by the hormone cortisol (Ironson et al., 1996), which becomes abundant with stress. High levels of cortisol can, however, be reversed by massage. Various research has shown that high cortisol levels, as well as the epinephrine and norepinephrine resulting from stress can, in most cases, be reduced through the relaxation offered by massage (Field et al., 1996b; Ironson et al., 1996; Acolet et al., 1993). This occurs through the limbic–hypothalamus–hormonal connection which can also be described as the hypothalamus–pituitary–adrenal (HPA) axis. There is also parasympathetic stimulation, e.g. that of the vagus nerve through the pressure of touch (Field, 2002). These associations are discussed in the psychogenic–autonomic effects of massage, later in this chapter.

PAIN REDUCTION

Pain sensation

Pain is perceived when a stimulus of some sort is causing, or about to cause, damage to a tissue. It is therefore a signal of tissue-damaging (noxious) stimuli and a protective mechanism from imminent harm. The quality and location of the pain sensation are indicators as to the severity and the nature of the causative factors so that conscious (in addition to the involuntary) avoidance action can be taken.

Pain impulses are transmitted to the CNS along spinal and cranial nerves. Impulses from pain receptors, as well as those from thermore-ceptors, are transmitted along the lateral spinothalamic tract in the spinal cord. As the sensory information reaches the thalamus there is some awareness of the quality of the pain. However, recognition of the intensity, type and localization of pain does not fully occur until the impulses reach the cerebral cortex. The location of pain perception occurs as the cortex projects the pain back to the stimulated area. This does not occur in all cases of pain arising in viscera, however.

The degree of perceived pain differs from one individual to another. Factors such as past experiences, suggestion and emotions (e.g. anxiety and fear) can alter the levels of pain and how it is perceived. The pain threshold is therefore very much the subjective tolerance of the person receiving the stimulus.

Reflex responses

A stimulus that gives rise to pain will also evoke a reflex response. This can be primarily a motor response affecting the skeletal muscles, e.g. a withdrawal of the hand when accidentally touching something hot. There are also other responses mediated by the hypothalamus and the sympathetic nervous system, as well as the endocrine system. One such outcome can be reflex skeletal muscle tightening which is protective.

Pain description

The classification of pain is based on the onset, duration, quality and location. Further subheadings can also be attributed to other factors.

- *Acute pain*. Impulses from acute pain are carried along A fibres and therefore travel very fast. The pain itself has a quick onset and is not generally felt in deeper tissues. It can be described as sharp, fast, pricking.
- *Chronic pain*. Impulses travel along C fibres and therefore travel more slowly than those of acute pain. Chronic pain has a more gradual onset, over minutes or days. It can still be excruciating but can also be described as burning, aching, throbbing, slow.

- *Superficial somatic pain.* Stimulation of receptors in the skin gives rise to superficial somatic pain.
- *Deep somatic pain.* Deep somatic pain occurs from stimulation of receptors found in the skeletal muscles, joints, tendons and fascia.
- *Visceral pain.* Visceral pain occurs from stimulation of receptors in viscera. The causes for visceral pain include distension, spasms or ischaemia of a visceral organ.
- *Referred pain.* In some cases of visceral pain the sensation is not projected back to the organ itself. Instead it is referred to the superficial tissue, usually overlying the organ. In some cases the referred pain is located in a surface area that is distant from the stimulated organ. Referred pain occurs when the innervation of a visceral organ shares the same spinal segment as that of superficial tissue. A typical example is the pain felt on the skin over the heart and in the medial aspect of the arm; the pain can be referred if there is heart dysfunction or pathology.

Sensory neurons

Sensory neurons are classified by the letters A, B or C. Another form of categorization uses Roman numbers I–IV, and a third classification uses the Greek alphabet: alpha, beta, gamma and delta (Lee and Warren, 1978, as cited by Walsh, 1991).

- Touch and vibration reception is transmitted along some of the Class A fibres (Groups I and II—alpha). These have a large diameter, 20 μm and 5–15 μm, respectively. Impulses along these fibres travel very fast. Touch and gentle pressure are typical sensations associated with these fibres.
- Class B fibres have a diameter of 3 μm and are found as preganglionic and autonomic nerves.
- Nociceptors (pain receptors) transmit their impulses along Class C (Group IV) fibres, which have a small diameter (0.5–1.0 μm) and are thinly myelinated. Impulses along these fibres travel slowly. Impulses travelling along C fibres can be associated with a dull aching type of pain, sometimes chronic pain. The

source can be a viscera or somatic structures such as skeletal muscles and tissues. Pain transmission starts with the pain receptors referred to as nociceptors or free nerve endings. To recapitulate, these sensory organs are located at the end of small unmyelinated or lightly myelinated afferent neurons (afferent neurons transmit impulses towards the spinal cord). Nociceptors are sensitive to any trigger that can cause tissue damage and, consequently, they can respond to a variety of stimuli. Some nociceptors are sensitive to intense mechanical pressure, some respond to mechanical and thermal stimulation, and others respond to irritant chemicals as well as to mechanical and thermal stimulation.

- Other sensory neurons that also transmit pain impulses are from the Class A (Group III—delta) fibres. In this case the fibres are myelinated and slightly larger in diameter (1–7 μm) than the Class C fibres. They travel fairly fast and respond to intense stimuli such as extreme or sustained pressure, and are believed to carry sensations of acute injury to the skin.

Irritants and proinflammatory chemicals

As already indicated, nociceptors are stimulated by irritants that are likely to cause tissue damage. An irritant therefore is a stressor and can occur, for example, as excess pressure, trauma or a noxious material. When the tissue is damaged, it releases chemical substances such as serotonin, bradykinin, histamine and prostaglandins. The release of certain chemical substances in response to tissue injury or metabolic activity was one theory put forward for the activation of the nociceptive pathways (Watson, 1981).

These chemicals play an important part in the inflammatory process and healing of tissues; they also irritate and depolarize nearby nociceptor nerve endings and in so doing initiate an action potential in the afferent nerve fibres.

As well as responding to chemical substances, nociceptors will themselves release chemicals that are inflammatory in nature. Substance P is an example (Walsh, 1991). Increasing the venous blood flow helps with the removal of such chemical irritants/proinflammatory agents and inhibits pain at the peripheral level (Walsh, 1991).

Massage is very effective in enhancing the venous blood flow; hence it has a significant role in pain reduction. Substance P is also seen as causing pain. It is found as a transmitter that is released at the synapses between the afferent nerves and interneurons in the spinal cord. The release of substance P, however, is reduced during sleep. In addition to the removal of substance P with the increased circulation, massage can also be seen as lowering the circulating levels of substance P, and therefore the intensity of pain, through its sleep-inducing effect. Another substance which is released during sleep is somatostatin. This is an inhibiting hormone (it inhibits the growth hormone) and a product of the hypothalamus. Its significance is that it has the effect of reducing pain perception (Sunshine et al., 1996).

A build-up of oedema results in the elevation of hydrostatic pressure within the interstitial tissues. If the pressure is significantly raised, it can irritate the nociceptors and produce pain. Massage helps to drain excess lymph from oedematous areas and, as the pressure on the nociceptors is reduced, the pain is relieved.

Pain can be caused by an impingement of nerve fibres, which may be precipitated by contractions or congestion in the skin and fascia (superficial or deep). Nerve fibres can also be confined by mechanical imbalances in the joints and their associated ligaments. Muscles that are tight, in spasm or contracted can have a similar effect on the nerve fibres (Greenman, 1989); for instance, pressure on the sciatic nerve is often caused by a tight piriformis muscle. Massage helps to free nerve entrapments by removing muscle tension, stretching the superficial and deep tissues, and loosening up the joints and ligaments.

Pain reduction

Reduction of pain, or more appropriately of pain perception, can be achieved in a number of ways. It frequently results from the interruption of the pain impulses along the pain pathway. Inhibition

through a reflex action is also likely and sometimes both mechanisms are in operation. Interrupting or modifying the transmission of afferent impulses is mostly carried out in one of three sites:

- At the periphery, and therefore at the site where irritation of the pain receptor takes place.
- In the spinal cord, where the afferent neurons enter the cord to join the CNS.
- At the higher levels or supraspinal area of the CNS, including structures such as the hypothalamus and the cortex.

Inhibition of pain impulses

Pain reduction can be achieved through inhibition of the sensory pain impulses. The mechanism of inhibition is based on the speed of the impulses travelling along the sensory pathways.

One method of inhibition involves stimulation of the painful site or of the peripheral nerves leading from it. Transcutaneous electric nerve stimulation (TENS) is one example of this mechanism where low-voltage electrical currents are transmitted via electrodes placed on the surface of the skin. The electric current stimulates nonpain, low-threshold afferent fibres, e.g. the touch–pressure receptors. Impulses from these receptors travel fast in A fibres and can therefore block the pain impulses travelling in the slower C fibres.

The diameter of the nerve fibre dictates the speed at which the impulses travel. As the diameter of the nerve fibres increases, the resistance to current flow diminishes (Walsh, 1991). This means that the larger the diameter of the nerve fibre, the easier and faster the conduction of the impulses. A simple comparison can be made to a water pipe; the larger its diameter, the easier and faster the flow of water through it.

Because some of the Class A fibres (Group I and II—alpha) have a large diameter, they carry impulses faster than some of the smaller Class C fibres (Group IV) and certain Class A fibres (Group III—delta). Applying a light touch to the skin during massage stimulates the larger and faster Class A (Group I and II—alpha) fibres. Impulses travelling along these fibres reach the spinal cord at a faster rate and, consequently, predominate over the slower stimuli. In so doing, they 'block' the slower pain impulses travelling along Class C (Group IV) fibres and other Class A fibres (Group III—delta).

The blocking mechanism is found in the substantia gelatinosa, which is at the periphery of the posterior horn of the spinal cord (Melzek and Wall, 1988). This grey matter has a 'gating mechanism', which controls the entry of all incoming sensory impulses and, in particular, those from nociceptors. The physiological blocking at the spinal segmental level is called the 'pain gate mechanism' (Fig. 3.4). It is very effectively achieved electrically by using such methods as interferential currents and TENS (Walsh, 1991). Because of this pain gate mechanism, impulses are modified or prevented from ascending along the cord to the brain. Pain is therefore reduced in intensity or not perceived at all. When massage is carried out for a period of time, the continuous flow of sensory impulses along the sensory nerves will help to keep the gates closed or in a

partly open position, and will therefore block the pain stimuli reaching the CNS.

The theory of the pain gate mechanism was applied many years ago by James Cyriax in his technique of cross-friction massage. Also referred to as transverse massage, this technique is applied over an area of trauma or inflammation to reduce adhesions and prevent excessive scar tissue formation (Cyriax, 1945). In addition, the technique is said to have pain-reducing properties. A blocking of the pain impulses has been given as one explanation. This theory may be disputed since the cross-friction technique in itself can be quite painful and therefore stimulate the pain receptors. Another likely theory is that the traumatic hyperaemia created by the cross-friction massage helps to remove the chemical irritant substance P (already described as causing pain by speeding up transmission of pain impulses). This is most probably achieved by the release of histamine (Chamberlain, 1982). Other research also confirms that the neurophysiological concept behind the pain gate theory is the 'diffuse noxious inhibitory control mechanism'. As already discussed, the mechanism is seen as a

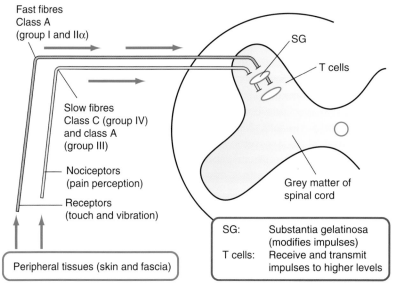

Figure 3.4 Pain gate mechanism.

blocking of the Class C (Group IV) fibres by the stimulation of 'faster' sensory fibres in other terminals such as heat, pressure and chemical receptors (Le Bars et al., 1979; De Bruijn, 1984).

Upper nerve centres

An instinctive reaction to pain is to rub the area where it hurts. Rubbing a painful site or pressing hard is a similar type of TENS that is often carried out instinctively in response to pain. The comforting and numbing feeling that is experienced when doing so is due to a blocking of the pain impulses along their route to the brain. Massage (such as continuous stroking) will likewise stimulate a great number of impulses from the mechanoreceptors. Consequently it exerts a similar inhibition on the pain impulses reaching the hypothalamus and the cortex. Inhibition through massage can be applied, for instance, to reduce somatic pain and chronic visceral pain.

With the reduction of pain impulses reaching the upper nerve centres in the brain, the sympathetic reaction to pain by the hypothalamus and the cortex is also reduced. One outcome is that descending pathways emerging from some parts of the thalamus and brainstem selectively inhibit transmission of impulses originating in the nociceptors. Some of these inhibitory neurons can also release certain endorphins that can exert a weakening influence on the sensory neurons transmitting pain impulses.

In addition to a reduction of pain, the inhibition helps to reduce muscle and tissue tension. Blocking of the impulses from the massaged area will result in a reduction of hypothalamic impulses to the cortex and subsequently to a relaxation of any protective muscle tightness and tissue tension in the same region.

Emotional influence

Emotional factors such as expectancy, anxiety and fear can influence the perception of pain. The greater the tension in the subject, the stronger the perception of pain; conversely, the more relaxed the subject, the less severe the pain appears to be. Stress can therefore be seen to exacerbate pain,

while relaxation, as achieved with massage, can be said to be instrumental in pain reduction.

Relaxation can influence the impulses travelling through the hypothalamus and to the cortex, and indirectly reduces the descending efferent impulses.

Reduction of pain through adaptation

Adaptation is a decrease in the frequency of action potentials in an afferent neuron despite maintenance of the stimulus at constant strength. Some receptors adapt completely so that, in spite of constantly maintained stimulus, the generation of action potentials stops. Pain receptors adapt only slightly, or not at all.

It is stipulated by some authors that, with the continual stroking of massage, the mechanoreceptors adapt and reduce the action potential in the sensory pathways. Gentle massage strokes have the effect of stimulating the mechanoreceptors (e.g. touch, pressure and temperature receptors) in the superficial tissues. This will initially create a reflex response via the motor centres in the cortex and the lower motor neurons in the anterior horn of the spinal cord. The result is protective tissue tension and muscle guarding in the area being massaged. If the gentle strokes are continued for a period of time the mechanoreceptors gradually adapt to the stimuli. Consequently, the number of afferent sensory impulses travelling to the cord and upper nerve centres is reduced. With the lowering of the action potentials in the sensory neurons there is also an inhibition of reflex responses by the hypothalamus and cortex nerve centres. The decrease in this sympathetic reaction leads to an easing of the muscle and tissue tension and to a reduction of pain perception. As the pain receptors are very slow to adapt, if at all, it can be argued that the pain inhibition is more likely to be caused by a weaker sympathetic influence than adaptation of the pain receptors.

Pain modifiers

Pain is consciously perceived in the brain at the level of the thalamus. In this supraspinal area, the cortical and brainstem structures are said to be involved in the release of endorphins and serotonin (Watson, 1982). A significant response to massage is said to be the production and circulation of such endogenous opiates. These naturally occurring painkillers are found mostly within the brain, but they also circulate in many other parts of the body. One painkiller group is the beta-endorphins, which are opioid peptides (opium-like compounds). Another painkiller is beta-lipotropin, which is a form of lipotropin. This is a hormone produced by the pituitary, and its function is to mobilize fat from adipose tissue. Beta-lipotropin contains the painkillers, endorphins and metenkephalins. These chemicals are said to inhibit or modify pain transmission at all three sites: the peripheral end of sensory nerves; the dorsal horn of the spinal cord; and the higher centres of the limbic system and cortex (Milan, 1986). By improving the circulation, massage can then improve the transport of these pain modifiers.

The influence of massage on painkillers has been disputed in a number of research papers. A study on the effects of connective tissue massage showed a moderate elevation of plasma beta-endorphins, which reached a peak 30 min after treatment (Kaada and Torsteinbo, 1989). Further research looked at the effects of connective tissue massage on severe chronic pain that developed after neurosurgical procedures. This type of pain is referred to as post-sympathetic pain, or reflex sympathetic dystrophy. It was found that massage compared very favourably with epidural injections and pethidine (Frazer, 1978). One trial revealed no change in the peripheral blood levels of beta-endorphins and beta-lipotropin after massage treatment, and a possible explanation for this was that the experiment was carried out on pain-free individuals (Day et al., 1987). Other research projects have compared the effects of massage to those of exercise, which has been shown to increase the peripheral blood levels of beta-endorphins and beta-lipotropin greatly.

The pain cycle

Massage is perhaps one of the oldest methods of pain relief. One possible mechanism by which massage causes analgesia is the disruption of the pain cycle (Jacobs, 1960). This can be described as a sustained muscle contraction, which leads to deep pain within the muscle itself. In turn, the pain results in a reflex contraction of the same muscle or muscles. It has been suggested that massage helps to break the pain cycle by its mechanical and reflex effects and by improving the circulation. In addition, the pain is blocked by the pain gate mechanism, which stops further reflex contractions.

Improved circulation

Sustained muscle contraction creates ischaemia and pain in the muscles. Increasing the circulation by massage helps to relieve this pain. The mechanism for the increase in circulation is, first, the mechanical pressure on the superficial venous and lymphatic channels and, second, a reflex dilatation through stimulation of the cutaneous afferent fibres mediated by touch and pressure (Jacobs, 1960).

Inhibition of muscle contraction

Relaxing and stretching the muscle tissue reduces the sustained contraction. Compression techniques such as petrissage and kneading have a stretching effect on the fascia and tendons of the muscle being treated. Stretching of the tendon has the effect of stimulating the Golgi tendon organs (stretch receptors), which in turn produces powerful central inhibition of the neurons controlling that muscle. This effect has been called the inverse myotatic reflex (Lloyd, 1955).

Massage techniques to reduce pain

Implementation of the various mechanisms of pain reduction necessitates the use of the appropriate massage movements.

These can include gentle effleurage, gentle kneading and vibration movements. Other techniques such as NMT, reflex zone and trigger point treatments are also applicable. Equally important are the different methods and routines of applying the techniques.

The various strokes. Gentle effleurage is perhaps the movement mostly associated with pain reduction. Gentle kneading is equally effective and can be applied as an alternative technique. For pain reduction the massage movements are carried out very slowly and are repeated for quite some time, i.e. some minutes rather than a few times. Heavy kneading or percussive strokes are not suitable for reducing chronic pain that is perhaps associated with a viscera. Many subjects, however, find the heaviness of a movement pleasant, especially when addressing severe tightness in muscles and tissues.

A vibratory movement is considered to be very effective in reducing pain. The most likely mechanism is one of blocking of the pain impulses through the 'pain gate'. The response by the hypothalamus and cortex is to send efferent inhibitory impulses to the pain receptors and pain perception is reduced. With the aim of pain reduction, vibratory movements are usually applied at an average rate of 80 times per min.

Pressure. As noted earlier, the pressure of the stroking must be very gentle when using stroking for pain reduction. Any increase in pressure has to be carried out very gradually. Pressure must never be strong enough to exceed the pain threshold of the subject.

Acute traumatic pain. Trauma to the superficial tissues and muscles, like a muscle strain, will lead to acute pain. Very naturally, the subject's pain threshold is likely to be lowered in this situation. A pain sensation is likely to originate from the tissue damage and also from an abundance of pain-inducing chemicals such as prostaglandins and histamine that are part of the inflammatory and repair mechanisms. Applying light stroking massage movements may induce some degree of pain reduction. However, it may be wiser not to apply any movements on an injured area so as not to disturb the clotting process. If light stroking is to be applied it needs to be carried out extremely gently and without exceeding the pain threshold of the subject. Light stroking can also be applied in mild cases of trauma, such as a bump on the head, where there is minor bruising and no tissue tears.

Acute visceral pain. In an acute visceral pain, however, the causative factors must be estab-lished before any massage treatment is carried out in the region of the organ. Inflammation, oedema and nerve irritation are amongst the contraindications that must be ruled out during the assessment.

Chronic pain. Chronic visceral pain or a deep somatic pain may be treated with a combination of effleurage, gentle kneading and the vibration technique.

Pain of ischaemia. Superficial somatic pain or deep somatic pain that is related to ischaemia can be reduced with the massage techniques already mentioned. Light pressure stroking brings in the mechanisms of *inhibition* and *adaptation*, as well as stimulating the *pain modifiers*. Slightly heavier movements increase the local circulation, thereby lowering the interstitial tissue pressure of the ischaemia and, in turn, the irritation of the nociceptors.

Mechanical and reflex effects on the blood circulation

Massage can have a direct as well as an indirect influence on the circulatory system. For example, it has an effect on cardiac function via the somatic–visceral reflex as well as a mechanical increase in blood flow. Studies show an increase in the rate of blood flow and cardiac stroke volume with massage; this in turn involves an enhanced venous return and improved circulation (Goats, 1994). A further example is simple congestion, which occurs when the blood vessels are subjected to severe and sustained compression. One causative factor is excessive pressure from surrounding tissues which themselves are in a malfunctioning state, e.g. contracted fascia and adhesions. Mechanically, massage helps to relieve congestion by freeing the soft tissues through manipulation and stretching. It also assists the venous return by mechanically draining the vessels.

Mechanical effect on the blood vessels

The pressure of venous flow is very low in both the superficial blood vessels and the deeper ones, where it is unlikely to exceed 5–10 mmHg

(Mennell, 1920). The average venous pressure is less than 10 mmHg (Vander et al., 1990), falling to 0 mmHg (negative) at the level of the right atrium of the heart. At the root of the neck, the same negative pressure is found in those veins draining the head. It follows that heavy massage of the neck, which may be used with the intention of relieving intercranial pressure, is neither effective nor necessary (Mennell, 1920).

Massage for the venous flow requires little effort and necessitates only light pressure to move the blood forward along the vessels. The easy drainage of the venous return can be observed in the rapid depletion of the lower limb when it is elevated with the subject in the supine position, provided no pathology is present. Increasing the venous return of a tissue area creates more space for the arterial blood to flow to the same region. Massage can therefore be seen as improving the circulation through the part being treated, and not only that to the tissue area or away from it. Heavy pressure will still result in the emptying of the venous vessels, but it may also affect the arterioles and small arteries, where the pressure is low. Applying heavy massage may push the arterial blood flow centripetally (against the arterial flow) instead of centrifugally (towards the periphery). This can happen in the deeper arterioles as well as in the superficial ones (Mennell, 1920). However, if this effect does occur it is likely to be minimal and shortlasting; the overall impact of the massage is an increased venous flow.

Reflex effect on the involuntary muscles of blood vessels

Manipulation of the tissues, the skin and fascia has a reflex effect on the unstripped muscles of the arterioles. The response is vasomotor and, hence, a toning of the smooth muscle fibres. Furthermore, manipulation of the soft tissues unavoidably includes that of the superficial arterioles. This in itself will activate a further reflex contraction of their muscular walls, which is then followed by a paralytic dilatation of the involuntary muscles.

As these arterial walls are temporarily paralysed and cannot contract further, there is vasodilatation and hyperaemia (Mennell, 1920).

The same rationale probably causes the vasodilatation that can be achieved by compression. In massage techniques that involve compression a degree of pressure is applied to the soft tissues and sustained for a few seconds. As the pressure is released there is a reflex vasodilatation of the superficial vessels.

It is also postulated by some authors that the vasodilatation in a somatic area can occur as a reflex response to massage and soft tissue manipulation of a corresponding reflex zone, i.e. in another region. A further theory is that the vasodilatation occurs through the 'axon reflex'. When somatic superficial tissues are manipulated, impulses travel along sensory nerves towards the CNS. Along the course of their pathway these nerves give off small branches that feed adjacent vascular vessels. Stimulation of the mechanoreceptors in the skin and superficial tissues leads to impulses (action potentials) being transmitted to these small extensions or branches, in addition to the impulses travelling toward the sensory neurons. An initial vasospasm in the adjacent blood vessels is created by the action potential, but this is soon followed by vasodilatation as the receptors adapt to the stimulus (Jacobs, 1960). A study on animals showed that stimulation of the sensory afferent nerves by massage creates local vasodilatation. This is brought about by inhibition of the vasoconstrictor fibres in the tissues close to the massage site, and by excitation of the vasodilator fibres in the local area (Bayliss as quoted in Jacobs, 1960).

The walls of the veins also contain smooth muscle innervated by sympathetic neurons. Norepinephrine, which is released when the sympathetic nervous system is activated, causes contraction of the smooth muscle in the walls of the veins, thereby raising the blood pressure (Vander et al., 1970). While an increase in blood pressure is necessary or desirable in some conditions, it is damaging when it is constant. The relaxing effect of massage can be used, for example, in situations of hypertension, to reduce sympathetic activity and in turn the blood pressure.

Influence on circulation

The enhancement of blood circulation, particularly venous return, with massage was observed in a number of experiments. Researcher and physician Von Mosengeil injected a rabbit's knee with India ink, which was soon cleared away with the application of massage (Tracy, 1992/3). The venous blood flow was monitored in another study carried out on 12 athletes aged 22–27 years. A contrast medium was injected into the veins of the lower limb, and X-rays were taken before and after massage of the area. These showed no traces of the contrast medium after the treatment (Dubrovsky, 1982). In another experiment, blood volume was observed to increase with massage. Deep stroking and kneading massage were applied for 10 min to the calf muscles of one leg, and changes in the blood volume were measured and recorded on a plethysmograph instrument. It was observed that blood volume and therefore the rate of blood flow had doubled. The effect lasted for 40 min; this compared very favourably with exercise, which caused an increase for just 10 min (Bell, 1964).

Research has also indicated that massage induces a fall in blood viscosity, haematocrit count and plasma viscosity. Viscosity is the state of thickness and stickiness of a fluid. If the blood or plasma viscosity is high, it can slow down the blood flow. Haematocrit refers to the volume of erythrocytes packed by centrifugation in a given volume of blood, and in this context it relates to the density or number of erythrocytes in the blood. A high density of erythrocytes means a slowing down of the blood flow. The blood and plasma viscosities together with the haematocrit count influence the blood rheology (fluidity); the lower their values, the higher the rheology. Blood fluidity is considered of clinical importance because it determines blood perfusion in certain pathological states. Pharmacological preparations are generally used to increase blood rheology in ischaemic diseases. Massage has been found to be a good alternative (Ernst et al., 1987).

One hypothesis is that massage affects the blood rheology by the mechanism of haemodilution, which is defined as an increase in the volume of blood plasma. Haemodilution is said to occur as a result of reduced sympathetic tone, which is achieved by massage. With the lowering of the sympathetic tone, the smooth muscles of the blood vessels relax and the blood flow is increased (the increased blood flow therefore is not caused by an increase in blood pressure but to a perfusion of blood in a local tissue). It is postulated that the plasma volume also increases. A high plasma volume also means a reduced concentration of red blood cells (Ernst et al., 1987) and, therefore, a lower haematocrit count.

An alternative concept is that the haemodilution occurs by the reactive hyperaemia which follows massage (Bühring, 1984). When the blood flow in the capillary beds of the skin and muscles is increased by massage, it is likely that circulation is also enhanced in microvessels within the general systemic circulation. This theory is supported by experiments which showed that, during massage, blood vessels with stagnant blood flow are invaded with cell-free interstitial liquid of low viscosity (Matrai et al., 1984). As a result of this fluid being added to the general circulation there is also an enhanced blood flow. Another theory is that improvement in the circulation is achieved by the mechanical manipulation of muscles with massage. This has the effect of decongesting microvessels so that stagnant plasma fluid within these vessels is reintroduced into the general circulation. One further idea is based on the flow of lymph. The compression of massage drains lymph from the interstitial spaces into the lymph vessels and ducts, and haemodilution is further enhanced as the lymph is returned to the heart and joins the general circulation as plasma.

The effect of massage on the circulation can therefore be interpreted as an increased perfusion of blood with plasma fluid. This in turn has the effect of improving blood flow and rheology. This increase in fluidity and improved blood flow might also benefit muscles when their circulation is disturbed, for instance when there is local myogelosis (hardening of a portion of a muscle). These actions contribute to the therapeutic efficacy of massage therapy in muscular disorders, and in any impairment of the peripheral circulation.

Influence on blood pressure

As a general rule massage has the overall effect of reducing blood pressure. Some researchers report a decrease in both systolic and diastolic pressure following massage treatment carried out on reflex areas like the occiput, upper neck, shoulders and arms. Bradycardia (slowness of heart action) and a decrease in blood pressure have also been recorded following massage to the mid-thoracic region of the back and also to the thorax. Research also indicates that massage therapy may be of benefit for cardiac and hypertensive patients (Yates, 1989). In subjects suffering from primary hypertension, the blood pressure in the peripheral arteries was observed to increase when there was tension in skeletal muscles. Both the systolic and diastolic pressures were reduced following relaxation of the patient's skeletal muscles (Jacobson, 1939). In the past, some authors had stated that massage to the abdomen increases blood pressure. However, more recent studies have indicated a decrease in blood pressure in response to abdominal massage. Studies carried out on rats, for example, have shown a decrease in blood pressure and a slowing down of the heart beat following a short massage on the abdominal region (Kurosawa et al., 1995).

The skeletal muscle pump

A beneficial compression on the veins is administered by muscles, primarily those that are in contact with the blood vessels. Contraction of certain muscles, particularly those of the lower limbs, exerts a pressure on the nearby veins. Veins within the muscles are similarly compressed. In the interim period of muscle relaxation, the pressure is released and applied again with the next contraction. The pumping action that is therefore applied to the blood vessels assists with the venous flow, particularly in the lower limbs, where it tends to be weak. A similar pumping action is provided by some massage techniques, which compress the muscles and their associated blood vessels.

Respiratory pump

Any congestion within the abdominal circulatory vessels can be alleviated by abdominal massage; in this region massage has the effect of enhancing the portal circulation. In addition to this direct consequence, massage helps to increase the flow of blood by its influence on respiration.

During inspiration, the diaphragm descends and pushes on the abdominal contents. As the abdominal pressure is raised it is passively transmitted to the intra-abdominal veins. Simultaneously, the pressure in the thorax decreases and this causes a lowering of the pressure in the intrathoracic veins and the right atrium of the heart. As blood flows from a higher pressure toward a lower pressure it follows that venous return is enhanced with inspiration. The relaxation provided by massage helps to reduce tightness in the respiratory muscles, thereby allowing for deeper inspiration and improved venous blood flow.

Mechanical and reflex effects on the lymph circulation

Lymph flows from the interstitial spaces to the collecting vessels (also referred to as lymphatic capillaries or terminal lymphatics). As fluid pressure builds up in the interstitial spaces, it forces the endothelial cells of the terminal vessels to separate and allow the fluid and other materials through. Lymph then flows from the terminal vessels into the larger lymphatic vessels which are divided into segments called lymphangions. These vary in size; the smaller ones can be 1–3 mm in length, while the larger ones measure 6–12 mm. In the thoracic duct the segments are the longest at 15 mm (Overholser and Moody, 1988). Situated at each end of the lymphangion is a valve, which opens in one direction only to secure a one-way flow of lymph. In its forward journey the lymph then enters the lymphatic trunks and ducts, and it is filtered along the way by the lymphatic nodes. The volume of lymph that is moved through the vessels is very low; the flow rate in the thoracic duct has been measured at 1–2 ml/min, which translates to about 3 litres/day (Yoffey and Courtice, 1970). Finally, lymph is returned to the cardiovascular system via the right and left jugular veins. An uninterrupted stream is vital to maintain the balance in the lymphatic system and, in particular, in the fluid content of the interstitial tissue. A number of irregularities, such as obstruction of the lymph flow, excessive leaking of proteins from the capillaries, and abnormal water retention, will interfere with the lymph circulation and, as a result, oedema can easily develop. The flow of lymph is different to that of the blood in that it does not have the assistance of the heart to create a back pressure. Its continuous movement is therefore dependent on a number of mechanical and reflex mechanisms.

Effective filtration pressure

One of the mechanisms controlling the lymph flow in the interstitial spaces is related to blood circulation. In turn, the blood circulation is dependent on pressure differences within the capillary bed and the interstitial tissues. Hydrostatic pressure is created by the volume of water in the blood vessels or in the interstitial spaces, which is greater at the arterial end of the blood capillary bed and therefore pushes fluid into the interstitial tissues. A second pressure is osmotic, and this is created by the protein mass in the blood or in the interstitial fluid. It is greater in the blood capillary bed, and therefore exerts a pull on the fluid from the interstitial spaces back into the capillaries. The difference between the osmotic and hydrostatic pressures dictates the flow of the fluid and its direction of flow. This is referred to as the effective filtration pressure (P_{eff}). In normal conditions there is a net outward force of 8 mmHg at the arterial end, which forces fluid out of the capillary into the interstitial spaces. At the venous end of the blood capillary there is a negative value of –7 mmHg, which is the net inward force moving fluid back into the capillary. However, not all the fluid is returned to the venous flow; some remains within the tissues or is returned to the cardiovascular system via

the lymph channels. An imbalance in the pressures can cause oedema.

The action of massage on the venous flow has an indirect effect on the movement of lymph. Congestion in the capillary network raises the blood hydrostatic pressure (BHP), which leads to excessive fluid moving into the interstitial spaces. Massage reduces the blood capillary congestion by enhancing the venous flow and, in so doing, it helps to lower the hydrostatic pressure and therefore prevents the formation of oedema. A high blood pressure within the veins can likewise cause an increase in hydrostatic pressure within the capillaries (BHP). This will lead to oedema formation. Conversely, improving the venous blood flow with massage reduces the blood pressure and, in turn, lowers the hydrostatic pressure. Oedema is therefore avoided or decreased.

Innate contraction of the lymphangions

The lymphangions (or segments of the lymphatic vessels) have a layer of smooth muscle, and it has been observed in research that these muscle fibres have an innate ability to contract. These spontaneous contractions are considered to be the primary driving force that propels the lymph forward from one segment to the next (Wang and Zhong, 1985). The contractions of the lymphangions appear to occur in a wave-like fashion; as one segment contracts it pushes the lymph forward, which increases the pressure and contractions in the segments ahead. If the contracting segments are not coordinated, the flow of lymph is said to be interrupted (Smith, 1949). The rhythmical movements of the lymph massage strokes can restore the rhythm of the wave-like contractions in the vessels and thereby improve the flow.

Lymphangions have been observed to contract at a rate of 1–9 contractions per minute in the human leg (Olszewski and Engeset, 1979/80) and 10–18 contractions per minute in rabbits (Zweifach and Prather, 1975). An average rate of 10 contractions per minute is quoted by Overholser and Moody (1988), who also compute the length of a lymphangion as 1 cm. Observations have shown that, with each contraction, the lymphangion is emptied of its fluid. This means that the lymph travels the length of the lymphangion (calculated as 1 cm) during each contraction (Smith, 1949). If the lymph is moved 1 cm and the rate is 10 contractions per minute, then the velocity of lymph is 10 cm per minute (as quoted by Overholser and Moody, 1988). The relevance of this calculation is that, for massage to be effective, it has to be carried out at an equivalent speed. It has also been postulated that the rate of lymph drainage in the skin and superficial tissues is more or less constant and is not affected by exercise (Bach and Lewis, 1973). On the other hand, the rate of flow in the deeper vessels that drain the muscles speeds up by 5–15 times during exercise (Guyton, 1961).

Reflex contraction of the lymphangions

The muscular wall of the lymphangion is also stimulated by a reflex mechanism. The process involves the pressure receptors (mechanoreceptors) within the muscular wall of the lymphatic vessel. Stimulation of these receptors leads to a reflex muscular contraction, which propels the lymph forward. In addition to pressure, these mechanoreceptors (or other receptors within the wall) will also respond to a stretching of the vessel. Stimuli for the mechanoreceptors are provided by the following factors:

1. A transverse or longitudinal stretch of the lymphatic vessel (Mislin, 1976). Some of the lymphatic massage techniques are specific in giving a longitudinal and transverse stretch to the lymph vessels. One of these techniques was first pioneered in France in the 1930s by Dr Emil Vodder (Wittlinger and Wittlinger, 1990).

2. An increase in pressure within the lymphangion. As it fills up with fluid, the pressure builds up and compresses the muscular wall outwards (Reddy, 1987).

3. Contractions of the adjoining muscles or arteries. As the muscle fibres contract they create an external force on the adjoining lymph vessels. In addition, the inward pressure applied to the vessel wall will cause it to stretch, thereby stimulating the mechanoreceptors.

4. Respiration, which creates a difference in pressure within the thorax. As the pressure increases within the cavity, it applies a force on the walls of the lymphatic vessels.

5. Peristaltic movements of the intestines within the abdomen. These can apply pressure on the adjoining lymph vessels by their intermittent contractions and movements.

6. Manual manipulation of the tissues, and passive movements. Massage techniques act as an external force on the superficial and deep lymphatic vessels. The reflex effect of these external forces is spontaneous contractions in the same vessels that propel the lymph forward (Wang and Zhong, 1985).

Superficial and deep lymphatic vessels

Two separate lymphatic duct or trunk systems have been identified. Although they start off as separate channels, the two systems merge together before they enter the lymph nodes. A superficial system drains the skin and the superficial tissues, while a second system lies deeper and drains the muscles (Grupp, 1984). It has also been observed in studies that the lymph flow in the interstitial tissues (superficial and deep) is under a different pressure to that in the muscular tissues. Other experiments have shown that light pressure can enhance the lymph flow of the superficial tissues, while a heavier pressure is required for the deep muscular tissue (Overholser and Moody, 1988).

The superficial lymph vessels

A mechanical and direct impact of massage on the skin and subcutaneous tissue is to push the lymph from the interstitial spaces into the collecting vessels. The cells that make up the wall of the collecting vessels are designed to separate and allow fluid to move into the vessel. Ligamentous filaments connect the endothelial cells of the vessels to the surrounding connective tissue (Fig. 3.5). When the fluid builds up in the interstitial spaces it causes the immediate connective tissue to stretch. The stretching causes the

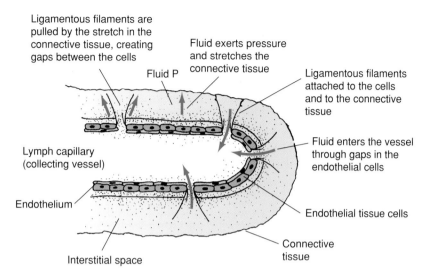

Figure 3.5 Direction of lymph flow from the interstitial tissues into the collecting lymph vessel.

ligamentous filaments to become taut, thereby exerting a pull on the endothelial cells. As a result, the cells separate and the junctions between them open. Research has indicated that massage creates sufficient pressure to push the lymph mechanically through the gaps between the endothelial cells of the collecting vessels (Xujian, 1990). As well as forcing the fluid through the open gaps, massage may itself increase the pressure within the interstitial spaces. A stretching of the connective tissue ensues, and the endothelial cells are pulled apart.

Another researcher observed that raising the temperature of the skin forced more junctions between the endothelial cells to open and, as a result, the effect of the massage was increased (Xujian, 1990). Heat can therefore be used alongside massage to reduce oedema. This is a very significant observation, because oedema reduction is generally associated with the use of cold packs. Two separate mechanisms must be in operation. The cooling causes vasoconstriction of the capillaries and therefore reduces the oedema of haemorrhage, while heat opens the junctions between the cells and allows the fluid to enter the collecting vessels.

Lymph flow in the skin was investigated using the isotope clearance technique (ICT). In this pro-

cedure, a colloid (a solution such as colloidal gold) is injected into the subepidermis and subcutaneous tissue and used as a tracer to monitor the movement of lymph. In one experiment the skin of a pig was used, as it is very similar to that of humans. The study observed the ability of lymphatic vessels to respond to massage, and this was investigated using the ICT. Significant changes in the lymph flow were observed when local gentle massage was performed. It is noteworthy that pressure did not play a vital role in the outcome. Variations in pressure did occur, albeit unintentionally, as the massage was applied with a hand-held massager. Also of interest is the difference in the rate of flow, which was noticeably faster in the subdermis than in the subcutaneous tissue. This was put down to the denser network of lymphatic capillaries in the subdermal area (Mortimer et al., 1990). One research experiment carried out on rabbits confirmed that the lymph flow is increased in the ear when rubbing (or massage) is used (Parsons and McMaster, 1938).

The deep lymph vessels

Exercise and the contraction of muscles play an important role in the movement of lymph, particularly in the deeper vessels. Muscle contraction exerts an external force on the lymph vessels, which directly pushes the lymph forward. The compression also stimulates the mechanoreceptors within the vessel wall, causing it to contract reflexively. One study showed that both massage and passive movements raised the proximal lymph pressure in dogs (Caenar et al., 1970). Other experiments were carried out on rats, with similar results (Wang and Zhong, 1985), and on human volunteers (Olszewski and Engeset, 1979/80).

Lymphatic pressure

Pressure within the lymphatic system is very low. At the interstitial end, the tissue pressure is said to be below that of atmospheric pressure. In the collecting vessels (terminal lymphatics or lymph capillaries), it is between 0.98 and 1.75 gcm^{-2} (0.014–0.025 $lbin^{-2}$). As it reaches the lymph nodes, the pressure increases to 30.02–37.96 gcm^{-2} (0.427–0.540 $lbin^{-2}$) (Zweifach and Prather, 1975). These pressures are sufficient to stimulate the mechanoreceptors and to cause reflex contractions of the lymphatic vessel wall. As the pressure increases slightly, the speed of contractions is also increased; however, too great a force has the opposite effect and the flow of lymph slows down or ceases altogether. This can result in the formation of oedema. For lymph massage to be effective, it needs to be of sufficient pressure to propel the lymph forward without impairing its flow (Mislin, 1976). The necessary pressure starts at about 4.39 gcm^{-2} (1 $ozin^{-2}$) in the terminal lymphatics, increasing to 35.15–52.73 gcm^{-2} (8–12 $ozin^{-2}$) in the lymph vessels and ducts. In chronic oedema, a slightly heavier pressure may be required. Longstanding lymph tends to thicken, and may prove difficult to pass through the fine opening (or stoma) in the lymphatic network.

Mechanical and reflex effects on the organs of digestion

Some authors would claim that massage on the abdomen has very little impact on the digestive and other viscera. Others would state that it has significant effects, mechanical as well as reflex. A common consensus is that massage improves the circulation to the viscera and, via a reflex pathway, causes contraction of the smooth muscles. It is also likely that, directly or indirectly, massage activates glandular secretions within the gastrointestinal tract. Applied anatomy and research findings support the claim that the reflex pathway linking the somatic tissues to the gastrointestinal tract is via the autonomic nervous system, primarily the vagus nerve. Stimulation of the pressure receptors by massage precipitates a barrage of sensory impulses along the peripheral afferent pathways and, through hypothalamic control, increased tone of the vagus nerve (Uvnas-Moberg et al., 1987). Studies on preterm infants found a very close connection between tactile/kinaesthetic stimulation and weight gain. One proposal for this correlation is that vagal nerve parasympathetic activation leads to a release of several peptide hormones, including gastrin. It can also cause acid secretions, glucose-induced insulin release, growth of the gastric mucosa and improved function of the gastrointestinal tract (Uvnas-Moberg et al., 1987). Although further research may be necessary on these characteristics of massage, some postulations can be put forward if they are based on clinical experience and applied anatomy. For instance, it is reasonable to deduce that manipulation of the tissues, and in some cases of the viscera, has a physiological influence. A case in point is that of the colon function, which is frequently seen to improve with massage in clinical practice. These observations are, however, in contrast to a study carried out on normal subjects and on patients suffering from chronic constipation. The study showed no significant difference in colon function when massage was carried out on both groups of volunteers (Klauser et al., 1992). While some reports support the theory of increased peristalsis with abdominal massage, others place more emphasis on the effect of massage on reflex zones to the digestive tract.

Mobility of the viscera

Within the abdomen, each viscus is attached to adjacent structures and/or to the peritoneum by ligaments or fascia. Any tightness or adhesions in these soft tissue structures can inhibit the movement of the viscus, and this has a knock-on effect on other organs. The visceral organs are also capable of spontaneous movements; furthermore, their inherent motility can be increased following the removal or lessening of any physical restrictions. Abdominal massage gently manipulates the viscera and frees up any limitations. By its action on the connective tissues it can therefore assist the overall mobility of the viscera.

Stomach

Massage on the abdomen has the mechanical and direct effect of moving the contents out of the stomach and into the duodenum. This is most effective when the stomach is dilated, as an empty stomach is almost hidden by the ribs. Manipulation of the abdominal wall also creates a neural reflex pathway, resulting in contractions of the stomach muscles. It is argued by some authors that such a reflex tends to be insubstantial, because a stomach that is already dilated (temporarily or permanently) is usually weak and therefore less likely to respond to reflex stimuli (Mennell, 1920).

Intestines

The portions of the gut which are fixed to the abdominal wall are the caecum, the ascending and descending colon, the duodenum and the iliac colon. It is therefore reasonably practicable to push forward the contents of these structures directly by massage. In addition, manipulation of the superficial tissues and of the visceral organs results in peristaltic contractions through reflex mechanisms. The small intestines, on the other hand, are very mobile and therefore more difficult to empty by mechanical means. Manual pressure on this region can easily move them and allow them to slip from underneath the therapist's hands. However, it is still feasible to propel their contents by the action of massage, and the peristaltic movement is quite often indicated by gurgling sounds. While this could be a reflex action, it is more likely to happen as a result of the mechanical and direct compression. The transverse colon is likewise difficult to locate, especially as its position is rather flexible; for instance, when the subject is supine the position of the colon is different to that when standing. If palpation indicates the presence of hard matter and gas within the colon, then it should be possible to effect their forward movement with massage.

Sphincters

Sphincters are influenced through a reflex action. A prime example is the pyloric sphincter, which is under the control of the autonomic nervous system. It is quite plausible that the sphincter opens as a response to sensory stimuli from the skin, or to relaxation. Both stimuli are provided by the massage movements.

Mechanical and reflex effects on the muscles

Change of venous flow in muscles

The venous blood flow in muscles has been measured using a technique called the 'xenon washout rate'. In this procedure, a fluid containing xenon (a radioactive isotope) is injected into the blood vessels and detectors then monitor the movement of the xenon. This technique was used in a study carried out to test the effect of massage on the venous flow of muscles. Petrissage has been shown to cause a significant increase in the xenon washout rate when there is venous stasis of skeletal muscles (Peterson, 1970). As the vascular bed is mechanically emptied by massage, it refills with a fresh blood supply and the stasis is reduced.

Tapotement (percussive movements) was found to cause a 5% increase in muscular blood flow, using the xenon washout rate technique. The increase in the rate of blood flow in the muscle was also worth noting. With tapotement, the rate of flow was comparable to the changes seen during active muscle contractions. An increase in the blood flow may have caused additional temperature changes in the muscle. However, a rise in temperature may also be a consequence of the mechanical friction caused by the tapotement. Superficial hyperaemia was also observed following the tapotement, and continued for up to 10 min (1–3 min in the arm and 4–10 min in the leg). This increase in superficial blood flow could also be seen as a tissue response to the trauma created by the tapotement. Cellular damage in the cutaneous and subcutaneous tissues leads to the release of histamine-like substances and intense vasodilatation. In this experiment petrissage also caused an increase in the tracer washout rate, but this change occurred during the initial stages and then stabilized (Hovind and Nielsen, 1974).

Removal of metabolites

Muscle contractions require adenosine triphosphate (ATP) energy, which is produced by glycolysis (the breakdown of the glucose molecule). During this process pyruvic acid is produced, which is either catabolized by the mitochondria into carbon dioxide and water or, in the presence of oxygen, into carbon dioxide and ATP. If oxygen is not available, the pyruvic acid turns into lactic acid (some energy is also produced in this anaerobic process). Eighty per cent of the lactic acid is drained through the venous return, while some accumulates in the muscle tissue and is subsequently converted into carbon dioxide and water. Muscles therefore produce by-products, including lactic acid, carbon dioxide and water. The presence of lactic acid in muscle tissue leads to fatigue. Lactic acid yields a high concentration of hydrogen ions, which affect the myosin and actin protein molecules and, as a result, the pulling action of the cross-bridges is weakened and the muscle becomes fatigued. The pain receptors (nociceptors) in the area are also affected and sensitized by the hydrogen ions, and stimulation of these end organs leads to the perception of pain in the region. By increasing the circulation through the muscles, massage has the effect of draining the metabolites, including lactic acid and water. Similarly, carbon dioxide is eliminated by the improved venous return. Stimulation of the pain receptors is also diminished by a lower concentration of hydrogen ions.

Uptake of oxygen

It is not clear whether massage assists in the uptake of oxygen when applied to skeletal muscles before or after exercise. Recovery after exhausting exercise with small muscle groups is, however, increased, and this has been ascribed to a quicker removal of substances responsible for the fatigue (Müller and Esch, 1966).

Influence on the muscle spindle—stretch receptor

Changes in muscle length and tension are monitored by stretch receptors embedded within the muscle (Fig. 3.6). One of these, the muscle spindle, encompasses a few of the muscle fibres, and these are the intrafusal or spindle fibres. The filaments of the receptor wrap around the muscle fibres and emit signals when the muscle length changes. One filament, the annulospiral or primary ending, is in the centre of the spindle. This filament is highly sensitive and fires rapidly and with a high velocity with the smallest change of length. Two smaller filaments, the flower spray receptors, are located on either side of the annulospiral filament. These are said to be slower in response, and are likely to respond more readily to the magnitude and speed of the stretch.

When the afferent neurons from the spindle enter the spinal cord, they divide and take different paths. One of the branches connects directly with a motor neuron in the cord; this link takes place without a synapse being formed with an interneuron. Efferent motor impulses leave the anterior horn by this monosynaptic connection, and travel along alpha motor neurons to the same muscle. They end in fibres (extrafusal fibres) outside the muscle spindle compartment, causing them to contract. Motor neurons (somatic efferent) have their cell body within the spinal cord or the brainstem; their axons are myelinated and have the largest diameter in the body. They are therefore able to transmit action potentials at high velocities. It follows that signals from the CNS can reach the skeletal muscle fibres with minimal delay. Inside the cord, the other branches of the afferent neuron connect with interneurons. When these are activated, they either feed the information to the brain or cause inhibition of the antagonist muscles. Others still cause contraction of synergist muscles.

Contraction of the intrafusal (spindle) muscle fibres is separate to that of the extrafusal fibres. The intrafusal fibres are under the control of the higher brain centres, and motor impulses to them pass along gamma motor neurons. When the intrafusal fibres contract, they pull on the annulospiral filament (receptor). Minimal contractions are needed to maintain a stretch in the filament. If the contractions are very strong or frequent, they cause the filament to become hypersensitive and to fire at random.

Relaxation, or the changed emotional state of the subject, is registered by the cortex, which relays the information to the cerebellum. It is very likely that relaxation causes the cerebellum to send out a reduced number of motor impulses (gamma efferent—Class A) to the intrafusal muscle fibres of the spindle. This has the effect of lowering the sensitivity of the annulospiral receptor and, in turn, of the muscle spindle itself. Afferent signals from the spindle become less frequent and, as a result, the reflex contractions of the extrafusal muscle fibres are also decreased. Consequently the muscle is able to relax, and the deeper the relaxation, the greater the accumulated calming effect on the subject.

Influence on the Golgi tendon organ—stretch receptor

A second receptor, located at the junction of the muscle and its tendon, monitors the tension exerted on the contracting muscle or imposed on it by external forces. The Golgi tendon organ has filaments wrapped around the collagen fibres of the tendon and, when the muscle contracts and the tendon is stretched, the filaments are distorted and stimulated to discharge afferent impulses (Fig. 3.6). These enter the spinal cord and synapse with interneurons connecting to the brain and to local motor neurons. As well as providing continuous information about the muscle's activity, the afferent neuron has another

function. Some of its branches also synapse with inhibiting interneurons, which bring about inhibition of the contracting muscle. This protective mechanism operates if the strain on the tendon is very high and the Golgi tendon organ is overstimulated. Massage can also cause inhibition by its action on the Golgi tendon organ. The pressure applied with some of the massage techniques overloads the Golgi tendon organ, and in turn causes the same reflex inhibition.

Relaxation by inhibition of efferent motor impulses

The inhibition of muscles involves other mechanisms, which are well researched and documented. Studies have shown that the pressure of massage has an inhibitory effect on the motor neurons innervating the muscle, and that inhibition can be inversely measured by the degree of muscle contraction. However, a direct evaluation of muscle tone may lead to erroneous interpretations. An alternative method is to measure the electrical activity across its tissue surface. This can be monitored using the Hoffmann reflex (H-reflex) test, which is a measure of the excitability of the spinal reflex pathway. Put another way, the measurement of the H-reflex peak-to-peak amplitudes evaluates the excitability of the motor neurons. The higher the H-reflex values, the stronger the excitability of motor neurons. A reduction in motor neuron excitability or activity is interpreted as low-level stimulation of the muscle; as a result the muscle tone is reduced. H-reflex amplitude testing has been used in studies to investigate the efficacy of therapeutic modalities such as icing, tendon pressure and cutaneous electrical stimulation. It has also been used in a variety of research projects to assess the effects of massage.

Reduction in muscle tone

A study using patients with a known history of hemiparesis (paralysis affecting one side of the body) secondary to a cerebrovascular accident (CVA) indicated that continuous or intermittent pressure on the Achilles tendon resulted in a

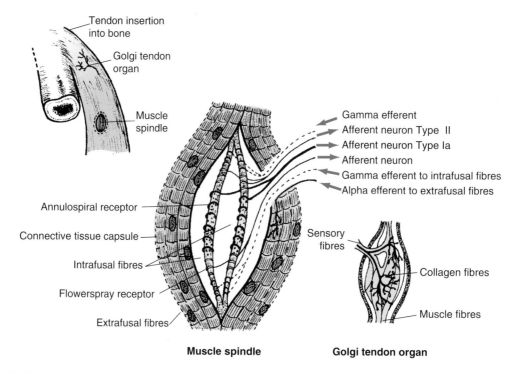

Figure 3.6 Muscle spindle and Golgi tendon organ.

reduction of gastrocnemius muscle tonicity (Leone and Kukulka, 1988). The study also evaluated the effect of two separate intensities (5 and 10 kg). These experiments showed that intermittent pressure was more effective than continuous, but that the 10 kg mass had no greater effect than the 5 kg. It was noted, however, that in healthy subjects the 10 kg mass was more effective than the 5 kg. The mechanism for this inhibition is a negative reflex arc in which the interneurons act as 'switches' and prevent the stimulation of motor neurons. This occurs in response to stimulation of the cutaneous mechanoreceptors.

Contrary to what is often suggested, hypertonic muscles do not necessitate excessive pressure. As previously discussed, a reflex contraction within the same muscle group will occur if the pain threshold is exceeded. The nature of the hypertonicity needs to be assessed. Emotional tension is also likely to maintain an involuntary contraction while the treatment is carried out. The therapist will then apply more pressure to coun-

teract this involuntary contraction. So once again it is best to apply the pressure only gradually and within a comfortable pain threshold.

Inhibition by varying pressure intensities

Another experiment measured the effects of one-handed petrissage on the triceps surae muscle (gastrocnemius and soleus). It was found that depression of spinal motor neuron activity was directly related to the intensity of pressure applied (Goldberg et al., 1992). The study was conducted on healthy subjects, and the pressure was applied to the belly of the muscle. Changes in the peak-to-peak H-reflex amplitudes were used to monitor the level of motor neuron excitability. It was observed that light pressure produced a 39% reduction and deep pressure a 49% reduction in H-reflex amplitude. Muscle relaxation was therefore produced with both intensities. It was proposed that this massage technique activated a wide spectrum of sensory receptors, including those mechanoreceptors in the cutaneous tissue and those found in muscular tissue. The study suggests that, based on available literature, stimulation of the cutaneous pressure receptors as well as those of the muscle mechanoreceptors (especially the secondary fibres of the muscle spindle) causes the reflex inhibition of motor neurons.

Inhibitory response

Some of the massage and bodywork techniques exert a passive stretch on the muscle tendon fibres and, in turn, disrupt the Golgi tendon organ. This is generally seen as being sufficient to inhibit the muscle temporarily and, by so doing, promote relaxation (Chaitow, 1987, p. 37). Several authors have suggested that passive stretching of muscle tissue (by tendon pressure, muscle tapping and other manual techniques) stimulates the secondary fibres of the muscle spindle and causes an inhibitory response. This seems to suggest that, while active stretching causes the muscle spindle to fire and cause a reflex muscle contraction, the opposite happens with a passive stretch. In this case, the spindle (or at least the secondary fibres) is either inhibited itself or causes inhibition when the muscle is passively stretched.

A similar hypothesis was offered in another study. It has been postulated that a reduction in the H-reflex amplitude, and therefore relaxation, occurs during passive muscle stretching and muscle tapping. Inhibition could well be mediated by the mechanoreceptors within the muscle (Bélanger et al., 1989). These findings support the theory that the passive stretch of the muscle spindle (particularly of its secondary fibres) and of the Golgi tendon organ can result in an inhibitory effect on the motor neurons.

According to other research, massage may also have a more generalized neurophysiological response. A reduction in H-reflex amplitude was recorded in the triceps surae muscle when massage was applied to other sites on the ipsilateral limb (Bélanger et al., 1989). A second observation was in contrast to the first. Petrissage of the triceps surae led to relaxation not only of that muscle, but also of other muscles on the ipsilateral limb. The generalized neurophysiological response may therefore extend beyond the muscle being massaged.

The same findings were reported in another study, which showed that H-reflex amplitudes of the triceps surae were reduced when it was massaged. Furthermore, massage to other sites on the ipsilateral limb resulted in a reduction in the H-reflex responses on the same triceps surae (Sullivan et al., 1991). The various findings seem to indicate that pressure and tapping are likely to stimulate the cutaneous pressure receptors, while massage techniques such as petrissage are more likely to involve the Golgi tendon organs and muscle spindles. Similar experiments confirmed the influence of massage on the motor excitability. A 71% decrease in H-reflex amplitudes was observed during massage to the triceps surae in healthy subjects (Morelli et al., 1990). It was also suggested that, based on the findings of other researchers, the deep lying receptors (including those in muscles and tendons) dominate over the influences of the superficial cutaneous receptors (Morelli et al., 1990).

A slightly contradictory theory is that tone can be improved if the stretch reflex concept is implemented (Ganong, 1987). According to this theory the stretching of the muscle, although passive, is registered by the muscle spindle and consequently an action potential is generated, causing contraction. This theory contradicts the findings of other researchers, who argue that stimulation of the muscle spindle with passive stretching causes inhibition.

4

The clinical application of massage

INTRODUCTION

Following on from the considerations of the mechanical and reflex effects of massage in the previous chapter it is now appropriate to consider the clinical applications. The proposals put forward for the use of massage in many conditions are either based on theoretical reasoning, research material or clinical experience. Research findings are sometimes controversial and at times inconsistent but they provide a sound hypothesis. Clinical experience is bound to differ amongst practitioners and this is also reflected in the theories put forward by different authors. The suggestions, therefore, for the application of massage are not prescriptive but are designed to provide the massage therapist information on which to base their treatment approach.

The applications of massage and therefore the pathological conditions for which massage is indicated are addressed in this chapter. Disorders that are frequently encountered are apportioned the relevant consideration, while a somewhat briefer discussion is offered for the less common ailments. The use of massage is determined by the indications for and contraindications to the treatment, particularly when it is applied for a specific therapeutic effect. As in other therapies, however, opinions about the application of techniques may differ. The indications and contraindications to massage that are discussed in this book are therefore considered with this in mind, and serve as a general guide rather than as a list of hard and fast rules. On the other hand, some precautionary measures are unquestionable. To enable the therapist to decide on the suitability of the massage, the following questions must be addressed:

1. Is the condition acute, subacute or chronic?
2. What is the purpose of the massage; for example, improved circulation, relaxation, removal of toxins?
3. Which region(s) of the body need to be addressed? Is the massage applied to the local area, or is it systemic?
4. Which organ function or body system is the massage influencing?
5. Which massage movements are safe to apply?

Indications

A pathological condition is an indication for massage if the condition is likely to benefit from the treatment. Invariably the massage is administered as an adjunct to other approaches, medical or complementary, and in some cases it is only carried out with the approval of a medical practitioner.

At this stage, it is important to consider the application of massage for different types of conditions.

• In the more generalized constitutional disorders, the role of massage is to enhance the elimination of toxins and waste products. These substances arise from infections, inflammation, muscle spasms and similar changes. Massage achieves this goal by its influence on the circulation, in particular that of the venous return and of lymph. Further benefits occur with the relaxation of muscles and, equally significantly, of the patient. An indirect yet relevant effect is the stimulation of the autonomic nervous system, which in turn improves the production of glandular secretions and organ function.
• All massage movements have a normalizing effect on reflex zones, whether these are areas of direct referred pain relating to organ malfunction or an indirect tissue change. In addi-

tion, some massage movements (such as neuromuscular technique) can be applied to specific zones related to a particular disorder or organ.
• In more specific conditions, such as pathological changes, massage is applied to help alleviate some of the symptoms associated with the malady.

Contraindications

While there is much to be gained from massage, it may be contraindicated in some pathological states. The reason behind this precautionary approach is to eliminate the possibility of exacerbating the severity or complications of the pathology. However, in the majority of cases massage is contraindicated only to those tissues or regions affected. Information obtained when taking the case history is used to assess the suitability of the massage treatment. In addition, each body region is examined for any signs or clues of possible contraindications, whether these are minor or of a more serious nature. Some conditions are perhaps more obviously contraindicated than others, while others still are best discussed with the patient's doctor. What is of relevance is that the massage practitioner is equipped with the knowledge of anatomy and pathology to make an informed decision about the appropriateness of the massage treatment (see also Chapter 1).

Reactions to the treatment

Reactions to the massage and bodywork vary from one patient to the next. Whereas one subject may have a positive response over a short period, another patient with the same condition may need a much longer treatment. Such a difference is unavoidable and only natural. It is worth remembering that it is the patients who are healing themselves, albeit with the guidance and assistance of the massage therapist. Disparity also exists in the immediate physical effects of the treatment. While the massage is intended to be pleasant, some of the strokes are more so than others. For instance, deep massage movements are more of a 'nice pain' when compared to the soothing feel of the light effleurage. A residual feeling of achiness can sometimes linger after the treatment, and this is invariably because of overstimulation of the sensory nerves. This form of reaction subsides in a few hours or less. However, any pain or bruising which persists or is significant is recorded, literally or mentally, as it conveys the need to make adjustments to subsequent treatments or to omit the area altogether. Patients may also report of a feeling of heaviness in the head, or the need to blow their nose immediately after the treatment; both of these symptoms are also transient, and indicate that the body is eliminating toxins. It is not uncommon for massage to the abdomen to be followed by defaecation, and lymph and kidney massage by emptying of the bladder, and this is indeed to be expected.

To complete the treatment, therefore, the patient is informed about the expected outcomes of the massage treatment and advised accordingly. In the unlikely event that a tissue or joint has been inflamed, a cool wet towel is placed on the area for about 15 min. A similar cold application is used if nerve inflammation is suspected. Aching of a muscle can be alleviated with a hot pack. In all events, the discomfort is monitored and, in the remote possibility that it is very persistent, advice may need to be sought from the patient's doctor.

CIRCULATORY SYSTEM

Anaemia

Anaemia is a condition where there is a reduction in the number of circulating red blood cells, or a deficiency of haemoglobin (the iron-containing and oxygen-carrying pigment of red blood cells), or in the concentration of the red blood cells per 100 ml of blood. A combination of two or more of these factors can occur simultaneously. The essential causes of anaemia are excessive blood loss, abnormal destruction of red blood cells, and decreased production of red blood cells. Symptoms include pallor, weakness, headaches, sore tongue, drowsiness, dyspnoea, angina, gastrointestinal disturbances and amenorrhoea.

Excessive blood loss is one of the more common causes of anaemia. It may be caused by factors such as heavy menstruation in women, coughing of blood (as in tuberculosis), blood loss in faeces (as in haemorrhoids, colon tumours, peptic ulcers, ulcerative colitis) and severe injuries.

Decreased production of red blood cells can occur, for instance, when there is aplasia (underdevelopment) of the bone marrow. One example is aplastic anaemia, where the production of red blood cells is affected, as is that of the platelets and white blood cells.

Abnormal production of blood cells can also occur from conditions that destroy the bone marrow, e.g. tumours, chemical agents and exposure to radiation. This also results in aplastic anaemia.

Low haemoglobin production may be because of a lack of proteins, iron, vitamin B12 or folic acid. These deficiencies can be related to conditions such as malabsorption syndrome (protein deficiency) and pregnancy (iron deficiency).

Increased destruction of red blood cells can take place if, for example, the spleen is malfunctioning and overactive. Destruction of the red blood cells occurs in sickle-cell anaemia, because of a hereditary or genetic defect in the haemoglobin molecule. In this condition, most of the red blood cells contain the abnormal form of haemoglobin which causes the cell membrane to distort into a rigid sickle-shaped structure. The red blood cell's ability to absorb oxygen is also reduced and the sickle-shaped cells create blockages in capillaries, with subsequent ischaemia to various organs and tissues. During an episode of sickle cell crisis the subject is likely to suffer from pain and infection in addition to the anaemia. The pain can be constant, severe and debilitating, and may even require hospitalization. It is common in the bones of the chest, back, jaw, legs and arms, and the abdomen. There may also be ulcerations of the lower limbs and an increased incidence of strokes.

When treating anaemia with massage it is vital that the cause of the condition is first established and that a patient is referred to a doctor should there be signs of anaemia that are not diagnosed. It is also important to bear in mind that massage is not aimed at curing the condition but at alleviating some of the symptoms and supporting the patient.

Cautionary notes

- Subjects suffering anaemia, especially from sickle-cell anaemia, are prone to infections, and therefore care and extreme hygiene in the treatment room are of utmost importance.
- Where there is an excessive bleeding disorder (such as mild forms of haemophilia) light stroking is essential so as not to cause any bruising. Massage is contraindicated altogether in severe cases of haemophilia or where the risk of bleeding is high.
- Anaemia related to nutritional deficiencies is best treated by a balanced diet, but referral to dietitian may be necessary.
- Patients suffering from sickle-cell anaemia can be safely treated during periods of remission, although even then using only a very light stroking technique. As with cancer patients, very light effleurage movements can be used to reduce the level of pain (Ferrell-Torry and Glick, 1993), but the treatment should only be carried out with the approval of the doctor. Improving the systemic circulation may also help prevent the formation of ulcers in the lower limbs.

Massage application

- As a general effect massage can be used to improve the systemic circulation and therefore the movement of the red blood cells, their nutrients and oxygen supply to the tissues.
- Heart and renal efficiency will also benefit from systemic massage. Their combined output is vital to the elimination of waste products, which is essential to patient health. To accelerate the removal of toxins, the massage is applied systemically as well as to the abdomen, colon and kidneys.
- Abdominal massage has the additional benefits of assisting the portal circulation and helping to improve digestion and absorption, especially of vitamin B12 and iron.
- Massage treatment for anaemia can be carried out on a daily basis, particularly as it promotes

the relaxation and rest that are needed in this condition. Warm baths can also be taken for care of the skin.

Hypertension

Hypertension refers to a raising of the blood pressure from its normal values of 115 ($\pm$20) mmHg systolic and 75 ($\pm$10) mmHg diastolic. Blood pressure is the force exerted by the blood on the walls of the arteries. The pressure is determined by the rate and strength of the heart beat in addition to the resistance offered by the blood vessels. It is reduced in the veins by the compression of surrounding tissues and intrinsic forces within the abdomen. As it reaches the right atrium, the venous pressure is at its lowest level (0 mmHg).

Hypertension can cause damage to the heart. This is largely because of the great effort required to push the blood against the resistance offered by the arterial pressure. The heart muscles thicken and enlarge as a result of the extra demand put upon them and, consequently, they require more oxygen and an additional blood supply; they are also susceptible to fatigue and weakness. Furthermore, hypertension can cause arteriosclerosis (see Secondary hypertension, below), which may even affect the coronary arteries; this can lead to heart failure, myocardial infarction, or angina. Degeneration of the blood vessels caused by the high blood pressure may result in severe damage to the brain, e.g. cerebrovascular accident (stroke), and also to the kidneys.

Essential hypertension

Essential hypertension, also termed primary or idiopathic hypertension, occurs with no known causes and is very common. One explanation is that individuals who are susceptible to this type of hypertension have an exaggerated response to afferent stimuli. These arise from the external environment, or from internal sources such as the higher brain centres, chemoreceptors and the viscera. Stress is said to be an influence, causing the whole body to be on edge and making its receptors hypersensitive. Additionally, it gives rise to motor impulses along the sympathetic nerves which bring about contractions of the arterioles and, accordingly, there is a higher and more sustained rise in blood pressure than would normally occur. This elevation of the blood pressure is closely associated with arteriosclerosis (see Secondary hypertension) and ischaemia. The kidneys are particularly susceptible to these changes and respond by releasing renin (a precursor of angiotensin), which further sustains the high blood pressure.

Massage application

- Massage is applied to reduce the stress levels that are frequently implicated in this condition. Relaxation elicits a reduction in sympathetic activity and, therefore, a lower intensity of vasoconstriction in the arterial walls. The resistance to the flow of blood is thereby reduced.
- Some authors indicated in the past that abdominal massage may cause a slight rise in the blood pressure by its reflex action on the heart muscle (Mennell, 1920). More recent studies have indicated otherwise, however, and massage to the abdomen is considered to lower the blood pressure (Kurosawa et al., 1995).

Secondary hypertension

The other type of hypertension is secondary to identifiable causes. Degeneration of the large and medium-sized blood vessels is one prominent factor, and is responsible for resistance to the blood flow. The deterioration is commonly associated with arteriosclerosis, in which the muscle layer of the blood vessels is replaced by fibrous tissue impregnated with calcium salts. Although the lumen of the artery tends to widen, the calcium deposits cause it to become very hard and inelastic, and this loss of dispensability in the arterial wall leads mostly to an increase in systolic pressure.

Massage application

- Massage can be used to aid the circulation along these conducting arteries. Resistance to the blood flow is thereby reduced and, in turn,

there is a lowering of the high blood pressure. It is worth noting that massage, while increasing the circulation, does not increase the blood pressure.

- Relaxation is another goal of the massage. It acts as an effective anxiolytic (relieving stress) as a result of its influence on the sympathetic nervous system and, in addition, promotes deep sleep, which is an essential remedy for high blood pressure. For the purpose of relaxation, some of the massage movements on the back are carried out in a caudal direction (towards the feet). This path does not follow the systemic venous return but, when relaxation is the main purpose of the massage, the soothing strokes can temporarily take preference over those for the circulation. Strokes for the venous return can be resumed afterwards if necessary.

Degeneration of the small blood vessels

Secondary hypertension may also involve the small branches of the arterial system, the arterioles. These vessels can be affected by hyaline arteriolosclerosis; the hypertension itself and diabetes are two predisposing factors to this condition. Hyaline arteriolosclerosis results when blood plasma seeps under the endothelium of the blood vessel. This is generally accompanied by protein deposition and a gradual conversion to collagen. The muscle layer is replaced by hyaline material in the medial and intimal layers and, in this hardened state, the muscle wall offers an increased resistance to the blood flow. As a result of this resistance, the pressure within the arterioles remains constant during the diastolic phase of the heart contractions, while in normal conditions it would be lower. Diastolic pressure is therefore said to be high. A further complication of the dysfunction is that the lumen of the artery narrows and ischaemia is nearly always present, especially in the kidneys.

Massage application

- Systemic massage can be applied to assist the flow of blood through the arterioles; this in turn lowers the resistance and the build-up of pressure.

Vasoconstriction of the arterioles

The diameter of the arterioles is controlled by the vasomotor centre in the medulla; it is also under the influence of sympathetic impulses. Changes in the diameter of the arterioles have a direct effect on the blood pressure; for instance, contraction of the arterial wall elevates the blood pressure while relaxation lowers it. Essential hypertension is generally associated with the overstimulation of sympathetic nerves and, therefore, with vasoconstriction of the arterioles. Contractions can also be caused by chemical or hormonal influences such as epinephrine and norepinephrine (from the adrenal medulla), antidiuretic hormone (from the hypothalamus and posterior pituitary), angiotensin II or histamine. Overproduction of these hormones occurs owing to malfunction of the pituitary gland, which in turn affects the adrenal cortex. Another possible aetiology is malfunction of the adrenal gland itself (Cushing's syndrome, Conn's syndrome).

Massage application

- The benefits of massage are limited in these conditions. However, relaxation has the effect of reducing the production of epinephrine and norepinephrine. This reduction in turn lessens sympathetic influences on the involuntary muscles and therefore reduces vasoconstrictions of the arterioles.

Renal disease

Renal disease is perhaps the commonest cause of secondary hypertension, and the increase in blood pressure is more likely to develop if ischaemia of the kidneys is also present. Ischaemia to the kidneys causes renin to be released. Renin is a chemical that plays a part in fluid retention; it catalyses angiotensin (a vasoconstrictor) and causes the release of aldosterone, which is an adrenal cortex hormone responsible for fluid retention. Water retention increases the blood volume and, therefore, brings about hypertension. Additionally, the ischaemia of the kidneys may cause a build-up of back pressure, which may extend to the heart and place it under further strain.

Massage application

- Systemic massage improves the circulation, which relieves the back pressure as well as the ischaemia. Provided that no inflammation is present, massage can also be carried out over the kidney area. Effleurage techniques, in particular those for lymphatic drainage, increase the circulation and speed up the elimination of fluids. Vibration movements on the back, abdomen and lower limbs are also used to assist the lymph drainage. The kidneys are stimulated to eliminate toxins, thereby lessening toxaemia (see also reflex zones for kidney inflammation, p. 138).

Coronary heart disease

The coronary arteries supplying the heart muscles are subject to the same degenerative changes that affect other arteries elsewhere in the body. A plaque of atheroma, for instance, can cause a gradual and progressive narrowing of the lumen of the coronary artery. When more than 70% of the artery is blocked there is a reduced blood supply, or chronic ischaemia of the myocardium. The ischaemia is nearly always caused by atheroma of the coronary arteries; it affects mainly the ventricles, particularly the left side. Chronic ischaemia can lead to angina pectoris and/or to heart failure. The presence of a thrombus will complicate matters even more because an acute occlusion of an artery or arteries can lead to sudden ischaemia, necrosis of the muscle tissue and myocardial infarction (heart attack). Frequently the condition is characterized by a sharp pain in the chest; the somatic sensation can also spread to one or both arms. In addition, the sufferer may experience a burning sensation in the anterior and posterior aspects of the trunk. Sometimes there are no symptoms, and the attack is said to be silent.

If the subject survives the attack, the condition prevails and can lead to an acute illness with heart failure, cardiogenic shock, arrhythmia and chest pain. Sudden shock is a rapid fall in blood pressure, with inadequate blood perfusion to vital organs. Arrhythmia refers to ventricular fibrillation, also described as cardiac arrest, which is most likely to happen at the onset of the infarction and during the first few days; it can also be fatal. Healing of the muscle tissue takes place, but there is always scarring (fibrosis). Leg vein thrombosis may additionally develop in the first few days after a heart attack. The thrombus can be caused by the recumbency of the patient and the venous stasis. If it becomes mobile and transforms into a pulmonary embolism, it can have fatal consequences.

Massage application

- Massage treatment immediately after a heart attack is very difficult, because of the seriousness of the condition. For this reason, it is only carried out in agreement with the patient's doctor. Massage is applicable during the early stages to improve the circulation, in particular that of the upper and lower limbs. Gentle effleurage is all that is recommended, and this is restricted to a few minutes at a time. A very brief effleurage to the chest area can help reduce the chest pain. Following the acute stage, the massage treatment is gradually extended.
- Reducing stress is another goal of the massage treatment and is likely to be of the most benefit during the first 2 months after a heart attack. Depression has been found to be a major problem after a heart attack; in some cases, subjects suffering from depression have further heart problems which prove fatal. Massage induces relaxation, helps to alleviate depression and builds up self-esteem. Gentle effleurage to the hands, face, feet and back is applied daily.
- A patient suffering from heart disease can derive benefit from regular massage as a preventative measure against a heart attack. Gentle effleurage movements are carried out to maintain a good systemic circulation and, in turn, that of the heart.
- Massage to reflex zones can be considered. Heart disease (and all conditions relating to it) can lead to tissue changes such as tightness, tenderness and swellings in the reflex zones to the heart. Massage of reflex zones is a controversial issue. Some authors consider massage to these areas to be contraindicated or that treatment has to be applied with extreme care

to avoid reflex activity. Others (including this author) would point out that normalizing these tissues helps to restore regular reflex pathways and therefore improves the function of the related organ. The effect of the gentle massage on these zones is seen as normalizing the visceromotor and somatovisceral reflex pathways between the heart and the somatic tissues. The areas affected include:

1. The left side of the neck and thoracic area of the back, including the dermatomes between C3 and T9. There is also increased tension at the levels of T2 to T4, extending laterally on the back. The tissues along the lower rib cage are similarly affected, including the lateral fibres of latissimus dorsi.

2. The cervical–thoracic junction at C7 and T1, where there may be congestion and tenderness.

3. The upper fibres of the trapezius, in the neck and upper shoulder area.

4. The posterior fibres of the deltoid.

5. The left intercostal spaces of T2 on the front as well as T6 and T7 may be tender to palpation.

6. Tightness in the tissues along the inferior border of the clavicle on the left, also the insertion of the sternomastoid muscle and the lateral fibres of the pectoralis muscle.

Angina pectoris

Angina is caused by ischaemia of the heart muscles, mostly of short duration. It is generally associated with arteriosclerosis and can be stable (on exertion only) or unstable (happens at rest). Pain is experienced primarily in the chest, but often radiates to the axilla and medial aspect of the arm, left or right. It can also occur in the epigastrium (upper abdomen), the side of the neck and the jaw.

Massage application

- Stress is one of the predisposing factors to an angina attack, therefore massage for relaxation is a good preventative measure.
- As the sufferer is not able to do much exercise, gentle massage can be applied for the general circulation and to eliminate toxins.

- The heart area of the chest is omitted at all times.
- It is usually assumed that no treatment is applied during an attack. Some researchers have reported, however, a reduction of angina symptoms following massage to the upper back, the neck, shoulders and arms. Although this positive effect is limited to certain patients it does appear that massage can help relieve the symptoms of angina and improve left ventricular function.
- On most occasions massage to the reflex zones of the heart can be a very effective treatment approach.
- Extreme weather conditions, or sudden changes in temperatures, can exacerbate the condition or render massage unsuitable. A warm environment is therefore essential if massage is to be carried out.

Cautionary note

- Should the patient show any symptoms of an angina attack during treatment it is vital that he/she is moved to a sitting or standing position. Medical attention may be needed in an acute attack and therefore called for without hesitation.
- Any medication which the patient is taking for the condition should always be kept at hand, in case of emergencies.

Heart failure

Malfunction of the left or right ventricle, or of both, causes the heart to weaken. The deficient pumping action is unable to maintain adequate circulation of the blood, and this leads to insufficient oxygen being delivered to the tissues. Ischaemic heart disease is the most common and most serious cause of heart failure. The myocardium becomes ischaemic owing to an atheroma or thrombosis in the coronary arteries. This is followed by the formation of fibrosis in some segments of the muscle tissue; consequently full contractions become ineffective. A worse outcome is a sudden infarct (tissue death) of the myocardium; if the necrosis is extensive it can bring about a heart attack. Other factors contributing to heart failure include conditions affecting the myocardium, such as myocarditis, inefficient nerve supply (which causes a weak pumping action and therefore cardiac arrhythmia), diseases of the valves and inefficient distribution of the blood caused by systemic or pulmonary hypertension, mostly caused by chronic lung disease.

It is not easy to treat acute heart failure, as this is instantaneous and there is no time for compensatory mechanisms to develop. Common effects of acute heart failure are rapid pulmonary oedema and ischaemic effects on the brain and kidneys. Massage is therefore contraindicated in this situation. Severe heart failure, particularly when bed rest is obligatory, can likewise be critical and difficult to treat. Terminal complications are likely to arise in this condition, including hypostatic pneumonia and pulmonary embolism from leg vein thrombosis. Massage is again contraindicated in such circumstances.

In progressive, mild or slow developing heart failure, compensatory mechanisms usually take place. There is an increased rate of pumping, together with dilatation of the ventricles, which causes the heart muscles to contract more forcefully. Another adjustment is hypertrophy of the myocardium, which enables it to contract with a greater force. The extent of the damage to the myocardium dictates the severity of the symptoms relating to the heart failure. Congestion and oedema of the lower limbs and lungs are common features. In addition, there may be fatigue, dyspnoea (breathlessness) and abdominal discomfort; the liver may also enlarge. Left ventricular failure is more common than right, and results in the overfilling of the left atrium. This leads to congestion in the pulmonary veins and in the capillaries. A low blood output ensues, with resultant hypoxia in the organs and tissues.

Right heart failure. Despite the fact that massage can help with the venous return and the lymphatic drainage, increasing the venous and lymphatic return can put an extra workload on the right ventricle. Should the right ventricle be very weak or diseased it may therefore be stressed by any sudden increase in the volume of blood. If there is a diagnosis of a diseased or very weak right ventricle, therefore, massage is contraindicated. The severity of the disease is also taken into consideration. In mild cases of right heart failure massage may be applied, with the approval of the patient's doctor. The treatment, if carried out, should be very light and of short duration. It is also worth noting that right heart failure can lead to portal hypertension, so massage to the abdomen would be contraindicated in this condition.

Left heart failure. Massage may be indicated if there is left heart failure. By assisting the venous blood flow massage helps to decongest the capillaries and the venules. Clearing these vessels creates more space for the arterial blood to flow into the arterioles and capillaries. Resistance to the blood flow is therefore reduced in the arterial system. An easier blood flow through the capillary beds reduces the demands on the left ventricle to generate additional pressure in the arterial circulation.

Cautionary note The application of massage and lymphatic drainage for congestive heart failure requires a cautionary approach. As a general rule, therefore, massage is only applied when there is no danger of putting extra demand on the heart. Right heart failure may present more of a problem when there is an increased volume of blood. In both situations, however, approval of a doctor may be needed prior to massage treatments.

Massage application

- Effleurage, carried out gently and with care, can be applied safely. This is a suitable technique because it encourages the arterial and venous flow and helps to reduce oedema. The massage should not be longer than 15–20 min but needs to be repeated often, even daily.
- The heart muscles contract as a reflex response to surface stroking, the reflex zones being in the upper regions of the trunk and the neck. Both the anterior and posterior sides contain reflex areas to the heart, albeit that the back is more likely to be ethically suitable for massage. Exercising the heart muscles via this reflex pathway maintains and improves their condition and aids the weakened heart. Reflex zone massage in the region of the ribs can also be helpful in reducing tachycardia (rapid heart beat).

- Enhancing the circulation brings about a number of benefits. The supply of blood and, therefore, of oxygen to the tissues and organs is increased. Restoring the oxygen supply lessens the effects of hypoxia (lack of oxygen) such as weakness and fatigue. Elimination of waste products is also improved with the increased circulation. This applies in particular to the kidneys; improving their blood supply increases their cleansing action and the elimination of toxins. If the toxins are allowed to build up they can cause fatigue in the skeletal muscles; fatigue due to toxins can similarly affect the heart muscles and intensify the heart failure.
- The peripheral circulation is improved with the massage movements. At the same time, venous congestion is reduced. These changes have the effect of lowering the peripheral resistance to the arterial blood flow, thereby decreasing the workload on the left ventricle. Assisting the circulation with massage movements therefore lowers the demand on the heart for stronger contractions.
- Massage to the lower limbs is of particular benefit. Light stroking only is applied for the first few sessions of treatment, deeper strokes can be introduced later on. Gentle kneading can also be used; this compresses the skeletal muscles against the veins, thereby pushing the blood forward along the venous return. An alternative or additional technique is the vibration movement, which can be applied on the lower limbs. As stated elsewhere, oedema is a common feature of right heart failure. Lymphatic massage movements can help drain excess fluid, particularly in the lower limbs (the most likely region for oedema in this condition). As noted earlier, however, this is contraindicated in severe cases of right heart failure.
- Massage to the kidney area can also be included. This helps to promote kidney function and, therefore, offers further aid in reducing oedema in the lower limbs as well as systemically.
- Dyspnoea is another symptom, in all likelihood precipitated by venous congestion and

fluid retention in the lungs. A person suffering from heart failure may find it difficult to do any exercise, and this lack of movement can further impair the circulation. Congestion in the lungs is likely to increase, together with an accumulation of toxins. As already discussed, the improvement in the systemic circulation can also help to decongest the lungs. Reflex zones to the lungs are found in the regions of the chest and upper back. Some of these overlap with zones for the heart, therefore massage in these regions (if ethically feasible) can be of benefit. In cases of less severe heart failure an appropriate exercise programme would be a suitable addition to the massage treatment.

- Constipation, especially in the elderly, can be a complication of heart failure. Abdominal massage may be indicated to assist the action of laxatives or as a substitute for them.

Contraindications

- Massage is contraindicated in life-threatening conditions such as fatty degeneration of the heart muscles. This condition affects the right ventricle more than the left. It is likely to render the heart muscles inefficient and weak; they are therefore unable to cope with an increase in blood volume.
- Massage is also contraindicated in endocardiac conditions, particularly endocarditis. This is a complication of rheumatic fever, an inflammatory disease with fever and migratory polyarthritis as the prevailing symptoms.
- Right heart failure may lead to portal circulation and, in this condition, massage to the abdomen is contraindicated.

Thrombosis

Thrombosis is the formation of a fixed mass (aggregation) within a blood vessel, mostly a vein. It is made up from the constituents of the blood, i.e. from platelets, fibrin, red blood cells and granulocytes. One of the factors leading to thrombosis is an alteration in the blood flow.

Slowing down of the blood flow, for example, causes the white cells and platelets to fall out of the main stream and accumulate close to the endothelium of the blood vessels. This can happen in cardiac failure. A similar dysfunction is venous stasis which can occur, for instance, during operations. It can also happen with prolonged bed rest, a case being the immobilization period following surgery or recovery from trauma. Pregnancy is another example of venous stasis, as the uterus can exert pressure on the iliofemoral vein thereby impairing the blood flow.

Interruption of the blood flow can also take place if there is turbulence within the blood vessels. Disturbance of the blood flow can be caused, for instance, when the wall of the blood vessel is distended. This type of expansion is seen in varicose veins, or in a segment of a blood vessel that is affected by an aneurysm. Turbulence can also happen if the blood flow is hindered around valves, particularly those of the veins.

Thrombosis can also be initiated by changes in the composition of the blood. A common occurrence is an increase in the platelets, fibrinogen and prothrombin following operations and childbirth. Furthermore, platelet adhesiveness increases in both these situations on about the tenth day after the event. The outcome is a higher risk of blood clotting and thrombus formation. Trauma will likewise lead to the clotting of blood but the threat of thrombus formation is not always so great.

Lower limb thrombosis is more common than that of the iliofemoral area; it is also less likely to instigate the formation of an embolus, and can heal spontaneously. On the other hand, thrombosis in the iliofemoral vein is more dangerous and tends to be the common factor for pulmonary embolism. The inferior vena cava is likewise susceptible; it has the largest lumen and consequently the potential for a very large thrombus to form. Another vessel that is also predisposed to thrombosis is the brachial vein.

In most cases, thrombosis requires instrumentation to determine its presence (ultrasound or phlebography). There is a high incidence of silent or asymptomatic thrombosis. Consequently the therapist, of whichever discipline, should be aware of the risk factors involved. The signs and symptoms of the condition can be present in isolation and in a mild form. If the symptoms are vague, or give rise to any doubt, the patient should be referred for further investigation before a massage treatment is administered. Massage is contraindicated in a known case of thrombosis.

The most important indicators are local pain, heat and swelling. These may become apparent suddenly or over a few hours, although sometimes the onset extends over a few days or even weeks. Often, the pain in the leg is misinterpreted as cramp by the patient. Pain in the calf, however, is one of the diagnostic signs of deep vein thrombosis. The pain occurs when the foot is dorsiflexed with the knee straight (Homans' sign). Tenderness on palpation can be elicited in the limb involved. There is also heat along the line of a superficial vein; a deep vessel does not necessarily transmit heat to the superficial tissues. The arterial pulse in the leg may be reduced or absent. There may be discoloration (or paleness), particularly in the lower leg or foot, albeit that these blemishes can be transient and would therefore be relieved by elevation. The thrombosis itself is sometimes palpable as a tender cord within the affected vein. Blood in the urine and small haemorrhage spots in the skin indicate an obstruction in the kidneys that may be caused by a thrombus. These signs can be accompanied by unilateral swelling of the calf and ankle. Chest pain is another symptom, caused by obstruction in the lungs or heart.

Massage application

- Any treatment for a patient who has had prolonged bed rest must be carried out with great caution, because of the possibility of a thrombus having already formed. Massage is best started soon after a patient is confined to bed. The treatment helps to maintain good circulation and prevent the formation of a thrombus. At this stage most massage movements are indicated, but particularly effleurage for the venous return.
- Massage can be contraindicated locally on areas of varicosity, where a thrombus may have already formed and could be dislodged. It can, however, be used to maintain good circulation throughout the body, and to prevent the blood flow from slowing down further.

- Massage on a suspected thrombosed vein is also contraindicated. If treatment is to be applied at all, it is to nearby tissues with the aim of increasing the venous return through the collateral vessels and reducing congestion.
- It is worth bearing in mind that treatment of thrombosis includes drugs that are used to inhibit clotting. Consequently, there is susceptibility to spontaneous bleeding, and massage, if administered, has to be light rather than deep to avoid haemorrhaging (even petechiae or ecchymosis under the skin).
- Treatment with massage is certainly contraindicated if the patient has been diagnosed as having an aneurysm. The blood flow can be additionally disrupted if the blood vessels are subject to a swelling or compression; this occurs mostly due to disease, and massage is not applicable in such a case.
- Following an operation or childbirth, massage can be applied to promote the circulation and to prevent the platelet coalition that may lead to a thrombus. Despite its preventative effect, the treatment may be disapproved by the medical team owing to the risk of thrombosis. Consequently, it is best applied with the consent of the patient's doctor.

Varicosities

In the lower limbs, blood flows from the superficial to the deeper veins. The main drainage junction is between the superficial saphenous vein and the deep femoral vein. Blood is prevented from flowing backwards by valves situated in both the superficial and deep veins; if the valves become inefficient they allow the blood to flow back into the superficial veins and cause congestion. Dilatation and varicosity of the veins ensues. Another common cause of varicosity is weakness in the venous walls; these can expand and the ensuing congestion weakens the valves. The aetiology for this situation tends to be idiopathic; in many cases it is familial and therefore difficult to treat. While varicosity mostly occurs in the lower limbs, it can also be seen elsewhere in the body. Varicose veins can also result from hypertension, which may be caused, for exam-

ple, by prolonged standing. The venous congestion associated with varicosity stresses the heart,
as it has to work harder to pump the blood
around the body. This in itself can lead to high
blood pressure and to heart problems.

Varicosity also occurs because of occlusion of
the vessels; compression may be exerted by the
fetus in pregnancy, by fibroids, an ovarian
tumour or a previous deep vein thrombosis.
Once the condition has been diagnosed, massage
on the varicosed vein itself is contraindicated; a
thrombus could be dislodged by the massage
and become an embolus. Another determining
factor for the cautious approach is the possibility
of spontaneous rupture of the venules. Furthermore, as the muscle walls of the veins are
stretched they do not respond easily to the reflex
stimulation of massage.

Massage application

- Massage is indicated as a preventative treatment, especially for those who are susceptible
to these conditions. When the treatment is preventative, techniques such as petrissage and
effleurage are used to compress the skeletal
muscles against the veins; this has the effect of
milking the blood forwards along the venous
return.

- Where varicosity is already present, massage
can only be applied in between the veins and,
therefore, without touching any of the vessels.
If the vessels are hard and tortuous, then the
primary aim of the treatment is to encourage
circulation of the collateral vessels. One or
more fingers can be used, placed on either side
of the vein. The easiest method is spreading
the fingers apart and massaging with the fingertips, applying light effleurage strokes in the
direction of the venous return. This technique
is also useful for reducing oedema. Vibration is
a similar technique, and is also carried out
between the veins with the fingers spread and
fixed in one position. If the veins are prominent without being deformed or painful, then
effleurage stroking can be applied over them;
in this case the aim is to empty the vessels and
de-stretch them, albeit only temporary. As the
patient is likely to suffer from impaired circulation, massage of the legs, proximal to the

varicosity, is indicated. In this instance the
massage movements are very light, and are
applied to the superficial tissues only.

Heart bypass operations

Massage application

- Certain massage movements can be applied
following open heart surgery, provided this is
done with the approval of the medical consultant. The massage helps to improve capillary
circulation and, in so doing, prevent any
peripheral resistance to the general circulation.
It also speeds up the healing of the wounds
and scar tissue.

- Oedema and general toxicity are common
symptoms after surgery, and massage is used
to drain the oedema and assist with the elimination of toxins. Light lymphatic drainage
techniques are applied to all regions, including
the chest area, as long as this is tolerated by the
patient.

- Gentle compression movements such as
kneading can be included to help relax the
muscles. The superficial fascia and muscles can
be gently lifted off the underlying structures to
break up adhesions and to improve the local
circulation.

- For the first 3 weeks after operation, no treatment is applied around the scar tissue areas
because of the fragility of the fibres. Light
effleurage strokes are the only strokes to be
carried out initially. These are gradually inter-
spersed with gentle kneading movements.
Thickening of the tissues is addressed with
friction techniques, and vibration movements
are subsequently performed close to the scar
tissue. The areas to be treated are found on the
lower limb, where the blood vessel (the great
saphenous vein) may have been removed for a
coronary artery bypass graft. Another common
blood vessel used for this operation is the
mammary artery from the left side of the chest.

- Relaxation is vital for the patient after the operation. To this end, relaxing massage may be
applied daily. Regions such as the hands and
the face are very practical to massage, even
while the patient is lying in bed or in a sitting

position. The treatment can extend to other areas in subsequent sessions. Foot massage is sometimes the only treatment the patient wants or can receive. It is none the less extremely beneficial in reducing anxiety and inducing relaxation in the patient.

LYMPHATIC SYSTEM

Oedema

Oedema is an excess of fluid in the extravascular tissues and, therefore, outside the blood and lymph vessels. The build-up can be intracellular (inside the cells) or in the interstitial tissue (between the cells). It can also be localized to one region, or spread systemically throughout the body (Table 4.1). Oedema is associated with tissue damage and organ malfunction, and its causes range from heart or kidney failure to lymphomas, infections and hypoproteinaemia (lack of proteins). While massage is indicated to remove any build-up of fluid, its application can be limited by the complexity of the oedema formation. The aetiology of the disorder needs to be established in all cases, and the doctor's approval sought if there is any apprehension about the treatment.

Massage application

- Some massage techniques, light effleurage in particular, help to drain the lymph by mechanically pushing the fluid from the superficial to the deep vessels. In addition, the lymph fluid is pumped forward by the contractions of the lymph vessels; the contractions occur as a reflex action to the massage stroke.
- Lymph massage movements have a more specific effect. One direct application of lymph massage is to reduce oedema around the ankle that broadly results from long periods of standing; a further case in point is oedema of the knee from overuse. Chronic oedema may require several treatments and additional movements such as vibration techniques.

Oedema and kidney failure

Oedema can be precipitated by kidney diseases such as glomerulonephritis and the closely

Table 4.1 Examples of oedema

Systemic and bilateral oedema

Primary sites:
● The legs	when standing or moving
● The lumbar region	when lying down
● The penis and scrotum	when lying down
● The labia	when lying down
● The eyelids and face	following sleep and lying down

Causes

- Kidney problems
- Renal vein thrombosis
- Diabetes
- Systemic lupus erythematosus
- Amyloid disease
- Sodium retention
- Action of antidiuretic hormone

Bilateral oedema of the legs
Causes

● Kidney failure	
● Cardiac failure	
● Cirrhosis of the liver	
● Anaemia	
● Venous stagnation	
● Faulty muscular tone	
● Premenstrual oedema	
● Prolonged standing or sitting	
● Hot climate	
● Carcinoma	
● Prolonged bed rest	
● Lack of movement	e.g. in the rheumatoid arthritic patient
● Obstruction of lymph flow	e.g. in cancer of the lymph nodes in lymphoedema
● Hereditary	e.g. in Milroy's disease
● Fatty deposits	e.g. in lipoedema
● Retention of sodium and water	due to: action of antidiuretic hormone from posterior pituitary
● Obstruction of the inferior vena cava	due to: tumour, ovarian cyst, enlarged uterus in pregnancy

Unilateral oedema of the leg
Causes

- Thrombosis
- Embolism
- Thrombophlebitis

Oedema of the upper half of the body
Causes

● Obstruction of the superior vena cava or its main branches	due to: tumour, chronic mediastinal fibrosis, thoracic aneurysm, thrombosis

related nephrotic syndrome. Such disorders lead to an excessive loss of proteins from the plasma, to be excreted in the urine. The decreased number of plasma proteins creates a low plasma osmotic pressure, and this fails to exert a pull on the fluid from the interstitial tissue into the venules. In this case, oedema is formed by the accumulation of fluid in the interstitial tissues.

- Fluid retention is reduced with the massage movement, although the treatment is palliative until the kidney infection is cured.
- Systemic massage is applied to assist the kidneys in eliminating toxins. More specific massage techniques to improve kidney function can be applied on reflex zones. Movements on the kidney area are contraindicated if there is inflammation and severe tenderness.

Oedema and heart failure

Systemic oedema that resolves when the subject is lying down is often a sign of cardiac failure. While cardiac failure can affect the right or the left side of the heart, oedema is often due to right heart failure. This condition is invariably accompanied by obstruction of the veins. Both malfunctions cause the blood pressure to rise in the capillaries, and a high capillary pressure leads to a greater filtration rate of plasma proteins from the capillaries into the interstitial spaces. As the proteins cause the fluid to move into the interstitial spaces, oedema is formed. Congestion in the veins is a further complication and occurs because of the weakened heart, which is unable to receive and process the venous blood. As a result, the hydrostatic pressure in the veins is elevated and this prevents the fluid in the interstitial tissues from re-entering at the venous end.

Massage application

- The application of lymphatic massage for this condition is slightly controversial. Although massage can be applied to assist with the drainage of the fluid into the lymph vessels and also to boost the venous return, in particular in the lower limbs, it can cause an increase in venous volume. This in turn can exert an additional stress on the right side of the heart.

If the condition is severe the treatment is best omitted. If it is not severe, massage is carried out for short periods only, but can, however, be repeated frequently.

Lymphoedema

A disturbance in the flow of lymph occurs in lymphoedema. The precipitating factor is a blockage in the lymph vessels or a mechanical insufficiency of the lymph system. Primary lymphoedema is either congenital or develops during puberty or adulthood; its causes are not known. A second and more common type is chronic lymphoedema, which frequently occurs after radiation treatment for cancer, especially breast cancer. It is also observed after the removal of lymph nodes, for example those of the groin, axilla or pelvis. Malfunction of the lymphatic system and the ensuing lymphoedema also arises from blockages in the lymph vessels caused by infections, injury to the lymph vessels, cancer and spasms of the lymphatics.

Massage application Lymphatic massage movements can be applied to assist with the drainage of the lymph fluid. The treatment is particularly useful as an adjunct to other procedures such as bandaging, support garments and exercise. Its beneficial effect can, however, be limited by the severity and duration of the condition. Furthermore, it is contraindicated if the patient is suffering from skin infections or any other type of bacterial or fungal disease. It is advisable that the treatment is carried out with the agreement of the patient's doctor.

DIGESTIVE SYSTEM

Dyspepsia

Although not a disease in itself, dyspepsia (indigestion) can be symptomatic of other conditions. These include excessive acid or intake of alcohol, insufficient bile production, heart or liver disease, faulty function of the stomach and the intestines, or malignancy. As a precautionary measure, underlying pathological causes must therefore be ruled out for the massage to be applied.

Massage application

- Abdominal massage movements may be carried out to promote the production of digestive juices and to assist the function of the organs.
- Stress increases the symptoms of dyspepsia; the relaxing effects of massage can therefore be of great benefit.
- Dyspepsia can also be caused by, or lead to, weakened contractions of the involuntary stomach muscles. These can be stretched from overeating, or do not fully contract owing to other disorders. Reflex contractions are encouraged by the massage on the abdomen and stomach region. Reflex zone areas (see Chapter 7) are included in the treatment for the same effect. Mechanical drainage of the stomach is also achieved with the massage strokes.

Obesity

Obesity requires little clarification, other than to mention its causes. There may be an hereditary factor; however, the obesity from such a cause does not necessarily have a detrimental effect on the health of the individual. The condition of obesity can be endogenous, and therefore brought about by some abnormality within the body; for example, endocrine or hormonal disturbances. Amongst these disorders, adrenal hyperfunction, testicular hypofunction and ovarian hypofunction are the most significant endocrine factors. Fat also accumulates when the metabolic rate is slowed down, e.g. in hypothyroidism, another endocrine imbalance. Obesity from overeating is sometimes described as a toxic and 'gouty' type. In this condition, excess fatty deposits accumulate in the subcutaneous tissues and around organs, including the heart and lungs. Other causative factors include emotional problems and some lifestyle routines, which are of great relevance and frequently give rise to the most common forms of obesity. These are caused by simple overeating, or an imbalance between the intake of food and the energy expended. Being overweight can have an effect on the overall body structure and may even cause back pain. Naturally, the best cure for obesity is a check on the diet, the lifestyle and exercise regimes.

Massage application

- Petrissage movements and other massage techniques can provide, to a very small degree, a mechanical aid to help break down the fat globules and encourage their passage into the lymphatic system. Of more importance, perhaps, is the psychological boost and encouragement that massage offers to the subject. Such support must not, however, obliterate the fact that the obesity problem needs addressing in other ways.
- Adipose tissue is highly vascular and requires a great supply of blood. An overabundance of fat therefore exerts great demands on the heart. Massage is applied to lessen the workload of the heart by improving the systemic circulation; however, it is contraindicated when the strength and function of the heart have deteriorated as a complication of the obesity. One such manifestation is fatty degeneration, in which the heart muscles are replaced by fat and are unable to function. In such a situation, massage treatment, along with exercise, is not advisable.
- It is often the case that an overweight person has a reduced lung capacity owing to the compression of the thorax by the abdominal structures. Techniques to improve rib excursion and breathing are included alongside the weight reduction programme.

Malabsorption syndrome

This is a general term pertaining to a series of symptoms that are a consequence of malabsorption. They include anorexia, abdominal cramps, abdominal bloating, anaemia and fatigue. Malabsorption has a number of causative factors, including the destruction of the villi and the intestinal mucosa. Sensitivity to foods is another cause; for example, coeliac disease. Other causes are diseases of organs such as the pancreas and liver, obstructions in the intestines, and disease of the mesenteric blood supply.

Massage application
- While massage is used to address the prevailing symptom, it may not be effective in treating the underlying condition. The aetiology of the disorder must therefore be established, and massage applied accordingly and in agreement with the patient's doctor. Massage to the peripheral tissues stimulates the digestive glands, and therefore massage to the abdomen and other reflex zones is indicated.

Hiatus hernia

In this condition, the cardia of the stomach protrudes upward into the mediastinal (thoracic) cavity through the oesophageal hiatus (or opening) in the diaphragm. The oesophageal mucosa is subjected to the acid secretions of the stomach, and irritation of the lining of the oesophagus produces inflammation and ulcerations.

Massage application
- Massage to the upper abdominal region is contraindicated, and even more so if ulcerations have developed in the oesophagus. However, this can only be established with endoscopy. As the massage is not indicated for healing the hernia, it is best omitted on the abdomen.

Gastritis

Acute gastritis involves inflammation in the superficial layers of the stomach lining, or mucosa. A more acute type can also develop, with tiny ulcers and small haemorrhages forming in the apex of the mucosal rugae (folds). In most cases these changes are superficial, and the tissues return to normal very quickly. Gastritis is activated by a multitude of causes, including alcohol and aspirin, which act as irritants, infections such as childhood fevers, viral infections and bacterial food poisoning. Chronic gastritis can also be a form of autoimmune disease, with a strong genetic component; more commonly, it results from a continuing irritation. In either case, there is damage and possible atrophy of the specialized secreting cells. Severe cases are often associated with an absence of hydrochloric acid, which is secreted by the parietal cells. There is also deficient secretion of pepsinogen and intrinsic factor by the chief cells; a lack of intrinsic factor can cause pernicious anaemia. Gastritis is accompanied by epigastric (upper central abdomen) pain or tenderness, nausea, vomiting, and systemic electrolyte changes (acids, bases and salts) if vomiting persists.

Massage application
- Abdominal massage to the epigastric area is generally contraindicated because of local inflammation. Systemic massage is, however, indicated. In addition, massage can be applied to the following related (reflex) areas:

   a. Latissimus dorsi muscle and the thoracic back on the left side.
   b. Infraspinatus muscle, on the lateral part of the infraspinous fossa.
   c. The tissues situated inferiorly and lateral to the sternum at the costal margins.

Peptic ulcers

Peptic ulcers occur most commonly in the first part of the duodenum, the distal lesser curve of the stomach, the cardiac end of the stomach or the lower oesophagus. All these structures are sites of acid-containing juices. The ulceration is marked by a small damaged area, less than 1 cm in diameter, which affects the mucosa and submucosa. In severe and chronic peptic ulcers the damage is more extensive, and is seen as a perforation of the muscle layer. Although ulcers generally heal, they do so by the formation of scar tissue; in some cases this can cause strictures (narrowing) as in pyloric stenosis. Acute gastritis can be related to severe shock, the condition being referred to as 'stress ulcers'. Chronic gastritis, on the other hand, is more akin to acute peptic ulceration of the stomach, the causative factor being an invasion of the microbe *Helicobacter pylori*. The pain of peptic ulcers occurs about 1 h after a meal, and radiates to the back; that of duodenal ulcers occurs mostly in between meals.

Massage application Taking into account the pathological features of the condition it would follow that massage is generally contraindicated in all types of ulcers because of the possibility of escalating the haemorrhaging. This possibility is increased if the base of the ulcer has reached the peritoneum, which separates the stomach from the peritoneal cavity. While this precautionary attitude is likely to be the safest approach to the treatment of ulcers, it is worth noting that one or two studies have claimed massage to be safe and indeed of benefit. In one study, for example, abdominal massage and liver pump techniques were found to be of benefit in the treatment of gastroduodenal ulcers. Other reports have also indicated the normalization of peristalsis and gastric secretions associated with gastric ulcers. Massage to the reflex zones rather than on the abdomen, however, remains the safest and perhaps the most effective method. A decrease in the symptoms of this condition were reported to have occurred following a programme of connective tissue massage by Maria Ebner (Ebner, 1978). The same reflex areas as for gastritis can be massaged to bring about healing and to reduce the pain. If stress is part of the underlying cause, then relaxation massage can also be of great benefit.

Constipation

This disorder of the digestive system is predominantly an acquired condition that is associated with common influences such as stress and dietary imbalances. Pathological causes are also determining factors, and these must be ruled out before any massage to the colon is performed. The sudden onset of constipation in an elderly person, for instance, is a cause for concern, and renders massage inappropriate until the doctor has made a diagnosis. Some of the possible malfunctions associated with constipation are considered in this section. In those conditions which are of a less serious nature, massage is applicable and indeed of great benefit. One experiment on the effects of massage was carried out on 10 patients who had chronic constipation associated with other conditions such as cerebral palsy, multiple sclerosis and irritable bowel syndrome. Daily massage treatments showed improvement in the bowel movements and in the regularity of the stools (Richards, 1998).

Sphincter contraction

Constipation is incomplete or irregular defaecation, and can be accompanied by other symptoms such as abdominal pain, headaches and flatulence. Anxiety is a prominent characteristic amongst sufferers of this condition. Stress, and the body's reaction to it, involves the sympathetic branch of the autonomic nervous system. Overstimulation of these fibres causes the intestinal sphincters to contract and, in so doing, block the movement of the intestinal contents.

Massage application

- The general relaxation induced by massage has an influence on the parasympathetic fibres. Increasing the parasympathetic predominance reduces the tension in the sphincters.
- The contents of the colon are pushed forward directly by the colon massage movements, which are carried out in a clockwise direction. Deep stroking of the ascending and descending colon, together with vibration movements (particularly on the iliac colon), is used. Techniques for the stomach and the intestines are also included. In addition to their mechanical effect, these movements create a reflex response that stimulates the involuntary muscles of the intestinal wall.
- Massage is indicated on the following reflex zone: an area of tissue which is about 7.5 cm wide, and runs from the upper third of the sacrum downward and laterally to the greater trochanter.

Atonic muscular wall

A major cause of constipation is a loss of tone in the muscles of the intestines. The caecum is particularly susceptible, as the muscles in this region need to contract almost against the force of gravity. Dilatation of the digestive tract is another causative factor, and often affects the wall of the stomach or the caecum.

Massage application

- Massage is indicated to improve the tone of the muscular layers reflexively; this helps to counteract any stretching of the intestinal wall and of the stomach. Reflex contractions of the involuntary muscles occur when the sensory nerve endings in the peripheral superficial tissues are stimulated. Most of the abdominal massage movements, including small circular frictions, will provide this stimulus.

- Additionally, deep massage work and percussive (tapotement) strokes are carried out on the gluteal/sacral region to strengthen the action of peristalsis reflexively.
- Effleurage and friction techniques can be used on other reflex zones, such as the iliotibial band and the lumbar muscles.

Dietary factors

Repetitive and excessive stretching of the stomach wall or of the caecum often occurs in obesity. Lifestyle can have a significant effect on the digestive system. A sedentary lifestyle weakens the strength of the diaphragm and, in turn, reduces its beneficial massaging action on the visceral organs. Irregular bowel movements will also contribute to an impaired function. Another factor is an imbalance in the diet, usually when there is an insufficient intake of fluids or fibre. A cautious approach is needed if sufferers of constipation are taking laxatives; these can irritate the lining of the intestines and massage can exacerbate the discomfort.

Massage application
- In this situation, the general massage techniques described for the other causes of constipation and for the digestive system, in particular those for obesity, are indicated.
- Percussive techniques can be applied almost systemically, especially pounding movements to the sacral area. They are likely to have a reflex and stimulating effect on the digestive system, and counteract the overeating and lack of exercise.

Muscular spasm

In some cases constipation is associated with a temporary muscular spasm of the intestines, synonymous with intestinal colic. Massage on the abdomen itself may be too uncomfortable to administer. The application of hot packs may alleviate some of the pain, perhaps sufficiently for massage to be comfortable.

Twisting of the intestines

Blockage and constipation can also be caused by kinking of the intestines. This disorder can only be established by investigative procedures such as a barium meal examination; massage is contraindicated owing to the physiological impairment.

Carcinoma

Obstruction of the colon by carcinoma is a further contraindication to massage. The constipation that is a feature of the disease is irregular at first, and may alternate with diarrhoea. In addition, blood and pus may be observed in the faeces. Laxatives do not have much of an effect in these circumstances. Progressive weight loss, anorexia and anaemia are further symptoms of the condition. Diverticular disease of the sigmoid colon can present with a similar picture, and a thorough examination is required to distinguish it from carcinoma. In both situations, massage is contraindicated.

Toxins

Reduced efficiency of the visceral organs may lead to decreased elimination of toxins, not only by the intestines but by other tissues and organs in the rest of the body. The build-up of toxins is systemic, and extends to muscles and other soft tissues; as a result they become weaker and susceptible to injury (Stone, 1992). Slow intestinal transit times and impaired bowel function have also been attributed to cancer of the colon.

Massage application
- Systemic massage and lymphatic drainage techniques are carried out to promote the elimination of toxins.
- Massage movements on the colon, the liver area and to the kidney are included, as is massage for the portal circulation.

Irritable bowel syndrome

This is a general term used to describe a disordered action of the bowels. The typical characteristics are diarrhoea or constipation, abdominal pain, flatulence and distension. Investigation generally fails to reveal any organic disease, although this may be different in those over 50 years of age. However, underlying emotional situations may be very relevant to the condition.

Massage application
- Systemic massage is indicated to induce relaxation and to promote a parasympathetic response; this helps to reduce spasms of the involuntary muscles. In cases where there is diarrhoea, massage on the abdomen is naturally contraindicated. The abdominal pain associated with irritable bowel syndrome (IBS) can be very severe, and massage to this region is very likely to exacerbate the discomfort. Massage can, however, be of benefit when it is applied to reflex areas such as the anterior and lateral thigh, the glutei muscles, the area around the navel and along the left iliac crest. The region of the middle thoracic spine, around the 5th to 9th vertebrae, is also related to the stomach and intestines and may therefore be subject to tissue dysfunctions and hypersensitivity. These areas are therefore assessed and treated with NMT.

Colitis

Colitis pertains to inflammation and irritation of the colon. Ulcerative colitis, on the other hand, refers to inflammation of the mucosa and to ulcerations, primarily of the sigmoid colon and the rectum. Its causes are unknown, but it may be chronic with periods of remission. The disorder starts with abscesses at the base of the mucosal folds, which progress to ulceration and destruction of the secreting glands. Symptoms include mild diarrhoea, blood and mucus in the stools, anorexia, weight loss, anaemia and back pain.

Massage application
- Local massage is contraindicated in active ulcerative colitis. This is because of the presence of lesions and haemorrhaging in the intestinal wall

and the risk of perforation. During periods of remission, some massage can be administered to the abdomen to improve the local circulation and relax the abdominal muscles.
- Massage to the back is indicated, and can be very beneficial for the back pain.

Enteritis

Non-specific enteritis is inflammation, mainly of the small intestine, but it may also extend to the duodenum, stomach, jejunum and ileum. The condition subsides quickly in adults, but may prove fatal in infants.

Massage application
- Massage to the abdomen is contraindicated.

Regional enteritis (Crohn's disease)

This condition is also referred to as inflammatory bowel disease or granulomatous colitis. It is a condition seen mostly in young adults. Causative factors include immunological abnormalities, allergies, viruses and chemicals in food. There is chronic inflammation, primarily of the terminal ileum. It may also extend to any part of the intestinal tract, including the colon, mouth, oesophagus and anus. Ulceration of the mucosa is always present. Further complications include adhesions to adjoining structures, ulceration into the bowel wall, infection and abscess formation. The outcome of the condition is a thickening of the submucosa, which leads to a narrowing of the lumen and to subacute or chronic obstructions.

Lymph congestion and therefore oedema is also likely owing to the blockage of lymph flow in the gut. In the early stages there is mild diarrhoea and abdominal pain. Other symptoms associated with this condition can vary from a fever and nausea to flatulence and blood in the stools. As the condition progresses there may be signs of malabsorption such as loss of weight, fatty and foul smelling stools. Pain in the lower right abdomen and the diarrhoea persist, with periods of remission and exacerbation.

Massage application Abdominal massage is generally ruled out for this condition. However, a light soothing effleurage may be tolerated and safe, provided the condition is not severe. Systemic massage may otherwise be used to assist the circulation, lymph drainage and the elimination of toxins. Relaxation is also important as stress can exacerbate the disease. It is also worth bearing in mind that patients with this condition are likely to be taking corticosteroids. In addition to reducing inflammation these drugs can also impair the immune system and the patient is therefore susceptible to infection.

Diverticulosis

About 10% of the adult population are thought to have this condition, in which diverticula (pockets) form in the wall of the colon (mostly in the sigmoid segment). These pouch-like cavities push into the muscle fibres of the intestinal wall and invariably trap faeces inside them. Inflammation of the diverticula (diverticulitis) ensues, more commonly in older people. In diverticulosis, when there is no inflammation the pain is mild and located in the left lower quadrant. There may also be alternating constipation and diarrhoea. In diverticulitis, there are acute attacks of inflammation. In addition to the pain, which is colicky and located on the left side of the abdomen, there may also be excess gas formation, nausea, low grade fever and irregular bowel habits. Chronic diverticulitis can heal by the process of fibrosis, but this can cause the lumen of the bowel to narrow, leading to obstruction.

Massage application

- Massage to the sigmoid colon is contraindicated in the presence of inflammation. During non-inflammatory and colic-free periods, a gentle abdominal massage is carried out to encourage the peristaltic action. In so doing, it prevents congestion in the colon and may also remove trapped masses within the diverticula. Abdominal massage on an elderly person, particularly if there is constipation, has to be carried out with little pressure as diverticula can rupture.
- When the condition is accompanied by irregular and severe constipation, investigations are needed to differentiate it from carcinoma. In such a situation, and if the diverticulosis is chronic, massage may be contraindicated. Massage can also be applied to prevent the onset of diverticulosis.

Diabetes mellitus

Diabetes mellitus is a disorder associated with insulin, which is produced in the pancreas by the beta cells of the islets of Langerhans. Insulin controls the passage of sugar from the blood stream and through the membranes of most cells. The disorder is also related to insufficient use or uptake of glucose by the target cells. Two distinct clinical varieties of diabetes mellitus have been identified, types I and II.

Type I—Insulin-dependent diabetes. This disorder is also referred to as early-onset or juvenile diabetes and usually develops in the first two or three decades of life. The disease is believed to be an autoimmune condition in which the body develops antibodies to the beta cells in the pancreas; the antibodies destroy the tissue. It is marked by a dramatic decrease in the number of beta cells (sometimes to less than 10% of the normal number) in the pancreas and a complete absence or reduction of insulin production. This leads to a marked fluctuation in blood glucose, which is particularly difficult to control. Insulin injections are needed to relieve the carbohydrate imbalance.

Type II—Non-insulin-dependent diabetes. This disorder is also known as late-onset or mature diabetes. It is a mild form of the condition and makes up more than 90% of all cases of diabetes mellitus. It has a gradual onset and occurs mostly in obese people over the age of 40 years.

In this case, the beta cells are normal but the production of insulin varies; it is frequently reduced but is sometimes very high.

In obese individuals, the food intake is substantially increased and, as a result, there is an excessive secretion of insulin. One likely mechanism is that, as a result of the insulation overload and through a negative feedback mechanism, the number of insulin receptors on the target cells is decreased. Consequently, the cells are not effective in taking up the insulin from the blood and using it.

One of the metabolic effects of diabetes mellitus is decreased utilization of glucose. As the cells that are dependent upon insulin can take in only about 25% of the glucose they require for fuel, the glucose remains in the blood. An increase in the blood glucose is referred to as hyperglycaemia.

An absence of insulin prevents sugar from being stored as glycogen (by the process of glycogenesis) in the liver. This leads to a further increase of blood glucose. Equally affected is the breakdown of sugar into simpler compounds (by the process of glycolysis). Carbohydrate metabolism is generally reduced, while that of fat and protein is increased. As the cells cannot utilize glucose they must turn to other sources (fat and protein) for fuel. Increased fat metabolism by the cells increases the formation of ketone bodies; these are acetone and other breakdown products of fat metabolism. Ketosis is a condition that occurs when the levels of ketone bodies rises. Acidosis can follow because of the imbalance in pH levels and this can lead to coma or death. The increased protein utilization leads to a loss of weight despite a good appetite. Amino acids are converted into glucose by the liver, increasing further the excess blood sugar levels.

The insulin:glucose balance is very delicate in diabetes, and increasing the circulation may cause the blood sugar levels to fluctuate.

There is therefore a need for these levels to be monitored closely before and after a massage treatment. Hypoglycaemia (low blood sugar) can occur in the diabetic patient, and the massage therapist must therefore watch for warning signs, such as rapid pulse, sweating and disorientation. Diabetic patients are usually well aware of these signs, and invariably carry a sugary snack with them; however, it may be useful for the massage therapist to keep something similar in the treatment room.

Long-term complications of diabetes include the development of neuropathy (nerve disorders), damage to the retina of the eye, degenerative changes in the blood vessels and increased susceptibility to infection. Impaired circulation is another symptom, and this is associated with the development of cardiovascular disorders and atherosclerosis.

The neuropathy of diabetes is a disorder of the peripheral nervous system that leads to reduced sensations of pain, temperature and pressure, especially in the lower legs and feet. A disorder may also occur in the autonomic nervous system, leading to alternating bouts of diarrhoea and constipation, to impotence and impaired heart function. Applications such as hot water bottles or infrared lamps should not be used because of reduced sensitivity and, for the same reason, heavy massage techniques are not appropriate.

Massage application

- Stress can be associated with diabetes because it causes the adrenal gland to release epinephrine. This hormone has the effect of increasing blood sugar levels, which can upset the delicate balance of plasma insulin and glucose. Slow and rhythmical massage movements are used to reduce stress levels. Using massage as part of a stress management regime can also prevent the onset of diabetes.
- Gentle effleurage massage movements are applied to improve the circulation, particularly in the lower limbs. Maintaining a good blood flow in this region helps to prevent the formation of ulcers, which can result from impaired circulation; worse still would be the onset of gangrene. Systemic massage is indicated to eliminate toxins and prevent degeneration of the blood vessels by atheroma. Lymph massage and abdominal strokes for the portal circulation are used to assist with the elimination of toxins.
- With the impaired circulation there can also be oedema, and massage is used to encourage lymphatic drainage.
- In non-insulin-dependent diabetes the diet is significant in the treatment regime, and obesity makes the condition harder to control. Massage does not reduce obesity, but can help to increase tonicity of the tissues.
- The muscles of the lower leg, and in particular the foot, may become atrophied, and would therefore benefit from the exercise of massage.
- Diabetic neuritis necessitates that the massage strokes on the limbs (especially the feet and

hands) are carried out with a gentle approach. Besides the obvious reason of consideration for the patient, gentle stroking is necessary to help alleviate the numbness, irritation or tingling which are symptoms of this condition.

Cirrhosis

Cirrhosis is a chronic disease of the liver that is characterized by the formation of dense connective tissue in and around the lobules. There are also degenerative changes in parenchymal cells, alteration in the structure of the cords of liver lobules, as well as fatty and cellular infiltration. The dysfunction of the liver cells leads to increased resistance to the flow of blood through the liver (portal hypertension). The aetiology of cirrhosis varies from alcoholism, nutritional deficiencies, poisons or drugs, and previous inflammation caused by a virus or bacteria, such as viral hepatitis. Heart failure can also lead to congestion of blood in the liver and eventual cirrhosis. The signs and symptoms include loss of weight, fatigue, jaundice, enlargement of the liver and spleen, and ascites (fluid in the peritoneal cavity). There are a number of serious complications of liver cirrhosis, including hormone imbalances, jaundice, portal hypertension, susceptibility to infection, digestive problems and bleeding tendencies. For instance, liver damage such as cirrhosis leads to obstruction and increased pressure in the veins of the abdomen. The pressure build-up causes fluid to seep out of the capillaries into the peritoneal cavity (ascites). In addition, the obstruction forces the blood to flow through the veins in other structures, such as the oesophagus, on its journey back to the heart. In certain cases, such as liver cirrhosis that is accompanied by portal hypertension, the oesophageal veins making up the substituted pathways are very dilated and susceptible to rupture.

Cautionary note The patient suffering from viral hepatitis can be a carrier and therefore massage may be contraindicated.

Massage application

- Massage to the abdomen is certainly contraindicated in this condition.

- Owing to the complications affecting the lymphatic and venous circulation in the abdomen, massage to reduce the oedema of the legs or the abdomen is also contraindicated.
- Increasing the venous return can also exert excessive pressure in the dilated blood vessels around the oesophagus, umbilicus and anus. Massage is therefore contraindicated in any of these areas. Effleurage stroking of the lower limbs will also increase venous pressure in the abdominal area and should be avoided.
- Any massage movements carried out on other regions need to be very light as the patient is susceptible to easy bruising. The sensory receptors are likely to be affected by the condition so that sensations of pressure, especially in the lower limbs, may be impaired.

Portal hypertension

In this condition there is an elevated blood pressure within the portal circulation which is responsible for delivering blood from the digestive organs to the liver. Having been treated by the liver the blood then flows to the inferior vena cava which empties into the right side of the heart. Blockage to the flow of blood in the hepatic or portal veins is the main cause of portal hypertension. The obstruction is due to thrombosis within the veins or to pressure from outside the vessel, e.g. by a lymph node or tumour. A history of thrombosis, alcohol intake and cirrhosis can be predisposing factors. The hepatic veins are the most commonly affected, the obstruction being due to the pressure exerted by the fibrous tissues of the cirrhosis. Another common cause of portal hypertension is right heart failure. Owing to the weakened heart muscles the venous blood flow through the heart is impaired and the subsequent back pressure affects the veins in the abdomen. The venous congestion creates ascites (fluid in the peritoneal cavity) as well as increased pressure in the vessels around the umbilicus, oesophagus and rectum. Oedema in the legs can also develop because of the right heart failure. In addition to liver failure and cirrhosis, portal hypertension is associated with jaundice and anaemia.

Massage application Massage can be carried out to most regions of the body except for the abdominal area. If right heart failure is present the patient is also likely to be suffering from oedema in the extremities or systemically. As the function of the right side of the heart is weak, it is unable to process the increased fluid return created by lymphatic massage techniques, which may therefore be contraindicated. As discussed elsewhere, the application of massage for right heart failure depends on the severity of the disease and, in severe cases, it is in fact contraindicated. Caution is also required as the patient may be prone to easy bruising or infection.

SKELETAL SYSTEM

Osteoarthritis

Although classified as arthritis (joint inflammation), this condition relates to the degeneration of the hyaline cartilage in synovial joints. The inflammation itself is secondary to the joint degeneration. In primary osteoarthritis there are no obvious causes; one likely factor is the abnormal metabolism of chondrocytes (cartilage-forming cells). Hereditary factors are common, while nutritional and chemical imbalances may also be involved. Secondary osteoarthritis results from any type of joint abnormality. A case in point is mechanical stress to the joint, which may be caused by alterations in the joint mechanics (for example, from misalignments of the bones). Another common trigger is a structural imbalance distant to the joint. For example, foot problems can lead to osteoarthritis of the hip. Other structural imbalances may be caused by obesity, postural patterns, sports or occupational activity. Joint abnormalities can also result from damage to the articular surfaces; for instance, if the joint is subjected to trauma.

In normal function, the wear and tear on hyaline cartilage is replaced by the activity of chondrocytes. The onset of osteoarthritis is marked by changes in the chemical composition of the matrix, which becomes soft and is easily damaged. Chondrocyte activity is impaired and cannot cope with the damage and the loss of cartilage, and the exposed bone underneath the damaged cartilage becomes hard with fissures. Synovial fluid enters the cracked bone surface and forms cysts within the bone. Proliferation and mineralization of bone ensues, with the formation of lipping and osteophytes round the joint margins or edges (for example, Heberden's nodes in the fingers). These contribute to the limitation of movement associated with arthritic changes.

Osteoarthritis (also referred to as osteoarthrosis) mainly affects the weightbearing joints such as the knees, hips and vertebral spine. An example of mechanical stress is that on the knee joint, which is said to carry a weight of 1.75 kgcm^{-2} (25 lbin^{-2}) during standing; this is doubled when walking and quadrupled when running. The condition of osteoarthritis leads to chronic pain and inflammation, and these are exacerbated by activity. Associated structures such as the ligaments, tendons and fascia can also become inflamed because of their proximity to the joint. Rheumatism is a term that describes the degeneration and inflammation of a joint and its associated soft tissues.

As already stated, arthritis is commonly accompanied by osteophytosis (the formation of spurs) around the joints. In the spine these can affect the vertebral bodies as well as the intervertebral facet joints. The osteophytes can cause neurological complications as they protrude into the intervertebral foramen or into the spinal canal and this in turn can lead to compression of the nerve roots and damage to the spinal cord.

In the cervical spine the osteophytic formation can encroach into the vertebral foramen and compress the vertebral artery, leading to vertebrobasilar ischaemia and to symptoms such as vertigo and ataxia. In this situation, gentle effleurage strokes and pick-up technique can be used to improve the circulation to the tissues. However, mobilization of the cervical spine, or passive stretching of muscles, need to be performed with extreme care and may be best treated by a manipulative therapist.

Spondylosis, which is defined as 'osseous hypertrophic spur formation at the vertebral end-plates due to disc degeneration' (Gatterman, 1990), is a typical example of arthritic degeneration of the lower cervical, mid-thoracic and the lumbar regions of the spine. It is often accompanied by intermittent periods of stiffness which are related to muscle guarding (Stoddard, 1969). Massage can be applied to help reduce the tightness and it can be followed by gentle mobilization.

Spondylitis. This is synonymous with osteo-arthritis of the apophyseal (facet) joints. It has a gradual onset and is found commonly in the over-60 age group. The pain of spondylitis does not abate completely and quiescent phases do occur. Inflammation and irritation of the joint surfaces are common, with movement as well as compression of the joints as in extension of the neck. Massage is used to improve circulation to the area. Passive movements should be limited to gentle traction (e.g. of the cervical spine) as rotational techniques may aggravate the roughened surfaces.

Massage application

- Massage is always used to improve circulation to arthritic joints. The only exception would be during inflammatory periods such as those of rheumatoid arthritis or spondylitis.
- Systemic massage is indicated to encourage the general metabolism and, in turn, the absorption of nutrients.
- Improving the systemic circulation eliminates systemic toxins, which can cause dysfunction and inflammation of the joint structures.
- Massage also improves respiration, thereby increasing the oxygen supply to all tissues.

Contracted muscles

A natural protective mechanism in chronic arthritic conditions is to accomplish movement by using an alternative joint to the one that is disabled. An example of this is the use of sacroiliac and lumbar spine movements rather than a chronically arthritic hip joint. The muscles involved in this compensatory joint movement become overworked, fatigued and painful, and the muscles that control the arthritic joint may also be contracted in their attempt to 'lock' the joint and avoid painful articulation. They are treated with massage and stretching.

Massage application

- Massage is used to increase the circulation of the muscles and ease any tightness. It is also applied to eliminate toxins within the muscles, improve their nutrient supply and alleviate pain.
- Hot compresses can be applied to help relax the muscles during or before the massage. Passive stretching can be used to provide a stretch to the muscle without inducing muscular contraction.
- All passive movements and massage strokes are carried out to the subject's pain threshold. If any of the techniques elicits pain or subsequent inflammation, it is either adjusted or omitted completely.

Adhesions

Adhesions (fibrous congestion) of the soft tissues can develop around the affected joint, and other nearby tissues are also susceptible to these changes. The reduced flexibility of the soft tissues restricts the mobility of the joint and exacerbates the pain on movement.

Massage application

- Cross-friction massage is applied across these fibres to free up any adhesions. The treatment is followed by passive joint mobilization (applied only to the limbs). Congestion around the spinal column is treated with thumb effleurage.

Flaccid muscles

As the arthritic condition progresses some of the muscles associated with the joint may gradually weaken, more so if the body should become less mobile or bedridden. Toning of the muscles is therefore indicated, and exercise is certainly one of the best options.

Massage application

- Rapid stroking or circular massage movements are used to improve tone of the muscles; these movements are repeated frequently. Gentle percussive strokes may cause some pain in the underlying joint and, consequently, they are carried out for a short period and restricted to the superficial muscles.

- Gentle joint mobilization helps to stimulate the joint proprioceptors and, in turn, to improve muscle tone; this passive mobilization is a procedure used mostly for the limbs.
- An effective toning method is isometric contractions, which are carried out with the joint in various degrees of flexion and extension. The therapist first supports and fixes the limb in a position. Next, the patient is instructed to contract a group of muscles (e.g. the adductors) while the therapist opposes the movement. In this manner the muscles are made to contract against the resistance offered by the therapist. All the muscles of the limb (for example, the ones associated with the hip joint) can be made to contract and tone up using this procedure.

Effusion

Effusion may be present in the joint space owing to inflammation of the synovium (synovial membrane). This local inflammation follows prolonged use of an arthritic joint, but responds well to the application of cold towels and lymph drainage massage techniques. Arthritic joints are very susceptible to changes in the weather; accordingly, in cold or damp climates hot compresses are of great benefit.

Referred pain

Malfunction and inflammation of the arthritic joint may give rise to referred pain areas, which are usually located in the nearby soft tissue structures. Such changes are treated with thumb effleurage and the NMT.

Rheumatoid arthritis

Rheumatoid arthritis is a systemic inflammatory condition affecting many tissues, most frequently the connective tissue and, in particular, the synovial membranes of joints. The disease also affects the skin, blood vessels, eyes, lungs and the lymphoid tissue (for example, Still's disease in children). It is considered an autoimmune disease, whereby the body's protective mechanism attacks the tissues it is designed to protect. The process involves the antibody IgM working against the smaller antibody IgG and attacking the various tissues of the body. It is also a complication of infection, where proteins in joints are damaged and are read as antigens by the immune system. Antigens are substances such as bacteria that induce the formation of antibodies.

Still's disease

This condition is also an autoimmune disorder that affects multiple systems in children. It is seen as being precipitated by infections from bacteria and viruses, emotional stress or trauma. The condition is synonymous with rheumatoid arthritis in adults and, in a similar way, produces degenerative changes in connective tissue and inflammatory vascular lesions. The attack on the lymphoid tissue causes the spleen and the lymph nodes to enlarge.

The onset of rheumatoid arthritis (and of Still's disease) is marked by inflammation and proliferation of the synovial membrane. This leads to the destruction of the hyaline cartilage and the formation of pannus (fibrous tissue) in between the joint surfaces. As the condition progresses to the chronic stage, fibrous adhesions across the joints and bony deformities are evident. Involvement of other tissues is associated with additional symptoms; for example, anaemia, subcutaneous nodules, breathlessness, carpal tunnel syndrome and even heart failure.

Massage application
- Massage is indicated in the absence of inflammation. It is used to increase the circulation, particularly as the patient leads a more sedentary life. The treatment is also applied to reduce pain and relax the patient. Stress can bring on an inflammatory attack, and massage is therefore used as a preventative measure. Furthermore, sleeping is greatly improved when there is less stress.
- Massage helps to maintain some tonicity in the musculature, which is subject to atrophy.
- Reflexively, massage helps to stimulate glandular function and this can improve the digestive processes. The function of the digestive

system is further stimulated by the direct mechanical effects of abdominal massage and other techniques. Kidney and bladder function, as well as respiration, can also benefit from massage treatment.

Dysfunction of the soft tissues

The inflammatory exudate in the joints tends to thicken and coagulate. It also spreads to the adjoining synovial tissues, including the ligaments and tendons, with resultant joint limitation.
Massage application
- Massage techniques such as deep effleurage and cross-friction generate heat and ease the rigidity of the exudate and the surrounding soft tissues.
- For the more superficial layers, kneading is used to break up adhesions and strictures within the tissues. These techniques also improve the blood supply to the area. All the movements are carried out during non-inflammatory periods.
- Mobilization reduces adhesions within the joint structures, and is therefore used in the early stages of the condition to help maintain mobility. This manoeuvre becomes increasingly difficult as the joint(s) become progressively more abnormal, but should be continued for as long as possible. Passive joint movements to the affected joint(s) are contraindicated during inflammatory periods; cold compresses are used instead to reduce the inflammation.

Ankylosing (rheumatoid) spondylitis

Ankylosing spondylitis is a progressive and painful disease that is similar to rheumatoid arthritis, but mostly affects the spinal column. Other tissues that may also be subject to changes are the heart and the eyes. Ankylosing spondylitis can be described as immobility and fixation of the joints (ankylosing), together with inflammation (spondylitis). Calcific and osseous ankylosis affects mainly the vertebral joints, the costovertebral articulations and the sacroiliac joints.

Although the cause of the condition is as yet unknown, one observation has been that most patients share the same genetic cell marker HLA-B27 (human leukocyte antigen B27). It could be that an otherwise harmless micro-organism sets up an inflammatory reaction when it comes into contact with HLA-B27.

Most of the inflammation occurs at the cartilaginous tendon and ligament insertions into the bones. A degree of bone erosion occurs as a reaction to the inflammation, and this is followed by a reactive bone growth in the soft tissues together with calcification; the process becomes cumulative with repeated inflammatory episodes. The bony union of the intervertebral discs gives rise to the bamboo spine appearance, while sclerosis of the sacroiliac joints leads to immobility and low back pain. Other common areas affected are the plantar fascia (leading to plantar fasciitis) and the Achilles tendon insertion into the calcaneus. Muscle stiffness and shortening are likely to occur, and these have a limiting effect on the joints, particularly the hips and the shoulders.
Massage application
- Massage is indicated to reduce any tightness in the muscles and to apply passive stretching. This treatment complements any exercise regime the patient may be following. Gentle mobilization of the joints is also included to maintain mobility; however, the procedure may be painful and is therefore contraindicated if the condition becomes chronic. Massage is also administered to improve the systemic circulation, to avoid fatigue and for relaxation. As the condition also affects the breathing, massage is used to relax and stretch the intercostal muscles and to keep the rib cage mobile; techniques that are used for the asthma sufferer can be applied for this purpose.

Osteoporosis

Osteoporosis refers to the condition in which there is a loss of the organic and mineral substances of skeletal tissue, leading to brittle and weakened bones. The condition is mostly related to old age and to hormonal changes (reduced levels of sex hormones) in postmenopausal women. It can, however, have hereditary factors and occur in early adulthood. Other predisposing factors include nutritional imbalances (high protein diet, poor nutrition), absorption dysfunction, prolonged use of corticosteroids and a lifestyle of inactivity, smoking or alcohol abuse. Conditions that may give rise to osteoporosis include hyperthyroidism, hyperparathyroidism, Cushing's syndrome, diabetes mellitus and rheumatoid arthritis. Pain that is felt in the bone tissue itself is one of the primary symptoms of this condition. Susceptibility to easy fracture owing to the brittleness and fragility of the tissue is also a principal characteristic. These changes can affect any bone, but the vertebral bodies are most susceptible and can undergo compression and collapse. In mild forms of osteoporosis the subject is able to move without discomfort; in more advanced stages there is pain on movement, and in severe cases the patient is unable to lie down.

Massage application
- Because of the fragile state of the skeletal tissue, heavy massage strokes are contraindicated in severe cases of osteoporosis. In most cases, however, massage is not applied to bony areas and therefore gentle techniques can be used on the muscles and for increasing general circulation. Careful positioning of the patient is critical in this condition. Lying in a prone position is sometimes difficult for the patient and, indeed, is not advisable if there is advanced osteoporosis of the spine. The sensitivity of the superficial and peripheral tissues may also be increased because of an accompanying condition such as diabetes mellitus, and this necessitates consideration and adjustment of the pressure. In milder cases of osteoporosis, general and gentle massage for circulation and relaxation can be applied.

MUSCULAR SYSTEM
Muscle fatigue

Fatigue develops when a muscle has been overworked or when its chemical balance is impaired, and these factors are interrelated. Fatigue upsets the muscle's physiological processes, while the resultant chemical disturbance causes the muscle to weaken. Malfunction of the muscle ensues in either case; the fibres do not respond fully to the nerve stimulation, and the strength of the contractions is progressively lessened. When the postural muscles are involved they become ineffective and can cause structural imbalances, which can manifest as misalignments of the spine; in this case, dysfunction of related organs may also occur. Common causes of muscle fatigue are shown in Box 4.1.

Massage application
- Muscle fatigue is very effectively reduced with massage. By improving the circulation to the muscles, massage removes any build-up of metabolites and supplies the muscles with nutrients and oxygenated blood.
- Some of the massage techniques are specific to the respiratory system. These are therefore applied to improve respiration and oxygen exchange.

Spasms

A spasm can be described as an involuntary sudden movement or convulsive muscular contraction. It can be clonic, where the contraction alternates with relaxation, or tonic, where the contraction is sustained. Spasms may affect the visceral (smooth) muscles; for example, those of the bronchial tubes in asthma and those of the ureter in renal colic. Skeletal muscles are equally susceptible to these involuntary contractions. A strong and painful spasm is referred to as cramp. Tonic contractions of the skeletal muscles frequently occur as a result of tissue damage. A spontaneous response to trauma is contraction of the nearby muscles, sometimes including the injured muscle; the contracted muscles act as splints and protect the body from further damage. Emotional stress is also a type of trauma and likewise may manifest as spasms. Sustained muscle contractions use large amounts of nutrients and oxygen and therefore cause an increase in the production of metabolites. The contraction of the fibres also compresses the blood vessels and causes ischaemia within the muscle itself.

Box 4.1 Common causes of muscle fatigue

- Malfunctions in the respiratory mechanisms can interfere with the oxygen supply to the muscle fibres
- Prolonged or sustained contractions will also deplete the oxygen supply. This is a common but transient aspect of exercise
- Cardiovascular disorders can impair the blood supply and the delivery of nutrients. The impaired circulation results in an increase of waste products within the muscle
- Inadequate nutrition leads to an insufficient supply of glucose and therefore of energy, adenosine triphosphate (ATP), for muscle contraction
- Reduced calcium intake or incomplete absorption has a limiting effect on the strength of the contractions. Calcium ions are used for the breakdown of ATP and therefore for the release of energy needed for the contractions.
- An accumulation of metabolic by-products are created by repeated or sustained muscle contractions. Biological processes within the muscle lead to such particles as hydrogen ions, lactic acid, carbon dioxide and fluid (catabolized lactic acid). These also result from the metabolism of other tissues and organs. All these products act as toxins to the muscle and weaken its contractions

---

This resultant congestion, together with a build-up of toxins in the muscle, irritates the nociceptors and leads to pain.

Massage application

- Massage is applied to improve the circulation, and in so doing it reduces the build-up of metabolites. Lessening the congestion has the effect of alleviating the pain by reducing the pressure on the nociceptors. The ischaemia within the muscle brings about micro-inflammation as well as tissue damage and pain. Further spasm develops by the muscle's reaction to the pain, and a vicious circle of spasm leading to pain and further spasm is created. Massage is therefore indicated to break the circle by easing the spasm and reducing the pain.

Contracture

Contracture is a permanent shortening or contraction of a muscle. One cause is a prolonged spasm or paralysis. A muscle is also said to be contracted when it cannot be passively stretched, and this is generally associated with fibrosis; that is, the laying down of fibrous tissue in or around the muscle. This process can be precipitated by a disturbance in the blood supply to the muscle due, for example, to tight bandaging elastic or cast. As a result, the cells atrophy and are replaced by fibrous tissues. Muscle shortening exerts an abnormal pull on the bones or joints to which it is attached. In Volkmann's contracture, for instance, the hardening and shortening of the forearm muscles forces the joints into a fixed position (flexion and pronation of the hand).

The fascia can also shorten or lose its full mobility if it is subjected to direct or reflex stress factors. As it covers the whole muscle, the muscle bundles and even individual muscle cells, any shortening within its fibres will prevent the muscle from reaching its full length, and also from contracting completely. A case in point is contraction of the palmar fascia in Dupuytren's contracture, which causes a flexion deformity of the hands and fingers. Restricted movement can also result from scar tissue, and from adhesions between the muscle and adjoining structures.

Massage application

- Deep massage to the muscles and their tendons is indicated, with the aim of reducing fibrous tissue and stretching the fascia. However, the shortening may be permanent or difficult to reverse if the condition is chronic. Bodywork techniques such as the NMT and passive stretching are also applicable.

Fibrosis

Fibrosis is defined as an abnormal formation of fibrous tissue (Taber's cyclopedia), and usually occurs as a reparative process following tissue damage and inflammation. The process can also be described as a reactive mechanism; for instance, as a result of repetitive strains to the tissues. Because skeletal muscle cells are mostly unable to multiply by mitosis, any injury or degeneration of the muscle fibre will lead to replacement by fibrous tissue composed mainly of collagen. Once these changes take place they are practically irreversible, and the muscle loses its full elasticity and contractibility. Fibrosis is common in postural muscles such as those of the back; this usually results from overuse or mechanical stress associated with postural patterns.

Massage application

- Massage is indicated to prevent the onset of fibrosis. As already noted, fibrosis can develop in cases of muscle overuse and postural imbalances. Massage is therefore used to improve the function of the muscles and to correct imbalances in the postural muscles. Tightness in the muscles is reduced and by-products of muscle activity removed. Effleurage and petrissage are used to increase the circulation and to loosen up adhesions within muscles. Deep thumb effleurage movements are used around joints. Passive stretching is applied to muscles to secure full extensibility.
- In the early stages of fibrosis, massage is indicated in an attempt to arrest the tissue changes by improving the local circulation and by stretching.
- In chronic fibrosis, massage is indicated to reduce the nodules that are also likely to be present. Deep friction or thumb effleurage are applied to stretch the fibres transversely. Bodywork techniques such as the NMT are also applicable. These are followed by passive stretching.

Fibrositis and fibromyalgia

Since the term 'muscular rheumatism' was first introduced in 1900 by Adler (as cited by Danneskiiold-Samsíe et al., 1982), many other names have been used to describe this condition of muscle pain. Among these are fibrositis, fibromyalgia, myofascial pain syndrome, myalgic spots and trigger points. Fibrositis is described as a syndrome, and is accompanied by symptoms such as headaches, exhaustion, abdominal discomfort and irritable bowel. The term fibromyalgia, like fibrosis, is frequently used to describe a group of non-arthritic rheumatic disorders characterized by pain, tenderness and stiffness. These are aggravated by physical or mental stress, trauma, exposure to dampness or cold and poor sleep.

Fibromyalgia therefore is also seen as a syndrome with pain all over the body but with no known aetiology. It involves not only the muscular system but also the central and peripheral pain mechanisms, neuroendocrine function (low levels of hormones such as serotonin and growth hormone). High levels of substance P in the cerebrospinal fluid is another common finding in this condition (Russell et al., 1993). Frequent sites for fibrosis or fibromyalgia are the lumbar region (also referred to as lumbago), the shoulder and the trapezium muscle, the sternocleidomastoid area, the chest and the thigh.

In clinical terms, fibrositis or fibromyalgia refers to muscle pain combined with nodular changes (Box 4.2). The disorder can be either secondary to joint diseases or a primary condition in itself. It has also been postulated that the pain of fibrositis is due to inflammation of the muscle cells, with the resultant general soreness, aching or stiffness. Particular foci of tenderness within the muscles are referred to as trigger points. One suggestion has been that the condition results from continued tension in the muscles. The typical person suffering from fibrositis is said to be one who leads a very busy lifestyle and is very likely a workaholic and subject to tension; the musculoskeletal structure is therefore under continuous stress.

As already noted, the condition of fibromyalgia arises from the muscle fibre or cell. Tension in the muscle produces hypoxia or lack of oxygen to the muscle fibre. Biopsies of muscle tissue by electronic microscopic techniques have shown that, in muscular rheumatism, there is degeneration of the mitochondria together with glycogen deposits. This is said to result from the hypoxia, and leads to a reduction of oxidative metabolic capacity within the muscle. Glycogen is not used up because of the mitochondrial degeneration and, as a result, the glycogen deposits within the muscle increase. The muscle fibres suffer slight inflammation and degeneration (Fassbender, as cited by Danneskiiold-Samsíe et al., 1982).

Myoglobin is found in muscle tissue. It is a protein, a respiratory pigment, with a high oxygen-carrying capacity. Furthermore, it is believed to improve the diffusion of oxygen into the

---

> **Box 4.2** Characteristics of fibromyalgia
>
> - Generalized aches and pains or stiffness in muscles which have continued for more than 3 months
> - The presence of five or more trigger points (hypersensitive areas), mostly in the muscle insertions
> - Tenderness on palpation of the superficial tissues, e.g. during skin rolling
> - Paraesthesia (tingling and prickling of the skin) which has no obvious causes such as a nerve root problem
> - Sleep disturbances
> - General fatigue
> - Irritable bowel
> - Anxiety
> - Headaches
> - An absence of arthritic factors (therefore a normal ESR and rheumatoid factors)
> - The condition is likely to affect women more than men
> - Onset is after the age of 30 years

muscle cell. Myoglobin can leak out of the muscle fibres into the plasma of the venous blood. It is not clear whether this leakage is associated with the destruction of muscle fibres; however, the rate of leakage from the muscle increases when there is tension and pain, or as the fibrositis progresses. In one experiment it was observed that, following a series of massage treatments, plasma myoglobin lowered while the symptoms of fibrosis simultaneously reduced. Although there was an initial increase in the plasma myoglobin after the massage, the slowing down in the rate of myoglobin leakage indicated that the muscle fibres were no longer tense and inflamed. By reducing tension in the muscles, massage can therefore be seen to reverse the process of fibrositis (Danneskiiold-Samsíe et al., 1982).

Another theory is that fibrositis is a disease of the connective tissue rather than the muscle cell. It primarily affects the fibrous connective tissue component of muscles, the tendons, ligaments and the periarticular tissues around the joints. The fascia within the muscle (i.e. that of the muscle fibres and bundles) is said to be particularly prone to the inflammation. This condition is known by such terms as intramuscular fibrositis, muscular rheumatism and interstitial myositis.

Fibrositis can also affect the subcutaneous fascia (panniculitis) and the fibrous sheath surrounding nerves (e.g. sciatica).

One study has shown that the fibres of those muscles with fibrositis are connected with a network of reticular and elastic fibres. This interconnecting network of thin threads in between the muscle fibres is said to be the cause of the pain. As one muscle cell contracts it exerts a pull on the other cells connected to it by these filaments, and the pull on the filaments may give rise to the pain. It may also cause the connecting cells to contract. This forced contraction of other cells will eventually cause the muscle to fatigue, which also leads to pain (Bartels and Danneskiiold-Samsíe, 1986). It is very likely that the fatigue causes hypoxia and inflammation, with the resultant formation of reticular fibres.

Massage application

- The most beneficial effect to be derived from massage is relaxation. As already noted, the person suffering from fibrositis or fibromyalgia is likely to be very anxious and tense. There also appears to be a strong link between anxiety, depression and the perception of pain (Sunshine et al., 1996). Relaxation techniques, together with stress management skills, a change of lifestyle and alterations in the sleep patterns, are needed as part of the ongoing treatment. Massage helps to reduce the .levels of anxiety and stress, as indicated by the lower levels of cortisol and norepinephrine. It also helps to reduce depression and promote sleep by raising the levels of serotonin. Studies in other conditions have indicated that disturbed sleep patterns, mood changes and increased pain sensitivity have been attributed to low levels of serotonin. Observations showed that pain, joint stiffness, fatigue and disturbed sleep (all symptoms of fibromyalgia) were reduced following a number of relaxing massage treatments (Field, 2000).
- Very gentle massage techniques such as effleurage are used to induce relaxation and relieve the pain. Petrissage and kneading techniques are included to help stretch the tissues and break up any adhesions in between the muscle fibres.

- Gentle thumb effleurage is applied to the origins and insertions of muscles to reduce any nodular and hypersensitive areas. Areas of referred pain or tissue changes are likely to be present, and these too are treated with thumb effleurage and the NMT. It is important that the patient is asked for feedback throughout the treatment, especially in the early sessions when a level of tolerance has to be established.
- Trigger points are treated with on-and-off pressure (which must be tolerable to the patient), followed by gentle passive stretching. Cooling of the tissues during the stretch helps to normalize the sensory nerve endings.
- If the fibrositis has progressed to the stage when the sufferer is very inactive because of the pain, the massage is used to improve the circulation and reduce any build-up of metabolites or toxins. The application of a heat pack helps to increase the blood supply and therefore reduce ischaemia in the muscles; this is particularly useful in chronic conditions. In acute situations ice packs may be more beneficial, particularly on trigger point areas.

Muscular dystrophy

Muscular dystrophy refers to degeneration of individual muscle cells leading to progressive atrophy. Voluntary skeletal muscles are most affected by this condition, whereas vital involuntary ones like the diaphragm are spared. Possible causes include inherited muscle-destroying diseases, genetic defects, faulty metabolism of potassium, protein deficiency, and an inability of the body to use creatine (produced by the liver to help store ATP energy). Orthodox treatment comprises muscle-strengthening exercises, surgical measures, braces and patient activity.

Massage application
- Massage is indicated to increase the systemic circulation, especially as the condition becomes more debilitating. Nutritional supply to the tissues, together with the elimination of toxins, is also enhanced.
- Massage is also carried out, in addition to exercise, in an effort to maintain muscle tone. The treatment is particularly indicated if flaccid paralysis is present.

Torticollis

Torticollis, or wryneck, presents with the head permanently tilted to one side, with perhaps some rotation to the opposite side. This structural change is caused by a shortening of muscles such as the sternocleidomastoid or scalenii. It may also have its root in skeletal abnormalities, i.e. in misalignments of the cervical spine.

It is generally seen as a congenital condition when there is shortening of the muscles with or without fibrotic changes. Before birth the predisposing factors include malposition of the fetus. During birth it could be caused by injury to the neck muscles by forceps delivery or other problems. There is a permanent contraction of the sternocleidomastoid muscle on one side, and this shortening and thickening causes the muscle to be prominent as a tight band. As a result of the same contraction, the face and chin are tilted towards the non-affected side.

Movement of the head and neck is restricted, not only because of the malfunction of the musculature but also the related curvature (scoliosis) of the spine. The restriction of the head movement and postural fatigue (e.g. from occupational tilting of the head) can result in pain in the contracted muscles. Trigger points can also develop and radiate pain to other regions of the head and sternum.

Massage application
- Relaxation of the subject is necessary to reduce any possible tension in the muscles related to stress.
- Muscle relaxation is also necessary, particularly to all the muscles of the neck and upper back. Effleurage with the fingertips or thumbs can be carried out on the sternocleidomastoid as well as the scalenii. Pressure is firm without being too heavy, and is certainly not applied on the carotid artery which is close to these muscles.
- Passive stretching is applied with the aim of releasing tightness in the sternocleidomastoid and scalenii. Stretching is best carried out as

part of post-isometric relaxation with the aim of increasing side bending and rotation.

- Gentle mobilization of the neck can be carried out provided it does not cause any pain or dizziness (some subjects can be susceptible to dizziness if there are circulatory problems).
- Treatment of trigger points is carried out before the passive stretching.
- The treatment can be carried out with the subject sitting, lying supine or on their side, whichever is the most comfortable arrangement.

FASCIA

Superficial fascia

Fascia is divided into the superficial and deep structures. The superficial fascia is referred to as the panniculus adiposus, owing to the fact that, in normal health, it contains an abundance of fats. Where these are absent, as in the scrotum and the eyelids, the fascia is simply areolar tissue. An excess of fats renders the fascia adipose tissue.

Adipose tissue

The benefit of massage extends to the adipose tissue. By exerting a mechanical pressure it may help promote, albeit to a small degree, the breakup of fat globules in these subcutaneous layers. It also creates heat and hyperaemia, which can influence the metabolism and may therefore activate the fat globules so they burn up and release their energy. In addition, massage aids the circulation in the abdomen and can therefore help the transfer of the fat molecules from the intestines to the lymph channels.

Another impact of massage is to lessen the stress that adipose tissue puts on the heart. Adipose tissue is highly vascular, and therefore demands an extensive blood supply. This tends to put a strain on the pumping action of the heart. Massage lessens the strain by assisting the circulation of the subcutaneous tissues as well as that of the systemic system. Another advantage is in the formation of fat. Fat formation in living

tissue develops primarily in regions where the circulation is moderate or sluggish. Conversely, when the circulation of adjacent blood vessels is improved, fat tends to diminish. Massage, along with exercise and local heat application, improves the circulation to most tissues, and in particular to regions such as the thigh, buttocks and abdomen. It therefore prevents or reduces any build-up of subcutaneous adipose tissue in these regions.

Massage application

- Petrissage can have a very significant effect on adipose tissue. When applied vigorously, it may help to emulsify the fat in the superficial connective tissue cells. The fat globules may therefore escape into the lymphatic system and be carried away.
- It is also feasible that some of the fat may be burnt up by the increase in temperature and the local hyperaemia. These claims are not scientifically proven and are therefore repeated only with caution; no guarantees are given to the recipient of massage therapy.
- The fact that the adipose tissues are being 'worked on' may be sufficient to give the recipient a positive psychological boost. Furthermore, some patients who are capable of exercising may be encouraged to do so by the feel of an increased tonus of the tissues. The experience of increased tone may be the result of a reflex action (Ganong, 1987), or it could be that the patient becomes aware of a 'tingling' feeling caused by the stimulation of the receptor organs and the hyperaemia.

Adhesions

Adhesions are composed of white elastic fibres, mostly around joints, or yellow elastic fibres in fascia layers. Inflammation or injury causes the fibroblast cells in the fascia to release fibronectins (adhesive glycoproteins), which provide 'scaffolding' and contribute to the progress of the repair process. Repair fibres are simultaneously laid down; this process is marked with the release of tropocollagen by the same fibroblast cells. The extent to which this fibrinous exudate is allowed to spread, and whether it remains acute or becomes chronic, determines the amount of scar tissue and adhesions formed. Microinflammation is common in myofascial planes, causing various stages of the 'adhesion process'.

Massage application
- Adhesions are reduced by the stretching action of some massage movements, in particular by the twisting component of the petrissage technique. Other strokes, such as friction movements, vibration and the NMT, have a similar effect of separating the fascia layers and breaking up the collagen microfilaments. Passive stretching of the muscle, tendon or ligament is necessary to secure the full expansion of the tissue. Sudden or rapid stretching manoeuvres are counterproductive, as they only irritate the tissues.

Scar tissue

Scar tissue is also made up of yellow elastic fibres and collagen. It is inelastic, and is associated with adhesions. Scar tissue may also function as a trigger point, and can therefore cause tissue dysfunction in a reflex zone. As noted earlier, such a dysfunction gives rise to symptoms and changes such as nodules, pain, tissue tightness and even organ malfunction. These in turn can cause or be associated with a condition that is either chronic or does not respond to treatment. Scar tissue is therefore palpated for adhesions and for hypersensitive zones that are exacerbated when the skin is stretched.

Massage application
- In addition to massage strokes like friction movements, scar tissue is treated with gentle stretching and the NMT. Vibration movements are also employed, particularly if the scar tissue is recent.

Cellulite

One simple description of cellulite is the hardening of the fat cells. It is sometimes wrongly referred to as cellulitis, which is inflammation of tissues just below the skin, and is rightly associated with hormonal activity in females. Apart from the fluid retention caused by the hormones, the problem is also caused by diets that cause too many toxins, accumulation of fat cells, and bad circulation which can be caused by lack of exercise. All of these factors need to be addressed if cellulite is to be reduced or prevented.

Cellulite is precipitated by an accumulation of fat globules or cells; these create a need for extra nourishment and, therefore, a bigger blood supply. To channel the blood to the tissues, new capillaries are formed and infiltrate the spaces. As the additional capillaries release more filtrate, the tissues become saturated with interstitial fluid; this build-up is exacerbated if the electrolytes are out of balance (for example, if there is an excess of sodium ions). Abundant reticular fibres in the interstitial tissues accumulate and thicken around the fat cells; they form capsules which gradually transform into collagen fibres and are felt as nodules. Collagen fibres are also laid down in the interstitial tissue spaces, rendering the connective tissue sclerotic (hard). The overall picture is of hardened tissue with a nodular feel, sometimes referred to as the 'orange peel' effect. Venous congestion is also likely to be present.

Massage application
- Lymphatic massage and effleurage movements are indicated to reduce the congestion and improve the venous return. Vibration movements are also used to help decongest the area. Kneading or petrissage techniques are applied to help break up the fibrous capsules, although this is a difficult task once the capsules have formed. Friction movements are also helpful in breaking up the fibrotic tissue and adhesions; they also improve the local circulation and drainage. Hard, percussive-type strokes such as hacking are contraindicated as they may traumatize the tissues.

Deep fascia

Deep fascia varies considerably in its consistency. Over the limbs it is well defined like a sheet of white fibrous tissue. It forms a non-elastic and tightly fitting sleeve, and has two functions: it keeps the underlying structures in position, and preserves the characteristic surface contour of the limbs. In some areas it forms a tendinous sheet or aponeurosis for muscle attachment. Fascial planes, compartments or sheets also form channels in between the organs, muscles and other tissues. As lymph is capable of flowing along or through these fascial layers, they can be seen as routes for lymphatic drainage; as such, they also provide paths by which infections can spread from one part of the body to another. In addition, the deep fascial structures have the important function of assisting lymph and venous drainage. They accomplish this task by forming a solid wall next to the lymphatic and venous vessels. When muscles contract, they compress the vessels against this fascial barrier (wall) and the fluids are squeezed forward.

Fascia is made up of a jelly-like ground substance and the various fibres: white fibrous (collagen), yellow (elastin) and reticulin. Both the matrix and the fibres are influenced by such factors as water retention, electrolyte balance and hormones. Reduced thyroxine, for example, leads to an increase in water retention in most cells, and in the quantity of the ground substance. One theory suggests that the minor 'pain' produced by the NMT acts as a stressor to the body. This leads to the production of some hormones, which cause a breakdown of the collagen fibres. Such a breakdown within the collagen will reduce any hardening or nodules in the tissues. A general decrease in water retention in the ground substance is also said to occur. The tissues are therefore decongested (Selye, 1984).

Massage application

- Some of the massage techniques can be seen as exerting the same level of 'pain' as the NMT, and can therefore cause a similar reaction in the connective tissue. In this process, any rigidity in the tendon and muscle fascia layers is reduced. Massage movements such as kneading and petrissage exert a considerable stretch to the connective tissue fibres of fascia.

NEUROLOGICAL DISORDERS

Introduction

This section looks at some conditions that are primarily dysfunctions of the nervous system (incorporating the brain, the central and peripheral nerves). In some of these disorders, however, the pathology involves more than one system. Cerebrovascular accident (stroke), for instance, is triggered by pathology of the vascular system but its symptoms are seen in the nervous system. Other conditions may have a degree of emotional aetiology or the illness itself can lead to emotional disturbances.

Spasticity

There are various terms concerned with the condition of spasticity that describe its variations or complications:

1. Spasticity itself denotes hypertension (extreme spasm) of the muscles, causing stiff and awkward movements. It results from upper motor neuron lesions and, therefore, malfunctions within the brain (motor cortex) or the spinal cord.

2. A spastic gait refers to stiff movements of the legs and the whole body. The toes appear to catch together and drag along the floor.

3. Spastic hemiplegia relates to partial hemiplegia (one half of the body) with spasmodic muscular contractions.

4. Spastic paraplegia indicates paralysis of the lower portion of the body and of both legs, owing to transverse lesions of the spinal cord and/or to paraplegic ataxia. In this disability there is sclerosis of the lateral and posterior parts of the spinal cord, and it is characterized by slowly progressing ataxia (muscular uncoordination) and paresis (partial or incomplete paralysis).

Massage application

- Massage is indicated to ease the tension in the muscles and gently stretch them, and has the additional effect of increasing the local and systemic circulation. It is worth bearing in mind that the easing of tension and the stretch provided by massage are of short duration; however, it is likely that a cumulative effect does also occur. More importantly, massage provides a caring touch and support for the spastic child or adult. For some subjects, this closeness is unquestionably of great emotional value.

Paralysis

A voluntary movement depends on the integrity of two motor neurons:

1. An upper motor neuron, arising in the motor cortex, travelling across the brain and ending in the anterior grey horn of the spinal cord.
2. A lower motor neuron, arising in the anterior horn cell and passing to the muscle.

Paralysis is a temporary suspension or permanent loss of function. It is caused by dysfunction of either an upper or lower motor neuron. To a great degree, paralysis manifests as reduced sensations or weak voluntary movements. There are two types of paralysis: spastic and flaccid paralysis.

Spastic paralysis

In spastic paralysis there is muscular rigidity accompanying a partial paralysis. It is usually caused by a lesion involving an upper motor neuron, as in a 'stroke'. The patient is unable to move the affected part, but other motor neurons may act on the muscle involved. Excessive muscle tone (spasticity) is common but is not always present. There is no atrophy of the muscle but some of the muscle bulk may be reduced because of lack of use.

Massage application
- Massage is used to increase circulation and drainage, and therefore improves the nutrition to the muscles as well as removing toxins.
- It is also applied to ease the spasms.
- Massage, together with some passive movements of joints, can also help to improve and stimulate nervous reflexes, i.e. the sensory and motor pathways in the brain.
- Local stimulation of the muscle fibres must, however, be avoided, to prevent further tension in the muscle. To this end the massage strokes are over a wide area, slow and rhythmically applied. Deep effleurage strokes are perhaps the most suitable; these can be followed by kneading of the whole muscle bulk rather than small sections. Passive stretching is also of use provided it does not overextend the muscle, as this may cause a reflex contraction.

Flaccid paralysis

The second type of paralysis, flaccid paralysis, is caused by a lesion of the lower motor neurons that travel from the anterior horn cell to the muscle. The affected muscle loses tone, atrophies and shows signs of degeneration. Muscular reflexes are absent.

Massage application
- Techniques for flaccid paralysis should be of short duration and very light, although the massage can be repeated daily.
- It is carried out for the purpose of improving the circulation, which is in a stagnant state because of lack of movement.
- The toxins that are present in the system may similarly be removed with massage.

Cautionary note
- Heavy pressure compresses the weak and fragile muscle tissue against the bone; it should therefore be avoided, together with any undue stretching of the degenerated muscle tissue. Atrophy has the effect of thinning out the muscle bulk, and this change in the muscle thickness diminishes the protective layer it provides to the underlying tissues. The arterioles are particularly affected and become susceptible to heavy pressure. While joint mobility needs to be maintained, passive stretching of the flaccid muscles is contraindicated owing to the fragility of the structures.

Cerebrovascular accident (stroke)

In a cerebrovascular accident (CVA), the injury to the brain results from a deficiency of blood and oxygen—ischaemia. A major cause is haemorrhaging (spontaneous intracranial haemorrhage). Hypertension, embolism, thrombosis or tumours are also closely associated with CVA. Other causes include obesity, heart disease, smoking, alcohol abuse and migraine headaches.

The brain receives 20% of the cardiac output via the paired internal carotid arteries and the vertebral arteries. Pathology of these vessels or malfunction in other components of the central circulatory system will curtail the blood supply to the brain. A diminished volume of blood, or a reduced oxygen and glucose content in the blood, will lead to brain damage. Restriction of the blood flow can result from atherosclerosis, which can also be diffused throughout the brain and cause dementia. Another common cause is thrombosis, which is exacerbated by oestrogens. The thrombus can be formed in a distant area and then become mobile to form an embolus. It may cause an attack during the night. If the embolism is composed of small platelets it will break up quickly, giving rise to the symptoms of a transient ischaemic attack, with temporary blindness and loss of speech.

The extent and severity of the symptoms of a cerebrovascular attack depend on the site and degree of the injury. Some of the after effects include visual disturbances, dizziness, confusion and speech impairment. Another prominent symptom is hemiplegia, or one-sided paralysis, resulting in loss of function of the voluntary and involuntary muscles. An additional feature is anaesthesia, i.e. partial or complete loss of sensation. As the damage is caused by an upper motor neuron lesion, the paralysis is also accompanied by spasticity; increased tonus therefore appears in the muscles supplied by the affected part of the brain. The spasms can affect the flexor muscles of the upper limb and the extensor muscles of the lower limb. Contractures of the muscles cause the joints of the upper limb to be fixed in flexion and those of the lower limb in extension; the antagonist muscles are usually flaccid. It is difficult to predict the speed and extent of recovery from hemiplegia, as this depends on the size of the lesion in the brain.

Following a stroke, massage treatment is applied primarily on the affected regions, i.e. the upper and lower limbs. The first few treatment sessions should be very short and are carried out with great care. If there is any doubt about the suitability of the massage, then approval should be sought from the medical team looking after the patient. Treatment generally starts at the proximal end of each limb, gradually moving distally to finish at the hand or foot. Stimulation of the palmar surface of the hand or the sole of the foot may elicit contractions in the same limb. While massage to these regions is necessary, the movements are none the less carried out with extreme care. In most cases there is a loss of sensation in the affected limb, and the patient is therefore unable to give any feedback about the pressure being applied. Consequently minimal pressure is applied, and this is only increased gradually as the patient recovers. At all times during the massage, the limb being treated is supported and the patient is held in a secure position.

Massage application

- A very significant effect of massage to the limbs is to help restore the sensations that are often affected by the stroke. Stimulating the nerve endings in the skin by different stimuli is said to improve these sensations. Massage acts as a very good stimulant and, to increase its effect, patients are encouraged to focus their attention on the tactile sense of the skin during the treatment. This exercise has a second valuable effect in that it helps patients to acknowledge the limb, which is sometimes 'ignored'. A stroke is extremely traumatic; it is often difficult for sufferers to come to terms with it and to acknowledge the affected limb or limbs. Massage can be used to help patients to accept their body and, in so doing, speed up the recovery.

- Massage helps to reduce the rigidity of muscles associated with the spasticity. Gentle effleurage and friction movements are applied to the spastic muscles to reduce the contractures. Friction movements are also included to decrease any spasm of the blood vessels; the resultant vasodilatation increases the skin temperature.

- Flaccid muscles are stimulated with gentle petrissage and kneading techniques. Rapid friction movements can also be applied; the treatment has the effect of encouraging the neuromuscular system within the flaccid muscles and thereby strengthening their contractions (Sirotkina, 1995). Following the massage, the patient is encouraged to contract the muscles to stimulate the motor nerves; these exercises should also be repeated regularly throughout the day.

- For the patient to regain full control and function of the limbs, there needs to be a reduction in the spasticity. This has to occur alongside the restoration of the controlled patterns of movement (Cailliet, 1980). To this end, gentle passive movements of the limb are carried out in all directions. These techniques stimulate the sensory organs and the proprioceptors within the joints, which results in improved coordination and toning of the flaccid muscles, and also helps to stretch the tight muscles. In the event that these passive movements elicit severe pain they are discontinued. Shoulder pain in particular is often a persistent symptom in residual hemiplegia or hemiparesis, and its cause has been attributed mostly to the spasticity of the associated musculature. While massage is therefore of benefit, the shoulder needs careful handling. As the patient shows some progress, gentle emphasis is placed on reversing the fixed joint positions resulting from the spasticity. For example, when treating the upper limb the shoulder is encouraged to move anteriorly; the humerus to abduct and externally rotate; the elbow joint to be extended; the forearm supinated; and the wrist and fingers to extend and adduct. The same passive techniques can be applied to the joints of the lower limb.
- The muscles of the unaffected side tend to be very overworked and tense as a result of their compensatory function. Massage is therefore carried out to the neck, trunk and shoulders of the unaffected side. If the patient is very tense, relaxation of these muscles can be a difficult task.
- Massage is also applied as a means of providing emotional support to patients, to improve their morale and reduce stress. Patients recovering from a stroke can become very anxious and frustrated if their speech is impaired, and these feelings of desperation and even depression are exacerbated if they are unable to use

their hand for writing and everyday activities. Inducing relaxation and repeating the massage regularly helps to restore their confidence in speaking, communicating and writing.

- As tension is often 'stored' in the abdomen, massage to this region may be indicated. It is also of benefit for the general function of the digestive system and, in turn, to the whole body. Treatment on the abdomen is not carried out until a few days after the stroke or until there is some recovery.
- Massage to the feet is always included, as it is very effective in reducing anxiety.

Parkinson's disease

Parkinson's disease is a highly complex neurological disorder and is not only progressive but is currently considered incurable. It is an upper motor neuron condition that affects skeletal muscles and leads to severe disability and irregularity in movement. Under normal circumstances muscle coordination is maintained by a balance of dopamine, which inhibits muscle contraction, and acetylcholine, which is an excitatory transmitter. In Parkinson's disease there is a reduction of the neurotransmitter dopamine to the basal ganglia, that part of the brain responsible for movement and muscular coordination. The disease affects mainly males, and starts at about the age of 50–60 years. As it progresses, the three characteristic signs of the condition become more noticeable: muscle spasm or rigidity, bradykinesia (slow movements and shuffling gait) and tremor at rest.

The term 'cogwheel rigidity' is used to describe the combination of rigidity and tremor in the upper limbs that is a feature of this condition. Rigidity of the arms is an early sign, as are contractions of the hamstrings and rounding of the shoulders. The slow and impaired movements are caused by the tightness in the upper and lower limbs. In addition, the stooping posture adopted by the patient creates tightness in the muscles of the back and those on the anterior region of the trunk. The muscles of the face are similarly affected, giving rise to an expressionless appearance. Muscle fatigue is a common outcome of the continuous spasms; it is also accompanied by pain.

Massage application

- Massage is indicated to ease the muscle tension and maintain the mobility of the joints. The treatment can be applied in the early stages and can continue as the condition progresses, provided it does not cause any discomfort. Gentle effleurage, petrissage and some kneading are mostly used, together with some gentle friction movements. The massage is generally carried out with the patient supine. Massage to the back can be applied with the patient in the sitting position or lying on the side.
- As the sufferer is unable to exercise, the circulation is likely to be impaired. Effleurage massage movements are therefore of benefit for the systemic circulation as well as for the rigid muscles. Techniques such as petrissage and kneading will further reduce the muscle tightness and passively stretch the tissues. Particular attention is given to the flexor group of muscles, which become shorter and tighter than the extensor group. Passive stretching techniques can be used to help relax and stretch certain muscles, such as those of the lower limb and the pectoral muscles. In addition, the joints are passively moved in their range of movement.
- Abdominal massage is carried out, primarily for assisting the portal circulation but also to relieve constipation. Although the involuntary muscles of the digestive tract are not generally affected by the disease, the progressing spasms of the abdominal muscles can make defaecation difficult.

Multiple sclerosis

This is a chronic, slowly progressive disease, which affects primarily the white matter of the CNS. It can affect the cerebral, brainstem–cerebellar or spinal areas. The disease is characterized by a random formation of plaques; these are areas of demyelination, where the myelin sheath is destroyed. While the causes of the disease are not well understood, one likely factor is viral infection. This is seen as causing the myelin to become abnormal (containing less fatty acids) and therefore susceptible to damage; the damage is exacerbated by an autoimmune attack. The primary symptoms of the disease relate to the white matter damage. Upper motor neuron signs include general muscle weakness and gait disturbances related to paralysis affecting one or both limbs. Exaggerated reflexes are accompanied by increased tone of muscles, lack of coordination, intention tremor, optic neuritis and visual disturbance, numbness, paraesthesia and scanning speech. Vertigo and incontinence may also occur. Although there are periods of remission in the early stages of the disease the symptoms become more severe and permanent with its progression.

Massage application

- Massage is indicated to maintain good systemic circulation. In so doing, it assists the delivery of essential fatty acids, the much-needed nutrients for the myelin sheath.
- The treatment also helps to ease the rigidity in the muscles, reduce any build-up of oedema in the limbs and alleviate the pain. These benefits may, however, be of short duration. Furthermore, there may be times when the patient is in considerable discomfort and the massage is not tolerated. At all times, therefore, the treatment is applied with great care over areas of numbness and loss of sensitivity.
- Stress is always very closely associated with an autoimmune disease; by inducing relaxation, massage can therefore help in promoting a remission.
- Abdominal massage may be indicated to help relieve the common problem of constipation.

Myalgic encephalomyelitis

This condition is also known as chronic fatigue syndrome, immune dysfunction syndrome, or chronic Epstein–Barr virus infection.

Myalgic encephalomyelitis (ME) is an acute inflammation of the brain and spinal cord. It may be caused by a virus, in which case it is referred to as viral encephalitis or postviral fatigue syndrome. Another possible cause is pancreatic malfunction. The condition is now being related to an abnormal immune response to a viral infection. The severity of the reaction is influenced by age, genetic predisposition, gender, stress, environment and previous pathology.

ME has an acute onset over a 2-week period; this is then followed by a long recovery period. Malfunctions of the immune system and of the body's metabolism are common features. If not already involved, the pancreas may be attacked, leading to periodic hypoglycaemia (reduced sugar levels). Neurological damage leads to abnormal muscle metabolism and, therefore, fatigue and pain. Other symptoms include depression and panic attacks (both in the acute stage), swollen glands and headaches. Paraesthesia in the extremities is also a symptom that is sometimes present, albeit that it is not always regarded as a major dysfunction of the condition. Paraesthesia refers to abnormal sensation without objective cause; tingling and prickling, numbness and heightened sensitivity.

Differential diagnosis for ME is more frequently based on the number of symptoms. One of the formulations states that, for a patient to be diagnosed with ME, they have to have two *major criteria* plus a minimum of eight *symptom criteria*. The *major criteria* are:

- Constant or recurrent fatigue which has a recent onset and is not relieved by bed rest. The normal daily activity of the subject is disrupted owing to fatigue in about 50% and for a minimum period of 6 months.
- Examination and laboratory tests show no other disorders or pathology.

The *symptom criteria* are:

- The least physical activity leads to extreme fatigue, more than would normally be experienced by the subject when they were free of the disease
- Mild fever
- Tender and painful lymph nodes
- Sore throat
- Headache
- Sleep disturbances
- Muscle weakness
- Muscle pain

- Joint pain that moves from one region to another, in the absence of inflammation or oedema
- Irritability
- Confusion
- Depression
- Photophobia
- Difficulty in clear thinking, concentration or remembering.

Massage application

- Although not always tolerable, massage is indicated for relaxation, calming down the patient in panic attacks and reducing muscle stiffness. It is contraindicated and is frequently unwelcome during episodes of severe fatigue, shortness of breath, diarrhoea and headaches, especially when two or more symptoms occur concurrently. As the patient recovers, massage is applied to remove the by-products of muscle activity (thereby preventing fatigue) and to help maintain tonicity in the tissues. Systemic massage continues to benefit the function of organs and glandular secretions.

Epilepsy

This is the most frequent neurological disease after stroke, and involves recurrent attacks of distorted brain function accompanied by excessive neuronal discharges. Epileptic seizures are of varying severity and symptoms, the main feature being loss of consciousness. There are many causes, including hereditary and nutritional factors, lymphatic lesions (Peyer's patches), digestive disorders, spinal problems, stress, the effects of drugs and alcohol, excitement, flashing lights, heat, allergies and trauma.

The many clinical states of epileptic seizures are described in a variety of classifications, none of which are standardized or universally accepted. The more common descriptions include the following. The *grand mal* (major) epileptic seizure invariably has an 'aura stage', when there is an apprehension of the oncoming seizure, which is followed by a complete loss of consciousness. There are muscular contractions and spasms of the mouth, jaw, body and limbs.

Biting of the tongue, foaming at the mouth and involuntary urination may also occur. This sequence of events is followed by deep sleep. The *petit mal* seizure (synonymous with childhood absence epilepsy) is characterized by a transient loss of consciousness with blank, staring eyes; this is frequently accompanied by some muscle jerks. Jacksonian epilepsy (synonymous with partial, focal, cortical and hemiplegic seizures) involves only parts of the cortex. Consequently the convulsions, if they occur, are mostly restricted to certain groups of muscles or are confined to one side of the body. There is not always loss of consciousness. For instance, in a temporal lobe seizure (a form of complex partial seizure) there is no loss of consciousness but a dreamlike state with hallucinations of smell, taste, sight or hearing and feelings of déjà vu.

Massage application

- Massage for epilepsy is slightly controversial as opinions differ about contraindications. On the one hand, massage is considered unsuitable because relaxation in itself can bring on an attack. Conversely, massage is seen as appropriate because the attacks are frequently precipitated by stress. Furthermore, the condition is very likely to be controlled with medication, in which case the benefits of massage (i.e. inducing relaxation and promoting sleep) may outweigh the risk of an attack. If massage is applied, then all necessary preparations should be taken to deal with a seizure should this occur while the patient is being treated. Immediately after an attack, when there is heat and swelling, massage is contraindicated and cooling packs are substituted.
- In the case of a severe attack such as a *grand mal* seizure, massage is only applied 2 or 3 days after the episode. At this stage, the purpose of the treatment is to reduce muscle spasms and to increase the circulation rather than to promote relaxation. Over the following days, relaxation techniques can also be included in the treatment.

Headache

A headache can be defined as pain felt in different regions of the head, and it is described in terms that reflect its location or its severity. An attack can therefore occur over the forehead, over the eyes, across the top of the head, etc. The ailment is also said to manifest as a 'splitting' headache, a throbbing pain or an intermittent ache. Similarly, it is expressed in terms of a tension headache, neuralgia-type headache or migraine. Its aetiology is very diverse, which accounts for its complexity and the frequency with which it occurs (Box 4.3). Some episodes of headache are transient and acute, resulting from factors such as infections, tension or dehydration. Others are chronic, and may underline serious pathology.

The actual sensation of pain inside the head can result either from pathological changes within the cranium itself or from abnormalities occurring outside it. Certain tissues inside the cranium contain pain receptors that are very sensitive, particularly to stretch and pressure changes. These 'pain-sensitive' tissues are the dural sinuses, the emissary veins (which carry blood from the sinuses to the outer side of the skull), the arteries, and the dura at the skull base. Intracranial pathological changes that stimulate the pain receptors include tumours (which

---

Box 4.3 Common aetiology of headaches

- Referred pain from nearby structures such as the eyes, teeth, sinuses, ear or throat
- Fevers
- Trauma to the head
- Muscle tension
- Psychogenic factors
- Anxiety
- Depression
- Psychosomatic factors
- Dehydration
- Migraine
- Inflammation of the temporal arteries
- Raised intracranial pressure
- Drugs
- Allergies
- Toxic fumes
- Constipation
- High blood pressure
- Low blood pressure
- Congestive heart failure
- Premenstrual tension
- Menopause
- Nervous exhaustion

stretch these tissues), fevers, intoxication and, possibly, hypertension (these last three factors cause arterial dilatation), meningeal inflammation, compression of the cervical vertebral artery and haemorrhage.

The second group is of extracranial pathological changes. All tissues outside the cranium are pain-sensitive. When the sensory nerve endings in these tissues are irritated, they refer the pain to the head via some of the cranial nerves (V, VII, IX and X) and the upper cervical nerves (C1, 2 and 3). Conditions that stimulate the pain receptors include inflammatory diseases (for example, in the sinuses, teeth, ears or eyes); other causes include prolonged muscle contractions in the upper back, neck and jaw. Compression of the cervical vertebral artery can similarly stimulate the pain receptors; another factor is distension of the blood vessels. Migraine is an example, caused by spontaneous contraction and distension of the extracranial arteries in the head and neck.

Tension headache

A very common type of headache is that caused by tension or stress. The connection between tension and headache is twofold. There is an elevation of blood pressure, which irritates the pain-sensitive tissues inside the cranium (e.g. the arteries and sinuses). Muscle tightness, on the other hand, irritates the pain receptors in the back of the neck and the jaw; the resultant pain is referred to the head along the cervical and cranial nerves.

Massage application
- Understandably, the underlying causes of stress need to be addressed by the appropriate remedial approach. Massage is concurrently employed for its beneficial effect of reducing anxiety. The levels of serotonin have been observed to increase with the relaxing effects of massage (Field et al., 1996b). Apart from promoting sleep, the raised serotonin levels may be beneficial in reducing the pain associated with headaches (in a similar manner that some headache medications are aimed at raising serotonin levels). Most of the massage techniques to the upper shoulder, neck, head and face can induce relaxation. In addition, trigger point techniques are applied to certain muscles. Muscle tension is often associated with trigger points that can exacerbate or indeed initiate the referred pain to the head. The more common muscles in which trigger points are likely to be found are:

a. The sternocleidomastoid muscle, just superior to the junction where the fibres divide into the sternal and clavicle segments.
b. The splenius capitis, below the mastoid process.
c. The temporalis, at the midpoint of the temples. If the tenderness is specific to the temporal arteries it could indicate cranial (temporal) arteritis, and massage on this area should therefore be avoided.
d. The masseter muscle, just superior to and over the temporomandibular joint.
e. The trapezius, anywhere along the lower, middle and upper fibres.
f. The levator scapulae, just superior to the insertion into the upper medial border of the scapula.

Neuralgia-type headache

Neuralgia manifests as a severe, sharp pain along the course of a nerve, and is usually due to compression, irritation by toxins, or malnutrition. It is described according to the part or organ affected; for example, cardiac neuralgia is synonymous with angina pectoris, and trigeminal neuralgia involves the trigeminal nerve. Occipital neuralgia is precipitated by irritation of the spinal nerves (sensory, motor and autonomic); the irritation is caused by abnormalities or degeneration of the cervical and upper thoracic spine. A neuralgia-type headache is often caused by a degree of misplacement and locking between two adjoining vertebrae, which leads to irritation and inflammation of the nerve roots emerging between the vertebral bodies. The outcome in this situation is a neuralgia-type pain radiating to the base of the occiput and possibly to other areas of the cranium. Spasms of the upper shoulder and neck muscles are invariably involved in this condition; they exert a pull on the spine and shift it into an abnormally fixed position. Conversely, spasms often develop if the spine is already out of line or locked. A vicious circle is therefore created whereby the muscle spasms sustain the locking, which in turn maintains the same muscles in spasm.

Massage application

- Massage is indicated to help break this vicious circle by easing the tension in the musculature and helping to restore the spinal movements. As the muscles relax the pain is alleviated, which encourages further muscular relaxation. In some cases, the most effective and quickest treatment for spinal misalignments or locking is that provided by a manipulative therapist such as an osteopath or chiropractor. This approach may be required if the headaches persist after one or two sessions of massage. Massage treatment is contraindicated when a headache is precipitated by certain pathological factors such as infections and viruses (e.g. fevers, meningitis) or the intake of narcotics or other drugs.

Migraine

Migraines are paroxysmal (sudden and periodic) and are characterized by recurrent attacks. They are usually accompanied by varying degrees of visual and gastrointestinal disturbances. The causes of migraine are not well understood, but evidence points towards vasoconstriction of the intracerebral arteries. A similar change also takes place in the extracranial arteries, which undergo episodic constriction followed by sudden vasodilatation. These alterations in the vessels and the intracranial pressure have a direct effect on the pain-sensitive tissues within the cranium. A cluster headache is a variation of migraine with severe neuralgic pain around the eye; it invariably returns every few months. Abdominal migraine is a recurrent abdominal pain together with vomiting, and occurs mostly in children. The most common symptoms of migraine include zigzags of light, vomiting and unilateral sweating. In addition, there can be a sharp stabbing pain in the temporofrontal region (frequently unilateral) and intolerance to light and sound. There may be a familial tendency to migraines, and they are often brought about by stress, hormonal changes, the contraceptive pill and certain foods.

Massage application

- During an attack, massage to the upper body is contraindicated. This precaution is taken to prevent massage from increasing the blood flow and hence the volume in the already dilated extracranial arteries, which would exacerbate the pain in the head. In any case, massage is unlikely to be tolerated by the sufferer. Massage may also cause a sudden rush of blood to the constricted intracranial arteries, which would lead to an increase in pressure. The cranial nerves may also be irritated by the sudden influx in pressure. Massage is, however, indicated in between attacks, for relaxation. By improving the systemic circulation massage also enhances organ function and, in so doing, additionally promotes the elimination of toxins and other materials that may cause the migraine attacks.

Sciatica

The pain of sciatica originates in the back and radiates down the posterior aspect of the leg. It occurs when a nerve root becomes irritated and inflamed, most commonly because of misalignment of any two vertebrae, degeneration of the spine and the intervertebral discs, or dysfunction of the pelvis. Structural imbalances or injuries can cause muscular spasms. A case in point is dysfunctions affecting the pelvic girdle that can lead to contraction of the piriformis muscle. As this is closely associated with the sciatic nerve, tightening of this muscle will often give rise to sciatic pain. Strains of the lumbar soft tissues as well as inflammation may be further complications of the sciatica.

Massage application

- Treatment of sciatica necessitates a thorough examination to establish the cause. Massage is therefore contraindicated until the predisposing factors are confirmed. Even when the cause is established, massage is avoided on areas of inflammation, particularly along the nerve route. While management of the condition with manipulative therapy or physiotherapy is the primary approach, massage can also be used as an adjunct to other treatments. If misalignment of the spine is causing the sciatica there are likely to be some protective muscle spasms in the lumbar region. Massage to the paravertebral muscles in this area can therefore be applied to help ease the pain of ischaemia and improve the local circulation. The benefit is of course temporary as the muscles resume their protective action. Should spasm of the piriformis be the primary cause then massage and passive stretching, as well as muscle energy technique, are likely to be of great benefit.

Intervertebral discs

A herniated disc, or worse still a prolapsed one, invariably gives rise to severe pain in the back. In simple terminology, a disc herniation refers to a tear of the outer covering (annulus fibrosus) of the disc whereas a prolapse involves the nucleus pulposus. The condition is nearly always accompanied by a radiating pain down one or both legs, depending on the extent of the damage. Paraesthesia and muscle weakness can also affect the lower limb. The acute pain can develop several hours or even days after a moderate strain. In a classic case the patient moves, perhaps to pick up a pencil from the floor, or just to sneeze, and then becomes aware that *something* has moved in the spine. A temporary sharp pain may be present but the subject may be able to continue with activities initially. The gradual increase in pain and the onset of the protective muscle spasms in the lumbar and gluteal regions are likely to result in very restricted movements. If the pain is very severe the patient is unable to walk, sit or lie down comfortably; this occurs in most cases of a disc prolapse. Disc herniation and prolapse are invariably accompanied by some deformity of the spinal curve, e.g. lumbar kyphosis or scoliosis, or pelvic shift. The patient may also need to lean to one side when standing.

Extreme tenderness on palpation is also likely in the regions of the spinous processes, the sacroiliac joints, the paravertebral muscles, and the tissues along the dermatomes.

Massage application

● Owing to the implications of the condition, massage is contraindicated and the patient is best referred to a doctor or to someone like an osteopath or physiotherapist. Cold packs may be beneficial until the patient receives the appropriate treatment. As the muscles are in spasm and therefore protecting the injury, any relaxation of these muscles will lead to an exacerbation of the instability and pain. Massage is therefore contraindicated, particularly on the area of the lumbar spine involved and along the path of nerve pain. Some massage can be applied to other regions, primarily to help the patient overcome the stress associated with the pain. However, the position in which the patient is massaged is critical. The patient must never be allowed to lie prone as this will further compress the affected disc and nerves. Side-lying is a possible alternative, provided the patient is able to lie down without too much pain. Alternatively, any massage, for example to the neck and shoulders, should be carried out with the patient sitting.

RESPIRATORY SYSTEM

Asthma

Asthma is characterized by intermittent attacks of dyspnoea (breathlessness) and wheezing, with periods of remission. It can also become chronic and develop into bronchitis and emphysema. An asthmatic attack is very traumatic. Difficulty in breathing is due to spasm of the bronchial tubes, so that the lumen of the tubes is considerably reduced. Inspiration remains comparatively easy, albeit short and shallow, but *expiration* becomes difficult. During an attack dyspnoea is also caused by inflammation of the mucus lining and the excessive mucus in the lumen of the bronchi and the bronchioles. Tightness in the chest muscles accompanies the breathlessness and wheezing, with the thorax being fixed in a position of inspiration. Breathing is facilitated by moving the rib cage, and with very little involvement of the diaphragm. Recruitment of the accessory muscles of respiration can be achieved if the subject holds on to some support and fixes the shoulder girdle. A bout of coughing usually brings about the end of an attack.

In between asthmatic attacks, there are periods of general good health. In chronic asthma conditions the mobility of the chest is reduced and the rib cage may become more or less fixed in a position of inspiration, accompanied by a shortening of the muscles used for forced inspiration (Wale, 1983). Respiratory muscles tend to be very tight and thoracic kyphosis accompanies the 'barrel-chest' and reduced chest mobility. Pulmonary function has been found to increase with regular massage treatments (Barr and Taslitz, 1970). In this study it is postulated that a sympathetic response to the massage causes a reflex bronchodilatation, and therefore an increased volume of air in the lungs. It is worth noting that in this case massage is seen as having a sympathetic rather than a parasympathetic stimulation of the autonomic nervous system.

Bronchial asthma is frequently caused by an allergy or hypersensitivity to pollen, dust or foods (e.g. egg, shellfish and chocolate), or it may result from drugs or irritants such as smoking and temperature changes. In some cases, asthmatic attacks may be brought about by exercise or by infections of the respiratory tract. The severity and frequency of the attacks can be influenced by endocrine changes at various periods throughout life. In a similar manner, emotional states such as tension, stress, anxiety and excitement can precipitate an attack.

Cautionary note

- Although gentle cupping on the upper region of the back can be applied to help release the build-up of mucus, it is vital to bear in mind that this in itself can exacerbate a spasm of the bronchial walls. It is therefore advisable only to carry out this treatment during remission periods and even then with the approval of the doctor.
- Contraindications to massage include an unrelenting asthmatic attack and respiratory tract infections.

- The treatment is also contraindicated if the sufferer has been taking medication that does not appear to have an effect. Referral to a doctor is essential in such a situation.

Massage application

- It is very unlikely that a sufferer would want or tolerate a massage treatment during a severe and traumatic asthmatic attack. On the other hand, if the attack is not severe and if it is comfortable for the patient, massage can be applied with the subject in the sitting position. Relaxing techniques such as effleurage and gentle kneading are carried out on the upper back muscles and lower cervical area. Circular thumb effleurage is applied alongside the paravertebral muscles of the upper back. The aim of the treatment is to induce relaxation, thereby reducing the involuntary muscle spasms in the walls of the bronchial tubes. Relaxation helps to reduce the number of sympathetic impulses being transmitted to the involuntary muscles of the respiratory tract, and as the muscle contractions become weaker the muscles relax and the airways open.
- Reducing the stress levels during remission periods can help delay or avoid an asthmatic attack. If the condition is exacerbated by emotional upsets, then massage is used on a regular basis to help the sufferer maintain a relaxed state.
- In between asthmatic attacks massage is also employed to treat the respiratory muscles (Table 4.2), which may be in spasm, fatigued or shortened. Particular attention is given to the pectoralis muscle, latissimus dorsi, abdominal muscles, scalene muscles and serratus posterior inferior.
- Passive stretching, muscle energy technique and gentle mobilization of the rib cage can also be applied (see Chapter 8). Mobilization of the scapulae further helps to free up the other muscles related to the rib cage, e.g. subscapularis and serratus anterior.
- Friction massage in the intercostal spaces helps to increase the local circulation and lymphatic drainage; furthermore, it has a relaxing effect on the intercostal muscles.
- Whole body massage is used to enhance the systemic circulation, particularly if the subject is unable to exercise.

Table 4.2 Muscles of respiration

Quiet inspiration—gentle breathing in:

Diaphragm	Draws central tendon downward, increasing the volume of cavity
Intercostales externi	Lifts the anterior rib cage upward
Intercostales interni	Draws the anterior rib cage downward
Levatores costarum	Raises the ribs upward
Serratus posterior inferior	Pulls the lower ribs down and anchors them against the pull of the diaphragm

Deep inspiration—the above muscles plus:

Scalenus anterior	Raises the first rib
Scalenus medius	Raises the first rib
Sternocleidomastoid	Raises the sternum
Serratus posterior superior	Raises the ribs
Sacrospinalis	Straightens the back

Forced inspiration—the above muscles plus:

Serratus anterior	With the scapula fixed, it raises the ribs
Pectoralis minor	Raises the ribs
Trapezius	Anchors the scapula for other muscles to work, e.g. the serratus anterior
Levator scapulae	Anchors the scapula for other muscles to work
Rhomboideus	Anchors the scapula for other muscles to work

Quiet expiration—gentle breathing out:

Elastic recoil of diaphragm	
Obliquus externus abdominis	Compresses abdominal viscera
Obliquus internus abdominis	Compresses abdominal viscera
Transversus abdominis	Compresses abdominal viscera
Rectus abdominis	Compresses abdominal viscera
Transversus thoracis (sternocostalis)	Depresses the ribs

Forced expiration—the above muscles plus:

Abdominal muscles	Greater compression of the abdomen; flex trunk
Latissimus dorsi	Depresses the ribs
Serratus posterior inferior	Depresses the ribs
Quadratus lumborum	Depresses the lower ribs

Referred pain

Conditions affecting the respiratory system, such as bronchitis and asthma, can refer pain to the left side of the neck and the medial aspect of the shoulder. Certain pathology, such as bronchial or oesophageal carcinoma, can also refer pain to the back. These areas of tissue changes can be treated with massage strokes as indicated. Hypersensitive areas may be trigger points, and are therefore treated with an on-and-off pressure followed by passive stretching. The massage treatment is, however, contraindicated in a number of conditions affecting the respiratory system, e.g. acute bronchitis and pneumonia; furthermore, it is only carried out in the absence of inflammation and infections.

Massage application

- Conditions of the respiratory system often lead to the following tissue changes, which are likely to be areas of hypersensitivity, tightness and congestion. In most of the disorders they can be effectively treated with effleurage, NMT and vibration movements. The reflex zones include the following:

  a. The whole region of the thoracic back, on both sides. Most tension is found along the paravertebral muscles.
  b. Increased tension between the scapulae and the spine.
  c. Increased tension along the occipital border.
  d. Tightness in the anterior fibres of the deltoid, left and right.
  e. The tissues along the lower rib cage and the lateral fibres of the latissimus dorsi muscle.
  f. The insertion and fibres of the sternocleidomastoid.
  g. The tendons of the latissimus dorsi and pectoralis major in the region of the axilla.

Pulmonary emphysema

Emphysema is a chronic disease of the respiratory system in which the air spaces distal to the terminal bronchioles are enlarged while the walls of the bronchioles are subject to degenerative changes. The principal feature of this condition is breathlessness on exertion. Some sufferers do not become breathless but develop right heart failure; others have a high respiratory rate. Bronchitis is nearly always a further complication, indicated by the presence of a cough and the production of mucus. As a result, the respiratory muscles are strained and likely to be tight and congested. The ribs are in a horizontal position and the diaphragm appears flat on X-ray. Movement and exercise are limited; consequently, systemic circulation is impaired and toxicity builds up.

Massage application

- In chronic emphysema patients are unable to lie prone or supine, and are therefore treated sitting up or lying on their side. Massage is indicated to increase the systemic circulation and also for lymph drainage. Rib excursion and breathing are assisted with massage to the respiratory muscles. The improved uptake of oxygen in the lungs reduces hypoxia and the need for oxygen therapy. Percussive cupping strokes on the back can help loosen the mucus. Whenever possible, massage to the abdomen is included to assist the digestion and portal circulation. Obesity is one of the exacerbating factors of emphysema, and massage can be included as part of a weight reduction programme.

URINARY SYSTEM

Inflammation of the kidney

Most pathological conditions relating to kidney malfunction involve some degree of infection and inflammation. Two representative cases are repeated cystitis and pyelitis (inflammation of the pelvis of the kidneys). The kidney area itself is generally very tender to palpation and, consequently, local massage is contraindicated. Malfunction of the kidneys can cause widespread pain to the loin area, which includes the regions of the lower back, both sides of the lower trunk plus the lateral borders of the buttocks and upper thighs. Pain in these regions is not always distinguishable from that related to disorders of the spine. Furthermore, soreness on the left or right side of the upper lumbar spine is easily

misinterpreted as muscle tightness instead of a kidney problem. Oedema (local, systemic or in the lower limbs) is another sign of kidney malfunction.

Massage application

- Systemic and abdominal massage movements are applied to improve the circulation to the kidney. Venous drainage of the organ is a further benefit of the massage and is equally vital to kidney function. Lymphatic massage is employed to drain the oedema, particularly in the lower limbs, that is associated with kidney disorders. It is important to bear in mind that, while massage is effective in supporting kidney function and promoting the healing process, it does not treat pathological conditions, some of which can have very serious complications.

- Abdominal and systemic massage can increase kidney output and micturition; this diuretic effect can also lower the blood pressure. However, due to the connection between kidney problems and high blood pressure, it is advisable to only treat with the doctor's approval. Any abdominal massage should be of short duration and applied mostly for portal circulation.

- Kidney disease can lead to the following tissue changes, mostly on the side of the affected kidney, and massage is used to treat these areas to effect a reflex response in the kidney:

  a. Increased tension in the pelvic and sacral areas, which may also radiate downwards to the iliotibial tract and upwards to the fascia of the latissimus dorsi along the spinal segment of T9 and T10. The tissue tension and tenderness can extend further, to the anterior region and the groin.
  b. Tightness in the lower rib cage area, along the dermatome of T10.
  c. A small area of hypersensitivity can be found at a point between the scapula and the vertebral column, at the level of T4.

Cystitis and bladder disorders

The inflammation of cystitis occurs mainly in the bladder. It is common in women, and is especially frequent during pregnancy. In men it is usually secondary to obstruction, generally that of an enlarged prostate or a urethral stricture. Blockage of any source encourages infection, exacerbates its effects and prolongs the inflammatory process. In non-obstructive cases the infection is usually caused by *Escherichia coli*; however, when there is an occlusion it is common to have mixed infections, such as *Proteus* and *Staphylococcus* spp.

Massage application

- Lymph massage is applied to help decongest oedematous areas, in particular the lower abdomen. As noted earlier, however, massage is omitted on areas of extreme tenderness and this may include the lower abdomen. Another effect of the lymph massage is to assist the immune system, which is likely to be weakened. It is worth bearing in mind that kidney stones may be a complication of cystitis and massage to the kidney area may therefore be contraindicated.
- Conditions relating to the bladder can lead to the following tissue changes. These areas are assessed for tenderness and are treated accordingly:

  a. Tension over the lower part of the sacrum.
  b. Tension along the iliotibial tract.
  c. Tension along dermatomes L3, S1 and S2, including the popliteal fossa.
  d. Tension in the area above the pubic bone and in the anterior region of the thigh.

Renal colic

Renal colic refers to pain in the abdominal area that arises from one of two circumstances. The first, a frequent factor, is a stone, which lodges in the bladder, urethra, ureter or in the pelvis of the kidney. Sometimes the stone is passed in the urine. The expulsion is accompanied by pain, which radiates from the kidney area to the abdomen and into the groin. The second cause of renal colic is malfunctions of the kidneys. These are associated with spasm in the region of the kidneys and towards the thigh.

Massage application

- Massage on the abdominal area is likely to be uncomfortable and is therefore contraindicated. The referred pain may extend to the back, which is likewise omitted. Some gentle massage may be tolerated and is carried out on other reflex zones (refer to zones for cystitis).

Urinary tract infection

Urinary tract infections are more common in women than in men because of their shorter urethra. An infection is more likely to occur during the sexually active years, and is highly related to sexual activity (e.g. honeymoon cystitis). Menstruation is another causative factor as it lowers the resistance to urinary tract infection. Common bacteria responsible for the infection include *E. coli* (a normal organism of the bowel), *Streptococcus faecalis, Staphylococcus* spp (rare), and *Proteus vulgaris* (associated with renal stones). Massage is not applicable in this condition.

REPRODUCTIVE SYSTEM

Premenstrual tension

Menstruation occurs when production of the ovarian hormones, especially progesterone, is reduced. This hormonal adaptation results from failure of the ovum to become fertilized. Menstruation itself is quite often preceded by premenstrual tension (PMT); this condition is in fact a syndrome and is therefore a combination of symptoms, ranging from water retention to backache and depression. Water retention is perhaps the most common symptom, and ensues from the cyclic increase in the steroid hormones. PMT can also be caused by endocrine changes such as progesterone deficiency, oestrogen/progesterone imbalance and raised aldosterone levels.

Pelvic congestion is a major feature of PMT and can refer pain to the back, over the sacrum, to the lower abdomen and down the thighs. Fluid retention is another common characteristic; this can lead to hypersensitivity and nerve pain in some regions, and even to headaches.

Alongside these changes are those which affect the fascia. In stable conditions, fascia is a flexible tissue that can expand with the increased fluid build-up. When it is subjected to mechanical stresses such as postural patterns and imbalances, the fibroblast cells within the fascia are activated and this leads to certain adaptations. Collagen fibres are laid down, causing the fibres to thicken and adhere to each other, and as the fascia becomes harder and unyielding it is unable to accommodate fluctuations of fluid in the interstitial spaces. The consequence of such a restriction is that any build-up of fluid creates additional pressure on the nerve endings, which exacerbates the pain. Malfunction of the fascia can also give rise to trigger points, which are sometimes observed in the cervical muscles. Trigger points can bring on or exacerbate headaches during the premenstrual period.

Massage application

- The relaxing effect of massage is very significant, as it helps to lessen the intensity of tension, irritability, depression and crying spells (Field, 2002). However, in some cases of PMT the abdominal area, or indeed the whole body, may feel too tense and tender for the physical contact of massage. In this situation massage to the feet, hands and the head may be tolerated and suitable as a starting point. With the effect of relaxation and the reduced pain sensitivity other movements can then be applied, provided the massage is always comfortable to the subject. Light effleurage techniques are mostly used, to soothe the pain, but movements such as kneading to some areas like the calf can also be used.
- Postural patterns and imbalances can complicate and increase the symptoms of PMT. Massage is used to address tightness and dysfunction in muscles and, in so doing, reduces mechanical stresses, spasms and fatigue. Passive movements to the joints can be carried out.
- Massage techniques for venous return and lymph drainage are carried out in between menses just prior to menstruation. The goal of the massage in this case is to remove congestion and to enhance the elimination of toxins

and excess fluid. The breast tissue is also susceptible to fluid retention and can, if appropriate, be treated with lymph massage movements.
- The application of massage techniques to deal with trigger points can be too painful during periods of fluid retention. Once the oedema is reduced, however, the area is treated with on-and-off pressure and passive stretching.

Pregnancy

The general effects of massage in pregnancy

Massage therapy can be of great benefit in pregnancy as it helps to relieve some of the discomforts associated with postural changes and additional weight. It also helps to maintain a good overall function of the body and provides relaxation and emotional support. The applications of massage during the second and third trimesters as well as postnatally are discussed further on in this chapter while some of the general benefits are given in this section.

Relaxation

- Anxiety is not usually an antenatal feature but should there be any apprehension associated with the pregnancy or any mood swings, massage is an excellent way of providing relaxation and support. If there happens to be stress that is related to psychosocial factors, massage can likewise be of benefit.
- Relaxation techniques can be applied throughout pregnancy and it is worth bearing in mind that the calming effect of massage can also be seen as extending to the baby *in utero*.
- Through its effect on the parasympathetic nervous system (Tovar and Cassmere, 1989) massage can stimulate the production of the body's natural endorphins; it can therefore be of great value in reducing pain (Jacobs, 1960).
- The sedating effect of massage helps with rest and relaxation and in turn lowers the levels of catecholamines. These compounds can interfere with oxytocin and other hormones during labour and they can also affect the baby *in utero* if they pass through the placenta.

Musculoskeletal

Hormonal changes, increase in body weight and postural adaptations are amongst the contributing factors to the back pain often endured during pregnancy (Cailliet, 1995; *French's Differential Diagnosis*, 1985). Massage can play a significant role, particularly during the later months of pregnancy, in alleviating pain in the lumbar area. In some cases, sciatica, which is often connected with tightness of the lumbar muscles and/or of the piriformis muscle, can likewise be eased with massage.

While not pertaining to the posture directly, carpal tunnel syndrome of one or both wrists does occur sometimes during pregnancy and may give rise to considerable discomfort. Increased fluid retention may be a contributory factor to the symptoms, and massage for venous return and lymph drainage on the upper limbs is therefore of benefit.

Circulation

During pregnancy the body increases its production of progesterone which may in turn cause hypotonicity in the peripheral blood vessels and consequently lead to a sluggish circulation, oedema and varicose veins. The circulation can be impaired further by the pressure of the uterine weight on the pelvic vessels. With a slow venous return in the iliac, femoral and saphenous veins the body's susceptibility to blood clot formation is raised. Blood clot formation increases four to five times during pregnancy while fibrinolytic activity (clot-dissolving) activity decreases dramatically to avoid haemorrhaging during childbirth. Massage movements, effleurage in particular (Dubrovsky, 1982), can be preventative in this respect as it helps to provide the 'back pressure' that is necessary to maintain the blood flow in the pelvic and peripheral vessels. Effleurage and lymph massage movements to the lower limbs assist the venous flow and reduce the build-up of fluid. Decreasing the congestion lessens the possibility of varicose veins, albeit that the massage is omitted if these have already developed.

Conversely, the pregnant woman may suffer from high blood pressure during the gestation period and, in such a situation, relaxation movements can be applied to help lower the readings.

An enhanced systemic circulation means there is also a good blood supply to the placenta and subsequently a good distribution of nutrients reaching this organ.

Improving the blood flow can help raise the number of red blood cells in the circulation. One possible pathway is the freeing up of any cells caught up in congested areas. An increase in the number of circulating red blood cells has the effect of preventing anaemia, or lowering its severity. In addition, more oxygen-carrying haemoglobin is released into the tissues systemically, and this helps combat fatigue.

Organ function

Another benefit of massage is the improved function of organs. An enhanced liver function, for instance, leads to the elimination of toxins (through the expelled bile) and subsequently to an elevation of the energy levels. Unless there is eclampsia (see Contraindications) the normal levels of toxins released by the liver are not likely to cause systemic toxaemia and therefore massage is safe.

Reduced peristaltic activity and constipation are often present during pregnancy. As pressure on the abdomen is best avoided, the massage treatment for improving peristalsis is applied by means of the stroking movements on 'reflex areas' to the digestive system; these include the thighs, the buttocks and the feet (reflex zones).

Connective tissue

To maintain tissue pliability and prevent the likelihood of stretch marks, extremely light massage strokes can be applied on the abdomen, using only the flat palm of the hand and with an appropriate body cream or oil.

The perineum too can be massaged during pregnancy to maintain the flexibility and elasticity in the tissues, thereby lessening the need for an episiotomy during childbirth. As it is not ethical for the massage therapist to carry this out, instructions can be given to the pregnant woman or her partner. A study to evaluate the effectiveness of perineal massage during pregnancy for the prevention of perineal trauma at birth was carried out at the Department of Family Medicine, Laval University, Quebec City, Canada. It was found that perineal massage is an effective approach to increase the chance of delivery with an intact perineum for women with a first vaginal delivery but not for women with a previous vaginal birth (Labrecque et al., 1999). No differences were observed between the groups in the frequency of sutured vulvar and vaginal tears, women's sense of control, and satisfaction with the delivery experience. A similar study, which looked at the effects of antenatal perineal massage on subsequent perineal outcomes at delivery, was carried out at the Department of Obstetrics and Gynaecology, Watford General Hospital, Hertfordshire, UK. The research concluded that antenatal perineal massage appears to have some benefit in reducing second or third degree tears or episiotomies and instrumental deliveries. This effect was stronger in the age group 30 years and above (Shipman et al., 1997).

Contraindications

While massage is beneficial and effective throughout pregnancy it can easily become contraindicated if certain disorders or complications arise, e.g. symphysis pubis dysfunction where massage is specifically ruled out in the pelvic area. Other possible contraindications listed here are meant to be pointers for the massage therapist and are not hard and fast rules. If the suitability of the massage is a borderline decision, then advice or authorization should always be sought.

- It is an essential precaution that massage is carried out without causing pain to the expectant woman. Adrenal stress hormones, released as a response to pain, have the effect of elevating blood pressure, respiration rate and heart rate; the immune function is also lowered and blood

flow to the uterus is impaired (Gorsuch and Key, 1974). It is easy to imagine how the same negative effects of the stress hormones can also diffuse into the fetal circulation through the placenta.

- As indicated earlier, massage on the pregnant abdomen is avoided other than very superficially for the purpose of applying creams or lotions. Abdominal massage is totally contraindicated if the linea alba is strained (diastasis recti) because of the increased pressure on the interior abdominal wall by the pregnant uterus.

- Compression is also avoided in the inguinal region as it can generate pressure on the iliac and femoral veins.

- Systemic massage is also contraindicated if complications arise during the pregnancy, particularly when there is a risk of increased intrauterine pressure. A case in point is an abnormality of the placenta (detachment or dysfunction) or irregularities in the uterus or cervix.

- Equally significant are disorders that can influence the blood supply to the fetus, such as high blood pressure and multiple fetuses.

- Pain in the abdomen that is not related to the later stage of pregnancy, and therefore to cramps or contractions, may have some underlying aetiology that requires investigation. Massage is therefore contraindicated until a diagnosis is carried out.

- Other precautions relate to persistent diarrhoea and gestational diabetes.

- Itching without the presence of a skin rash may be indicative of obstetric cholestasis and is a further contraindication to massage. Obstetric cholestasis is a liver disease which manifests in pregnancy and which completely resolves within a week or two of delivery. It tends to start around the 28th week and is likely to be caused by the high levels of oestrogen hormones causing a reduction in the flow of bile. An excessive amount of bile acids accumulate in the liver and leak into the blood, causing itching of the skin and in some cases jaundice. A deficiency of vitamin K may also be present as a result. The itching of obstetric cholestasis is often in the palms of the hands, the soles of the feet, and can spread to the limbs and trunk. It is different, however, to the normal itching of pregnancy which can occur around the breasts and abdomen. Massage in the region of the liver is not only difficult but is also not advised during pregnancy; it can cause discomfort and the increased circulation may even exacerbate the symptoms.

- Eclampsia is another contraindication to massage. This condition refers to severe toxaemia of pregnancy accompanied by high blood pressure, albuminuria (serum proteins, especially albumin, in voided urine, which are indicative of kidney impairment), oliguria (diminished amount of urine formation), tonic and clonic convulsions, and coma. A very gentle and short massage for relaxation may be possible with the aim of reducing the high blood pressure. This is best carried out to the upper back and shoulders, for example, and with the patient in a sitting position. Oedema does present in the lower limbs, but this is more likely to be a result of kidney and liver failure than lymphatic blockage. In any event, owing to the seriousness of the condition it is best to avoid any drainage massage movements on the legs.

- During the middle and later months of pregnancy, massage with the subject lying supine is best avoided as the weight of the fetus presses on the major blood vessels such as the inferior vena cava (supine hypotensive syndrome). If the supine position is the only feasible option then cushions and bolsters may be used to prop up the subject in a semi-sitting posture. This reduces some of the pressure on the abdominal vessels and allows for massage to certain regions such as the lower limbs.

- Massage in the prone position should be avoided after the twelfth week of gestation or much earlier in the case of multiple fetuses. Even with the use of special cushions or equipment, the prone position may increase the intrauterine pressure and will inevitably intensify the tension on the over-strained uterine and lumbar ligaments.

- Because of the laxity in the ligaments more or less systemically, extreme caution is required if passive movements to joints are carried out. Traction techniques, especially to the lower limbs, are contraindicated.

- Persistent or severe backache may need referral to a 'manipulation therapist' such as an osteopath, physiotherapist or chiropractor.

- In some cases, pain is felt in the lower abdomen, the pubic area, the groin or radiating down the inner thighs. This type of pain is usually made worse by walking or climbing stairs and is likely to be that of diastasis symphysis pubis (DSP) or symphysis pubis dysfunction (SPD). DSP and SPD are two conditions of pregnancy which certainly require the attention of a doctor or manipulative therapist. Fortunately these conditions only affect a small proportion of women.

DSP means an abnormally wide gap between the two pubic bones at the symphysis pubis joint, situated at the front of the pelvis. It can only be diagnosed conclusively by investigation such as X-ray, ultrasound or MRI scan. In the non-pregnant woman the normal size of the gap is 4–5 mm. Under the influence of the pregnancy hormones the pubic ligaments slacken and this gap increases by at least 2–3 mm during pregnancy. Therefore, it is considered that a total width of up to 9 mm between the two bones is normal for a pregnant woman. Following delivery, this natural extra gapping decreases within days, although the supporting ligaments will take 3–5 months to return to their normal state, making the symphysis pubis a strong joint again. An abnormal gap is considered to be 1 cm or more, sometimes with the two bones being slightly out of alignment, and remains evident after the time that the joint should have regained the normal non-pregnant width.

SPD refers to a dysfunction of the symphysis pubis joint. The symphysis pubis, along with the sacroiliac joints at the back of the pelvis, plays an important part in holding the pelvis absolutely stable during movements involving the legs and pelvis. Laxity of the pelvic ligaments may cause instability in the sacroiliac and symphysis pubis joints, and may give rise to the symptoms of groin and pubic pain. Although less serious than the DSP condition, symphysis pubis dysfunction necessitates appropriate attention.

The first trimester

In early pregnancy, usually the first 3 months (first trimester), many hormonal and physiological changes are taking place in the body.

Massage is unlikely to harm the fetus or disturb the natural processes. However, being such a delicate and important time for the expectant mother and bearing in mind that miscarriage (spontaneous abortion) is most common during the first trimester, it is advisable that any possible complications are avoided. Low back pain or pelvic pain may be one of the symptoms of spontaneous abortion and must not be mistaken for simple muscular ache. Consequently, lumbar massage for back pain is contraindicated. It is postulated by some authors that massage on the sacrum can lead to contractions of the uterus and to spontaneous abortion, and this is therefore specifically contraindicated. Support for this hypothesis is not readily available but this cautionary note to the massage is worth bearing in mind. Musculoskeletal pain in the lumbar area that abates with a change of posture or lying position may indicate that the pain is not referred from a contracting uterus. However, a cautious approach is necessary in all cases of back pain during this stage even if other possible causes such as soft tissue strains, spinal dysfunctions or urinary tract infections are ruled out. Massage on the abdominal area is certainly not recommended during this phase. Care may also be needed while there is still morning sickness or vomiting. Relaxing massage movements are otherwise of benefit.

Second and third trimesters

Changes to the posture and structure occur mostly during the second and third trimesters of pregnancy. Studies have shown that 48–56% of all pregnant women experience backache during pregnancy, mostly in the sacroiliac region but also in the lumbar and thoracic spine (Ostgaard et al., 1992). Understandably, there is an exacer-bation of discomfort, particularly in the pelvic area, during the last few months of pregnancy. Some studies indicate that the most uncomfortable period is between the fifth and ninth months (Ostgaard et al., 1992). The aetiology for the musculoskeletal pain involves a number of interrelated structures and postural changes:

- Backache is caused by several adaptations in the posture, which occur as the pregnancy progresses. To begin with there is an average increase in body weight of 30 pounds. The extra load is mostly at the front of the abdomen and chest, and is caused by the enlarged breasts, the uterus and the fetus. There is, however, systemic fluid retention as well as systemic weight gain and these all add to the extra stress on the structure.

- As the pelvis tilts forward from the additional abdominal weight the lumbar curvature deepens, creating a lordotic back and a shortening of the lumbar muscles and iliolumbar fascia. Weakness of the abdominal muscles is also a feature of these postural changes. With the anterior tilting of the pelvis the uterus also tilts forward and presses against the wall of the abdomen. If the pressure is excessive, or if the abdominal walls have weakened, a separation of the rectus abdominis at the linea alba (diastasis recti) may occur. Irritation of these tissues as well as other structures within the abdominal cavity can lead to myofascial trigger points referring pain to the lumbar and pelvic regions.

- Discomfort or pain can be felt in the region of the breasts, owing to the systemic weight increase and water retention. Massage to the pectoralis major and minor muscles can help reduce contractions, while gentle lymphatic drainage movements can help lower the fluid congestion.

- With the weight gain at the front of the body there is a shift of the centre of gravity, also in an anterior direction. For the pregnant woman to maintain her upright posture against this shift in the centre of gravity she has to recruit all the major postural muscles on the posterior side of the body. The paravertebral muscles in particular are used to counterbalance the weight at the front. Consequently the postural muscles of the back and neck become overworked, fatigued, nodular and likely to house trigger points (hypersensitive zones which are the source of radiating pain to other regions).

- The imbalance is compounded further by the pregnancy hormone relaxin, which softens the ligaments, the fascia and the tendons and, in so doing, causes instability of the lumbar and pelvic structures.
- Malfunction of the iliopsoas and of the piriformis muscles can occur if the pregnant woman walks with both legs laterally rotated in an attempt to steady her posture.
- Cramping may occur in the calf muscles, similarly related to the pregnant woman having to adjust her stance, in this case by hyperextending the knees to counterbalance the weight at the front.
- The body weight tends to be transmitted to the medial arches of both feet, causing pronation of the feet (a dropping of the medial arches). This biomechanical imbalance is often reflected in other joints of the lower limb as well as those of the pelvis and spine.
- The upper rib cage may be in a more posterior position to counterbalance the tilting of the pelvis anteriorly. This may then cause the head to shift anteriorly with perhaps some forward bending.
- A fetus that favours one side, left or right, exerts additional mechanical strain on that same side. This can lead to one-sided backache and the likelihood of functional scoliosis.

Several joints and structures are put under mechanical stress because of the weight gain, ligament laxity and postural changes:

- The intervertebral joints of the lumbar spine as well as the lumbosacral joint are susceptible to compression and restriction of movement. Entrapment or irritation of the sciatic nerve may result and this can lead to sciatica down one or both legs.
- The facet joints of the lumbar spine are likewise susceptible to mechanical strain.
- Ligamentous strain may affect the sacroiliac joints, owing to the anterior tilt of the pelvis,

and is exacerbated by walking (particularly with high heels), standing for too long and sitting without good back support. Hypermobility of one or both sacroiliac joints may develop. A disparity may also exist between the left and right sides, whereby hypermobility is found on one side and hypomobility is present on the other side. Dysfunction in the sacroiliac joint can lead to pain in any one of these regions: the upper medial buttock, the iliac crest or the posterior superior iliac spine. Weakness of the ligaments as well as inflammation of the cartilage is likely to lead to pain in the pubis symphysis (see Symphysis pubis dysfunction).

- The hip joints may become tender owing to the laxity of the ligaments, the resultant hypermobility, and the tendency for the lower limbs to be laterally rotated.
- Pain in the lumbar area, the sacrum, the glutei region, the thigh or the groin may be referred from the stretched uterine ligaments. These ligaments (two broad ligaments, two round ligaments, and the sacrouterine ligament) support the pregnant uterus and are subject to considerable stretching as it increases in size. Overstretching and mechanical stress of the ligaments can refer pain to other regions. The broad ligaments can refer pain to the lower back, the buttock and the sciatic pathway. Stretching of the round ligament can refer pain in the lateral region of the abdomen and the groin, sometimes extending to the pubic area and upper thigh. The pain is likely to occur on one side only, depending on the position of the fetus. Discomfort on either side of the sacrum or inferior to it may be referred from the sacrouterine ligament and is more likely to occur in the last 3 months of pregnancy.

Massage techniques

During the second and third trimesters massage to the back and legs is perhaps the most needed of all movements as it helps to ease the pain of overworked and fatigued muscles and to reduce trigger points. Several postures can be adopted when massage is given during pregnancy. The movements can be carried out with the subject lying on her side on the massage table. Cushions and bolsters are necessary to help support her and to ensure comfort and safety. If the pregnant woman lies supine the weight of the fetus is likely to exert pressure on major blood vessels such as the inferior vena cava; this posture is therefore best avoided. As discussed elsewhere, massage is also contraindicated with the patient lying prone. A large beanbag is a very good substitute to the treatment couch. The pregnant woman can lie comfortably on her side and the therapist can sit or kneel on the floor while carrying out the massage. Another posture of choice may be with the subject sitting on a stool or a chair and resting her arms on the massage table; this arrangement is very restful, albeit that it limits the massage to the back and neck.

The frequently used massage movements are effleurage (with the palms, the thumbs or effleurage *du poing*), petrissage and kneading. Percussive-type stroking such as tapotements are not applicable. The massage movements that can be applied during pregnancy are described in this section, with instructions and illustrations for some of the techniques. Other movements that are similar to those carried out on 'non-pregnant' subjects are referred to here but depicted fully later in the book (Chapters 5–10).

Massage techniques with the subject sitting

The lower and upper regions of the back can be massaged with the recipient sitting on a stool or chair (Fig. 4.1). In this posture she can also be leaning forward to rest her head, shoulders and arms on the treatment couch or an ordinary table of suitable height. A comfortable 'leaning angle' is adopted while ensuring that this posture does not create undue contractions in the muscles of the back. Cushions, folded towels and bolsters can all be used for additional support and comfort.

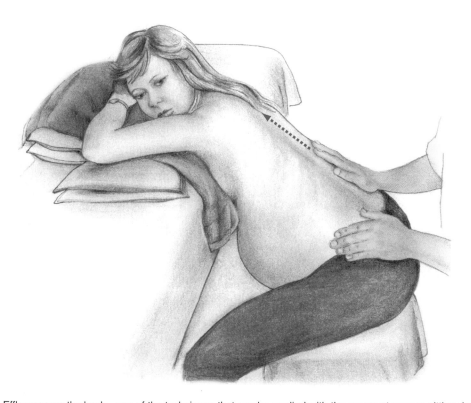

Figure 4.1 Effleurage on the back—one of the techniques that can be applied with the pregnant woman sitting down.

- Effleurage to the back is carried out with the massage therapist kneeling on one or both knees. It is applied to the lumbar and thoracic regions, moving in a cephalad direction, using one hand at a time or both hands simultaneously (see Fig. 4.1). Instead of kneeling, a standing posture can be adopted; this does, however, involve forward bending with some stress placed on the spine. An alternative is seated on a chair next to the patient.

- A slightly deeper and more local stroking on the muscles can be applied with the thumbs placed on each side of the spine (Fig. 4.2). The effleurage is carried out as simultaneous short strokes (5 cm) in a cephalad direction and is repeated several times on the same area. While the pressure is applied with the thumbs, the whole hand is moved in a cephalad direction, the stroking being applied with the thumbs in a slightly curved line rather than a circular movement. This technique is described as effleurage with the thumbs on the paravertebral muscles in Chapter 5.

- A variation to this technique is for the thumb stroking to be applied on one side of the spine at a time. Both thumbs are positioned on the side of the spine and the stroke carried out in a similar manner to that on the paravertebral muscles. When the treatment on one side of the spine is complete, the thumbs are placed on the other side and the procedure repeated.

- To stretch the lumbar muscles and fascia the effleurage *du poing* technique can be used. The hands are held in a 'fisted' position and a stroking action from the upper lumbar area is applied in a caudad direction, covering also the sacral area. The technique is described as effleurage *du poing* on the back in Chapter 5 (Figs 5.54 and 5.55).

- An alternative effleurage technique can be carried out in a caudal direction. The practitioner stands next to the patient and uses the fingers and palm of one hand, re-enforced with the other hand, to apply an effleurage stroke from about the middle of the back, downward toward the sacrum. The stroke is continued as far down as the sacrum or wherever is most ethically suitable. Can be repeated on the same side a few times before moving to the other side.

- The upper region of the back, the neck and upper shoulders can be treated with thumb effleurage. The thumbs are placed one behind the other, and on one side of the spine. Pressure is applied equally with both thumbs and a series of very short strokes is carried out (no more than 5 cm). The direction of the stroking can be along the fibres of muscles, for example the rhomboids. Massage can be performed across the fibres, for instance across the erector spinea muscles. The strokes are repeated as necessary and the practitioner moves their standing position as well as that of the hands to treat all the regions of the upper back.

- A kneading movement can also be used; this combines compression with the thumbs as well as a cross-fibre stretch. Compression is applied with the thumbs (lying flat to the skin surface) while counterpressure is exerted by the fingers on the anterior aspect of the trapezius and levator scapulae muscles. The tissues are held in this grip as the muscles fibres are rolled forward with the thumbs and stretched transversely, pinching of the tissues being avoided. The grip is then released and the sequence repeated. This technique is described as kneading of the upper side of the shoulder in Chapter 5 (Fig. 5.56).

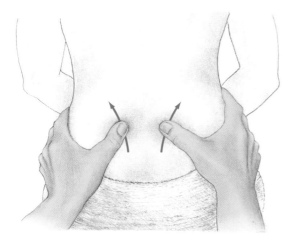

Figure 4.2 Effleurage with the thumbs in the lumbar region—simultaneous short strokes applied on each side of the spine.

• Passive stretch to the rhomboids. The practitioner stands on one side of the patient and reaches across to the contralateral scapula. The thumbs are placed along the medial border of the scapula, ensuring that no excessive pressure is exerted. The palm and fingers are placed on the upper and lower borders of the scapula so that a grip can be applied between the two hands. The thumbs are kept flat to the skin surface as the scapula is pushed away. It is possible to sense the stretch in the tissues after the slack has been taken up. The stretch is maintained for a few seconds and is then eased off; the procedure is repeated a few times.

Massage techniques with the subject side-lying

When the subject is in the side-lying position cushions and bolsters are needed to prop her up and prevent her from rolling onto her abdomen (Fig. 4.3). The uppermost leg should be supported in a horizontal alignment with the hip to avoid excessive side bending or rotation of the spine. A further consideration is that the side-lying patient may also require support underneath her trunk to prevent excessive scoliosis. Treatment procedures are planned so that the subject does not have to change position too often; this minimizes any painful stretching of the softened ligaments; for instance, those of the symphysis pubis. Some techniques that can be applied on the lumbar region in pregnancy are described in this section. Further methods for both the lumbar and the thoracic areas and which are also carried out in a side-lying posture are described in Chapter 5.

Effleurage is used to increase the local circulation, to reduce muscle tightness and to apply a longitudinal stretch to the muscle fibres and the lumbar fascia. Although a firm pressure is applied with these strokes, the massage is none the less relaxing and should not cause any discomfort. The movements are carried out very slowly, allowing about 6 seconds to complete each stroke. The thoracic, upper back and cervical areas are also massaged in this side-lying position, using effleurage and petrissage kneading techniques.

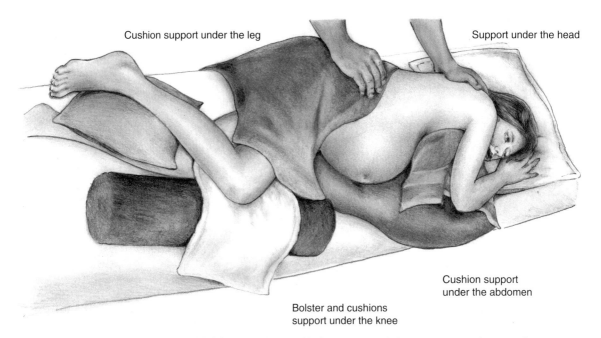

Cushion support under the leg

Support under the head

Cushion support under the abdomen

Bolster and cushions support under the knee

Figure 4.3 Massage with the patient side-lying—cushions and bolsters are needed to ensure a good support for pregnant women.

- *Palm effleurage movements.* The practitioner stands behind the patient at the level of the pelvis. One hand applies the massage and the other hand stabilizes the pelvis (Fig. 4.4). Effleurage is applied over the lumbar area and the stroke extended to the thoracic region. The direction of the movement is cephalad, commencing in the sacral region. The stroke is applied on the upper side of the spine but both sides of the spine may need to be massaged if the patient is not going to switch sides and lie on the other side. As well as straight longitudinal strokes, effleurage can be applied in a circular motion to increase the circulation (see also Fig. 5.37). An additional palm effleurage starting at the thoracic area and moving in a caudal direction over the lumbar and sacrum can also be included. This movement is particularly beneficial when stretching the lumbar tissues.

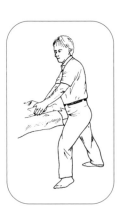

- Effleurage *du poing* (Fig. 4.5) can be used instead of palm effleurage, either to increase the pressure or to facilitate an easier stroking action. It is ideally suited to stretch the lumbar and sacral fascia as well as the muscles, thereby easing the stress of lordosis. In this case it is applied in a caudal direction. Effleurage *du poing* is applied by making a fist with the hand, with the fingers straight, and with the fingertips resting on the 'heel' of hand (see Fig. 5.38). The stroke is carried out with the flat surface of the phalanges and not with the knuckles. Pressure is applied by leaning onto the body, using body weight behind the movement. An upright posture is maintained as effleurage is carried out from the lumbar region in a cephalad direction. This is repeated several times. This technique is used on the upper side of the spine, being careful not to apply pressure on the spine itself. The movement can also be repeated on the lower

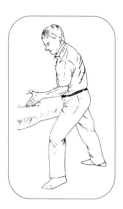

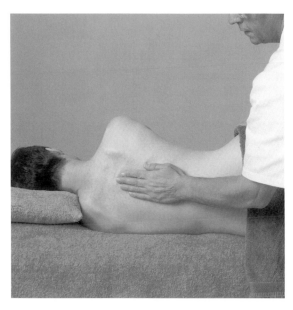

Figure 4.4   Palm effleurage on the back—the strokes can be carried out towards the head or as circular movements.

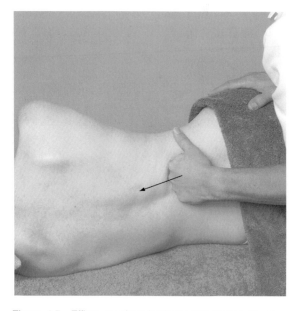

Figure 4.5   Effleurage *du poing* is used to apply a deeper stroke and to stretch lumbar fascia.

side of the spine, taking care to maintain good posture and applying the movement with ease. An additional and useful method is to apply the effleurage *du poing* in a caudad direction. The practitioner stands at the level of the thoracic region and uses the outermost hand, held in a fist, to effleurage the erector spinea muscles on the upper side of the spine, in the direction of the sacrum. The hand nearest to the body (i.e. the innermost hand) is placed on the pelvis and the body weight used to exert an equal pressure with both hands in a caudal direction. In this way a stretch can be applied to the posterior and lateral muscles and fasciae of the lumbar spine as the effleurage is carried out. The stroking is finished with the fisted hand on the sacral area to stretch the lumbar fascia (see Fig. 5.39).

- *Thumb effleurage*. An additional technique to ease the tightness in the muscles on either side of the spine is thumb effleurage (Fig. 4.6). The method is best applied on one side of the spine, using one hand. The thumb is kept flat to the skin surface and some pressure is exerted as the practitioner leans slightly forward. A short stroke is applied with the thumb, moving the whole hand at the same time. The pressure is eased and the procedure repeated. The thumb (and the hand) is moved very slowly along the muscle fibres. The stroke is repeated several times over the same region before the hand is placed on another area for the effleurage to be carried out again (see also Fig. 5.40).

Post-isometric relaxation   Two muscles that are likely to need addressing are the piriformis and the psoas. Both of these muscles are susceptible to tightness because of the postural changes and therefore benefit from easing off and stretching. Owing to the laxity of the ligaments it is therefore advisable that stretching is minimal or avoided altogether. Post-isometric relaxation (PIR) can produce sufficient relaxation without the need of a passive stretch. The method involves an isometric (static) contraction of the muscle against a resistance offered by the operator, which is held for about 6 seconds. This is followed by complete relaxation of the muscle and,

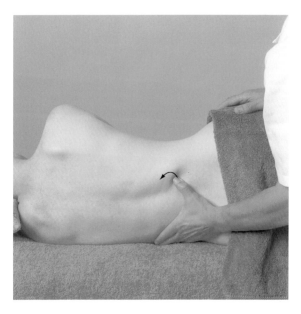

Figure 4.6   Thumb effleurage is used as an alternative method for treating small areas of tightness or dysfunction.

if necessary, by passive stretching of the same muscle. Muscle energy technique is described in Chapter 2. Two or three repetitions of the procedure may be required to achieve the desired relaxation. Treatment of the pelvic muscles, including PIR and stretching, is contraindicated in the case of symphysis pubis dysfunction (see Contraindications).

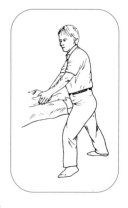

Massage techniques to the lower limbs

In the side-lying position the massage movements are carried out on the lowermost leg, which rests on the treatment couch. If desired, effleurage and petrissage movements can also be applied to the uppermost leg in a similar manner, without the subject having to turn over.

As well as being very relaxing, effleurage massage movements to the lower limbs assist the venous flow and reduce the build-up of fluid. The movements are generally carried out very slowly and with minimal weight. Sustained or deep pressure should be avoided at all times and in particular on the medial aspect of the thigh (bearing in mind the risk of blood clots in the great saphenous and femoral veins). Decreasing the congestion in the lower limbs lessens the possibility of varicose veins, albeit that the effleurage is omitted on areas where these have already developed. Effleurage and gentle kneading movements are also applied to the legs to ease cramps in the calf muscles.

Lymphatic techniques help reduce any build-up of fluid in the lower limbs. All the movements that are applicable during pregnancy are similar to those carried out on any subject. These are described in Chapter 6, in the section on Supplementary techniques for the lower limb (Figs 6.36–6.42). Passive movements of the hip joints can also be carried out, to maintain the suppleness, which would be of benefit during labour. It is vital to bear in mind, however, that, due to the laxity in the ligaments caused by the relaxin hormone, all joints can be potentially unstable. Any mobilizing technique, therefore, should only be carried out within the range of movement.

First stage of labour

- While some women prefer not to have any massage at all during labour, others find it beneficial. A sequence of massage movements can be pre-planned but more often than not the movements are applied according to the needs of the recipient; sometimes she may prefer deep pressure, while at other times only light stroking is requested, or no massage at all but assistance with the breathing. If applied, the massage treatment, whether carried out by the massage therapist or the subject's partner, has to fit in with the usual labour procedures and with the work of the midwife and doctors.
- During this stage massage is used first and foremost to reduce the anxiety and apprehension associated with labour and parturition. Sympathetic responses to anxiety, for instance,

can lead to increased tension in the uterine and cervical fibres (Read, 1972), subsequently giving rise to discomfort or pain. Relaxation on the other hand promotes the release of the opiates (endorphins and encephalins) while limiting the production of catecholamines.

- Massage also helps to relieve the pain of contractions, eases muscular tension and alleviates cramps (Chamberlain et al., 1993). Soothing techniques are carried out in between contractions to enhance relaxation and recovery.
- The areas where massage is applied can also vary. In the first stage of labour it may be the back, neck, legs (especially the thighs), hands and feet. Firm stroking is applied to the site of the contraction or pain, or as indicated by the subject. Slow and rhythmic movements are used, applied with the heel of the hand, with the distal phalanges held flat to the skin surface, with the flat palm and fingers or even with the thumbs and fist. Pressure can also be applied to the sacrum and buttock and is generally very effective in relieving the pain of contractions. It is worth noting here that this is in contrast to some viewpoints, as mentioned earlier, when massage on the sacrum is seen as causing uterine contractions. However, the massage is applied wherever it is needed, even on the abdomen. It can be performed early in labour, prior to and even following the first 5 cm of cervical dilatation. Gentle effleurage and circular stroking on the neck, back, hands and feet can be carried out for whatever duration is seen fit and repeated as necessary.
- Massage does not have to be contraindicated if a labour-inducing drug has been administered. It is vital to bear in mind, however, that if an epidural anaesthesia is used to ease labour pains the pressure of the massage stroking has to be carefully applied owing to the reduced sensitivity of the pain receptors. Some sensation can still be present, particularly in the feet, and foot massage therefore can be easily applied and very relaxing. It may also be indicated if the back and abdomen are not available, as can happen if fetal monitoring is taking place.
- Finding the best posture to carry out the massage may prove a challenge but not an

insurmountable task. Lying on the side is one choice, with the recipient propped up on cushions or a beanbag. Sitting on a low stool is good as it favours the pelvic position, the pregnant woman can rest her head and shoulders on cushions or a beanbag placed on the massage table or, if this is too high, on an ordinary bed. The massage practitioner can be standing or kneeling behind the subject. Kneeling on the floor is also a useful arrangement, with the subject leaning forward and supporting herself on a beanbag or cushions.

Second stage of labour

- In the second stage strong uterine and abdominal contractions are needed to expedite delivery. While this places great demands on her energy the subject is unlikely to want to have massage other than perhaps some soothing strokes to the forehead. Massage to the back would, in any case, be ruled out if she is lying supine. This option would be different if she is squatting or sitting on a birth chair. Furthermore, stimulation of the uterine muscles, rather than relaxation, is the main objective during this stage. Some gentle stroking on the abdomen may be tolerated and may be of use to help with the contractions.

Postnatal period

General application

- Provided that no complications occur, massage continues to be applied during the puerperal period (the first 6 weeks after childbirth).
- Systemic massage is carried out for the circulation and the elimination of residual fluid retention. Effleurage techniques as well as lymphatic drainage movements are applied on all regions. These are described in later chapters.
- Improving the systemic circulation has the additional benefit of improving tissue metabolism and oxygen supply, thereby renewing the energy levels.
- Emotionally, massage helps the mother to relax and adjust to her new role in life. Reducing

stress levels is also instrumental in stimulating the production of milk.

- Gentle colon massage techniques can be included if constipation persists, provided there is no abdominal tenderness. Massage to reflex areas such as the thigh and buttocks can also be carried out in addition to or as a substitute to abdominal movements (see Chapter 7, Figs 7.9 and 7.14).
- Back pain may persevere for some time following childbirth so treatment to this area is continued using deep thumb effleurage, effleurage *du poing* and the neuromuscular technique (see Chapter 5). In the case of severe back pain or sciatica, the postnatal patient may require treatment for misalignments of the pelvic, sacral or lumbar regions. Referral for spinal manipulation is therefore advisable.
- Effleurage and kneading movements are also carried out to the lower limbs to reduce cramps (see Chapter 6).

Precautions If there has been a caesarian birth, massage techniques on the abdomen are contraindicated until scar tissues are completely healed and the tenderness has abated.

Owing to the stretching and weakening of the abdominal muscles during pregnancy, the abdominal tissues must not be stretched during this period; stroking to these tissues is carried out from a lateral to medial direction only (see Chapter 7, Fig. 7.8). Petrissage on the abdominal muscles helps to improve the circulation to those muscles. When petrissage is applied to flaccid muscles and tissues it can help improve the tonicity.

Mastitis refers to inflammation of the breast and is common in women during lactation. The earliest sign is a triangular flush, generally underneath the breast, but there may also be a high temperature and increased pulse rate. This condition needs to be treated by a medical practitioner, while massage is contraindicated if there is a high temperature.

Menopause

The symptoms associated with the menopause, whether premenopausal, menopausal or during the late stages of menopause, can be alleviated by systemic massage. As abdominal massage tends to increase the blood pressure, it is omitted if it causes the patient to have hot flushes. On the other hand, trigger points can be housed within the abdominal wall which, when treated, provide considerable relief. Musculoskeletal pain is a common characteristic of the menopause, and is often persistent and severe. Gentle massage strokes are applied to help relieve the pain. In addition, treatment is applied to active and dormant reflex points. These are likely to be found in the occipital, cervical, interscapular, sternal and epigastric regions.

PAEDIATRIC

Premature infants

Premature infants are born as early as 26–28 weeks' gestation and, thanks to modern medical techniques, they often survive very well. At this early stage in their gestational life the infants need isolation in intensive care nurseries to help them overcome the dangers of disease. They are frequently susceptible to apnoea (pauses in the breathing lasting longer than 15 seconds) and bradycardia (slowing down of the heart beat); these symptoms can easily be caused or exacerbated by stress.

Handling of the baby in the neonatal intensive care unit was restricted in the past and indeed a 'minimal touch' policy still prevails in some departments. The therapeutic benefit of tactile stimulation is received more positively in certain hospitals and consequently it is encouraged and practised. A great deal of the research in massage for the preterm infant has been carried out by Dr Tiffany Field of the Touch Research Institute. Trials carried out as early as 1985 by Dr Field proposed that the use of tactile and kinaesthetic stimulation can have a profound effect on the development of the premature infant. It was found that infants who received massage and simple flexion/extension exercises did much better than those in a control group who received the standard nursery care. This and other subsequent research confirmed that the infants who received the tactile stimulation had a daily weight gain from 28% to 47% (Dieter, 1999; Field et al., 1986; Field, 2000). Explanations for the weight gain vary from stimulation of the vagus nerves, improved hormone activity and better food absorption. Activation of the vagus nerve enhances gastric peristalsis and is essential to the release of food absorption hormones such as insulin. The massaged infants were also more alert, and their behaviour matured at a faster rate than that of the control infants. Furthermore, attacks of apnoea and bradycardia occurred less frequently in the massaged infants. Stress was reduced in these infants, as determined by the low levels of the stress indicator cortisol. Improved alertness and activity in the preterm infant, demonstrated by increased limb movements and facial expressions, and resulting from the tactile and kinaesthetic stimulation was also reported in other research papers (Scafidi et al., 1986; 1990). It is apparent from these findings that the induced relaxation did not hinder the increased activity and alertness.

Supplemental stimulation for preterm infants is aimed at stimulating the sensory systems, and can be applied in a number of protocols such as tactile stimulation, kinaesthetic stimulation (e.g. passive movements of the limbs) and auditory stimulation (e.g. music and maternal speech). It was observed in some of the research that tactile stimulation such as massage, alongside other forms of stimulation, has been very effective in reducing stress. Evidence for the reduction in anxiety has generally been confirmed by a lowering in the stress indicators plasma and salivary cortisol, and urine levels of the catecholamines, norepinephrine and epinephrine. Reduced levels of serum cortisol, for instance, were recorded after tactile/kinaesthetic stimulation (Acolet et al., 1993). The changes in the levels of catecholamines are met with differing interpretations among researchers. As stated elsewhere, some researchers suggest that an increase in urine catecholamines in the adult are indicative of stress, whereas raised urine catecholamines in the preterm infant are significant of a normally developing brain. None the less, a general agreement does prevail about the reduction of stress from tactile stimulation. Other changes in the biochemistry of the preterm infant following supplemental stimulation were found to be an increase of bone mineral density, content and width (Acolet et al., 1993; Kuhn et al., 1991; Moyer-Mileur et al., 1995).

Contrary to the earlier fears of causing hypoxia, the touch of massage was found to have a tonic effect and increased oxygen consumption. The speedier improvement in these infants meant that they left hospital a week earlier than the control group (Field et al., 1986; Scafidi et al., 1990). Additionally, those pre-term infants who had received massage by their parents during the intensive care periods formed better bonds with them later on. Parents also showed greater interest in their children, and had better parenting skills and confidence.

Massage application
- Massage for the preterm infant is generally carried out to the head, shoulders, back, arms and legs (Field et al., 1986). Some areas, such as the chest and abdomen, can be too sensitive to touch. The feet can also be very sensitive owing to medical procedures; for instance, the insertion of needles to obtain blood for testing. However, most of the discomfort in these areas is caused by memory of the procedure rather than the massage itself. As babies get used to the idea of being touched, they will react more positively to it. In certain areas of research a positive pressure of stroking was found to be the most effective, particularly for vagal stimulation (Scafidi et al., 1986). In other studies, the only protocol of tactile stimulation was that of gentle stroking (Adamson-Macedo et al., 1994). An even less invasive procedure of tactile stimulation used in other clinical trials was the laying on of the hands upon the infant's head, lower back and buttocks (Harrison et al., 1996). Various research has compared the outcomes of tactile/kinaesthetic stimulation and those of other protocols such as gentle human touch. Reaching a conclusion as to what is the most effective is not important, taking into consideration that all research findings are significant and that data is frequently renewed. One suggestion is that the suitability of the protocols will vary from one infant to the next and throughout the treatment period for a particular infant.

Full-term normal infants

Of course, massage is not restricted to the preterm infant since it can equally be of benefit to the full-term baby of normal weight. One study looked at the effects of massage on babies who were under 3 months old and of normal weight and whose mothers were single, adolescents and suffered some degree of depression. Infants whose mothers suffer from depression generally show some degree of growth delay. The massage was carried out by a trained massage therapist during the time the infants were at a day nursery and the protocol, unlike that for the preterm infant, included massage to the abdomen, chest and face. Findings included increased alertness, weight gain, improved temperament and better sleep. A reduction in stress was confirmed by a fall in the levels of urine cortisol, norepinephrine and epinephrine and an increase in serotonin (Field, 2002).

Drug-exposed infants

Massage has been beneficially used for infants who have been exposed to drugs during their life *in utero*. These infants are born addicted to the drugs, with physiological and psychological problems. For example, they are unable to interact with others or receive comfort. They are also very irritable, are neurologically disorganized, poor eaters, and spend most of their time sleeping or crying. Making contact through the touch of massage helps them relate to another person and to relax slowly. In accepting the comforting touch of massage and feeling secure, these infants can release their emotions and heal.

Massage application
- The choice of massage techniques is dictated by the response of the infant. By 'listening' with their hands and feeling for reactions, the massage therapist can adjust the strokes accordingly. In addition, the therapist needs to be alert for any distress signals from the infant, and terminate the massage session if necessary.

Stress signals that can be observed include high-pitched crying, yawning, sneezing, frowning, gaze aversion and repeated extension of the spine (Griffith et al., as cited by Webner, 1991). Positive results have been achieved with preterm drug-exposed infants. A 10-day massage programme carried out on cocaine-exposed preterm infants who were still in the neonatal intensive care unit showed an increase in weight gain (with elevated insulin levels), improved motor function and orientation performances and fewer stress behaviours (Field, 2000). Similar results were also obtained with HIV-exposed infants.

The hyperactive child

The disorder of hyperactivity, which affects many children, is very saddening to observe and frustrating to deal with. There are a number of very distinctive and characteristic features in this disorder. Among these are aggressive behaviour, extreme emotional behaviour, lack of concentration, constant movements, anxiety traits (such as biting the finger nails) and a low pain threshold. The children themselves are generally unaware of their own behaviour, and are therefore unable to make changes. They end up feeling frustrated and rejected by their peers. Depression is also common, as is low self-esteem and, therefore, lack of self-confidence. Massage can be effectively applied, in conjunction with other modalities such as visualization and biofeedback technique, to help induce relaxation.

Massage application
- Gentle soothing effleurage is used to ease tension in the muscles and to fulfil the child's need for touch and closeness. In this way, the child does not feel isolated. The touch and closeness may lead to the child being able to verbalize feelings, rather than acting them out (Stewart and Wendkos Olds, 1973). As the child becomes used to the massage and is more trusting of the therapist, the massage techniques can address the deeper muscles and other areas where emotional tension is held. Releasing the deeper tensions helps to reduce fatigue. The massage is usually given by the

massage therapist, but the parents can also learn to use some basic movements. These can be applied as optional methods for calming the child during periods of agitation. In addition to reducing the stress levels of the hyperactive child, massage can do the same for carers and, in particular, the parents.

MULTIPLE SYSTEM CONDITIONS
Cancer

Cancer refers to the unregulated and disorganized proliferation of cell growth. It has many forms and is described in different terms, such as a malignant tumour, carcinoma or sarcoma. The exact cause of cancer is not yet established, but contributing factors include a weak immune system and certain carcinogens. Cancer tends to spread, or metastasize, to other areas; it can invade the surrounding tissues or disseminate to distant sites through the circulatory and lymphatic systems. Symptoms relating to cancer may come to light before a diagnosis is made; for instance, while taking the case history or during the massage treatment. Undoubtedly this eventuality necessitates tactful advice from the massage practitioner.

Warning signs include:

- Changes in bowel or bladder habits
- A superficial sore that does not heal
- Unusual bleeding or discharge
- A fixed lump in the tissues (mostly commonly found in the breast)
- Difficulty with swallowing or unexplained indigestion
- Unexplained loss of weight
- A wart or mole that becomes irregular in shape or bleeds
- Persistent coughing or hoarseness
- Unrelenting pain
- General malaise
- Temperature changes
- Unexplained heat or inflammation
- Unexplained weight changes.

Traditionally, massage has been contraindicated in cancer patients because of the risk of metastasis through the lymph, and in some cases the vascular, systems. Despite the great concern that massage may encourage the spread of cancer, no evidence has thus far been presented to confirm that this actually happens. Caution is still necessary, however, and prevention of any complications must always be a primary goal.

Massage is seen less of a risk in the terminally ill patient or following mastectomy.

The appropriateness of massage therapy for the cancer patient is dependent on several aspects of the condition, including the type of cancer, whether it is active or in remission, and whether it is terminal. Also to be considered are the types of massage movements to be carried out, the purpose of the massage and whether the massage is local or systemic. Obvious prerequisites for massage treatment are that the massage practitioner is well-trained, and that consent has been given by patients, their family and doctor. Furthermore, the massage therapist must be well aware of the various cancer treatments (surgery, chemotherapy or radiotherapy), their side-effects and the necessary precautions.

Situations where extreme vigilance is necessary:

- A person living with cancer may have a very weak immune system caused by the condition or, indeed, by the treatment itself. Leukopenia, for example, is a side-effect of cancer treatment that leads to an abnormal decrease in the number of white blood cells and, consequently, the patient can be very susceptible to viruses and bacteria. It follows that, if a massage practitioner is suffering from any form of illness (even a cold), massage on a cancer patient is ruled out.
- The cancer patient can suffer from thrombocytopenia (low platelet count) following treatment with chemotherapy and radiotherapy. This condition causes the tissues to bruise easily and, accordingly, heavy massage movements are omitted. If need be, the massage is limited to one or two regions—for example to the hands, face and shoulders or feet.
- Massage movements that would be used for increasing circulation are best omitted in

patients with cancers that metastasize easily through the lymphatic system and blood vessels, like melanoma and Hodgkin's disease.
- Alopecia, or loss of hair, is another common side-effect of cancer treatment, and this can naturally be very disturbing to patients. They may therefore benefit a great deal from the support during this emotional period, and may even find comfort in the massage to the scalp itself.
- A similar situation arises if the treatment involves surgery. Some surgical procedures are less traumatic than others. Needle biopsies and bone marrow aspirations, for instance, are easier to deal with than mastectomy and amputation.
- In the former two cases, massage can be resumed a day or two after the procedure, although the site of the needle biopsy or bone aspiration is avoided.
- Massage after surgery involving removal of a larger amount of tissue, such as lumpectomy (removal of a cancerous mass from the breast) or mastectomy, requires a very cautious approach. The trauma is caused not only by the physical discomfort that follows surgery, but also by the person coming to terms with an altered self-image. The gentle emotional support provided through massage can help facilitate this process.

Massage application

- As a general rule, massage is applied to help relieve the perception of pain, reduce anxiety and increase relaxation. Another benefit of massage is the emotional support it provides for the cancer patient. This is the same whether massage is given over the whole body or to a small region like the hand. Clinical research has indicated that touch is extremely important in the healing process, as it invariably creates a feeling of caring and wellbeing in the patient. Emotional support for the person living with cancer is invaluable from the very onset of the condition. For instance, great anxiety prevails while the person is waiting for test results; this increases considerably if a positive diagnosis is made.

- Provided that no contraindications are present, massage can be applied carefully during the treatment period and afterwards, when palliative care commences. It is used to relieve some of the symptoms, such as fatigue and pain, and to continue the emotional support. Gentle massage techniques, primarily effleurage, are used on the patient living with cancer. As noted earlier, pain reduction is one objective of the stroking; emotional support is another. Consultation and approval of the patient's general practitioner is always advisable.
- One study showed that techniques of effleurage, petrissage and trigger point work were found to reduce the levels of pain perception by an average of 60%. Anxiety levels were also reduced by 24%. The patients' subjective reports (measured by visual analogue scales) indicated an increase of 58% in the enhancement of their feelings of relaxation. Physiological measures such as heart rate, blood pressure and respiratory rate were also found to decrease from baseline readings. These changes provided a further indication of relaxation in the subject (Ferrell-Torry and Glick, 1993).
- Massage can be of benefit in the treatment of cancer because of its effect on the natural killer (NK) cells and their activity (cytotoxicity). Studies with HIV patients showed that daily massage treatment can increase the number of NK cells and killer cell cytotoxicity (Ironson et al., 1996). A similar positive effect is likely to occur with cancer patients. A study on the effects of massage on women with breast cancer was carried out at the Touch Research Institute (USA), headed by Tiffany Field. The study was conducted on women who had undergone mastectomy and completed chemotherapy and radiation treatments. Data collected during and after the 5-week massage programme indicated a very positive effect on immune function, with an increase in NK cells (NKJH1). It was also reported that the mechanism underlying the improvement in immune function may be related to a lowering of cortisol levels (Field, 2000). NK and other immune cells can be destroyed by the hormone cortisol (Ironson et al., 1996) which becomes abundant with stress (Zorrilla et al., 1996). Various research has shown, however, that the high levels of cortisol, as well as epinephrine and norepinephrine resulting from stress can, in most cases, be reduced through the relaxation offered by massage (Field et al., 1996a; Ironson et al., 1996; Acolet et al., 1993). In the study carried out on women with breast cancer, anxiety and depression were reduced following the programme of massage treatments (Field, 2000).

Contraindications   As with other conditions, massage has its limitations and contraindications. These include:

- Directly over a tumour or over nearby lymph nodes that may connect to it.
- Areas that are receiving radiotherapy become very sensitive to touch, and stroking the skin can therefore cause discomfort. Accordingly, massage is not put to use on irradiated areas. Another reason is that irradiated skin is very fragile, and is liable to be damaged with the massage. The areas of treatment must also be kept free of oils and lotions, which could interfere with the radiation.
- Chemotherapy can lead to nausea and vomiting; if this is the case, massage is unsuitable.
- Massage in the areas of lymph nodes is avoided.
- As a general rule, areas where there is active disease are best avoided so as not to increase the blood flow or metabolic rate. Other regions of the body may be massaged, particularly to promote relaxation.

Acquired immunodeficiency syndrome

Acquired immunodeficiency syndrome (AIDS) is caused by infection with the human immunodeficiency virus (HIV), which attacks the immune system by infecting the human T lymphocytes. The weakened immunity has a devastating effect on all the systems of the body, with resultant multiple infections and conditions. In the acute stage, the sufferer is subject to fever, rigors, arthralgias, myalgias, rash, abdominal cramps and diarrhoea. Subsequent problems range from meningitis to pneumonia. Advanced treatment with drugs has reduced the death rate from this disease, and has reduced the severity of some symptoms. The application of massage is indicated, provided the patient is not suffering from any condition that contraindicates treatment.

Assisting the immune system by removing toxins is, beyond any doubt, the most essential need for the AIDS patient, and massage can therefore be used for this purpose. It does, however, need to be applied very gently, and with constant feedback from the recipient. Relaxing massage techniques are also of great benefit to reduce anxiety and promote healing. Studies carried out on HIV patients indicated that positive improvements in immune function were recorded following a programme of massage treatment (Ironson et al., 1996).

Systemic lupus erythematosus

Systemic lupus erythematosus (SLE) is an autoimmune disorder that leads to the production of autoantibodies and immune complexes. Their effect is seen on a number of systems, including the muscular, integumentary, pulmonary, cardiovascular and renal.

While the aetiology of this condition is not quite established, it is more common in women, especially those still of childbearing age. Oestrogens are seen as favouring its development, while androgens tend to protect against it. There may also be genetic factors and triggers such as ultraviolet light, chemicals, drugs, food allergies and infections.

Apart from the characteristic 'butterfly rash' over the nose and cheek which is seen in the acute stage, the symptoms of SLE are similar to other disorders. For instance, joint pain and chronic inflammation of the joints as well as joint deformity are similar to those of rheumatoid arthritis, and indeed this can be a further manifestation of the condition. Inflammation of the kidneys (glomerulonephritis), fluid collection in the lungs (pulmonary effusion) and inflammation of the membrane surrounding the heart (pericarditis) are further complications of the disease. Mental–emotional disorders, such as depression or dementia, are also possible in the advanced stages.

Massage application

- People with this condition are often very keen on self-help programmes and are therefore agreeable to massage treatments. Relaxation is always of great benefit and therefore a whole body massage can be carried out. Gentle joint mobilization can also be included provided that there is no joint inflammation. Massage is also contraindicated on any tissues that are inflamed or hypersensitive. It is also important to bear in mind that the patient's drug regime can impair their immune system and make them susceptible to infections. Most massage movements, except percussion strokes, can be used to induce relaxation, improve circulation and reduce adhesions around joints. Petrissage and friction movements help to improve muscle tone and prepare the muscles for exercise.

MASSAGE IN SPORTS

Massage has a notable history of efficacy in the field of sports, and is consequently sought by the majority of athletes. The methods used to address muscle fatigue and tightness in the field of sports are the same as those in any other situation. Any divergence exists only in the application of the techniques for well developed muscles, and a number of these techniques are included in the massage for particular areas of the body in the following chapters. A further prerequisite for massaging the sports person is an awareness of the psychological aspects of competing. It is important to bear in mind that some aspects of the treatment, such as injuries and rehabilitation, fall into the realm of sports medicine and, consequently, require the expertise of a sports therapist. Massage in sports has now become a specialism for those interested in this field of work and this is too vast a subject to cover within the scope of this book. It is, however, good practice for those massage therapists not specializing in sports massage to be familiar with the basic principles and the common injuries associated with sports. Such knowledge is necessary to provide adequate treatment for the sports person. For the same reason, it is important that the aims of massage in sports are well defined.

The common injuries in sports involve one or more structures, depending on the type and extent of the injury. Some of the most likely tissues to be damaged are:

- *Muscles*. Muscle strains are common in most sports and occur if the tissues are over-stretched, contracted and stretched at the same time, or worked for long periods without sufficient rest.
- *Fascia*. This connective tissue forms the protective layer around the muscle fibres, the muscle bundles, and the whole muscle. It also goes on to form the tendons and the aponeurosis that acts as an insertion. Because of its close association with the muscle, fascia tears whenever there is a muscle strain. It can also become quite contracted and then prevent full stretch of the muscle. The level of pain and disability that results from a muscle strain is dependent on the degree of the injury.
- *Ligaments*. These tissues are used to maintain the tightness between the bones that make up a joint. They can strain from traumatic contact during sports or from twisting of the joint (as in an ankle sprain).
- *Tendons*. A muscle strain is sometimes located not in the belly of the muscle itself but in its tendon. An example of this is tennis elbow where the tendon insertion into the lateral epicondyle of the humerus is irritated, inflamed or torn.
- *Bursae*. The function of these structures is to prevent friction between two surfaces, mostly a tendon and bone. Unless inflamed they are two flat layers of tissue with synovial fluid in between. Bursitis (inflammation of a bursa) is the most common sports injury and is often related to overuse of a joint or muscle. A frequent example is supraspinatus bursitis, which is related to any sport where there are repeated arm movements.
- *Menisci*. These structures are located between the femur and tibia. Their function is primarily as a shock absorber and they are susceptible to tear when there is excessive torsion in the knee joint.
- *Bone fractures*. Although not very common, fractures can result from traumatic injuries. A hairline fracture can also occur in sports but this is mostly associated with overuse.

Treatment of injuries

Massage can be applied for the treatment of injuries and during the rehabilitation period. Muscles, ligaments and tendons can be treated as early as a day or two after the injury, although the type and duration of treatment depends on the severity of the injury. It may therefore be the case that the massage therapist has to work closely with a sports therapist during such times.

Massage application
- As a general rule, effleurage strokes are employed to increase the nutrients and repair materials in the injured tissue and thereby promote healing. Venous and lymphatic massage techniques are used to drain away the oedema associated with the injury. These movements are employed to alleviate pain by reducing the pressure within the tissues and removing the products of inflammation.
- Muscle tightness is a common compensatory mechanism to trauma. Sustained spasms cause fatigue and give rise to further pain. Massage techniques such as kneading and petrissage movements are used to ease the tension and free up the tissues as well as the associated joints.

Massage during training

- During periods of training and between sports events, massage is used to help maintain the peak performance of the muscles.
- Effleurage techniques are essential to remove metabolites and toxins produced by muscle activity.
- Deep thumb effleurage is applied to reduce nodular formations.
- Petrissage and kneading are employed to ease muscle tightness, and to free up any adhesions within the muscle or between adjoining

structures. Flexibility is maintained with passive stretching.

Pre-event massage

- Before a training session or sports activity, the muscles are first warmed up with the accelerated movements of effleurage and friction.
- Petrissage is also applied as a toning and warming up technique, carried out with little pressure but with rapid movements.
- Further stimulation of the muscles is next achieved with percussive strokes.
- All these methods are alternated with one another, and are repeated several times.
- Passive stretching of the long muscles, such as those of the upper and lower limbs, is included once the muscles have warmed up.
- Athletes must also carry out their own active stretching routine.

Post-event massage

- After the vigorous activity of exercise, the muscles are congested with metabolites such as lactic acid, carbon dioxide and water. These by-products can exacerbate fatigue and impair muscle function. Massage movements, mostly effleurage, are used to assist with the elimination of these toxins and to restore oxygen and nutrients to the muscles. It is, however, advisable that massage treatment is not carried out immediately after a training or sports activity. This precautionary approach is taken because the blood vessels, particularly the veins of the lower limbs, are engorged with blood following the exercise. As the walls of the vessels are stretched by the high pressure of the blood, they are susceptible to damage when handled. About 30 min should elapse before the massage is applied, although this time lapse is more relevant in some sports than others.
- Cramps are also common during or immediately after exercise. In marathon runners, for instance, cramps are often seen in the lower limbs. These are best reduced by a resisted contraction of the antagonist muscles rather than with massage.

PSYCHOGENIC DISORDERS

Introduction

Some of the 'psychogenic disorders' that are covered in this section are essentially manifestations of emotional angst such as depression and stress. The symptoms of some other conditions can be more complex and may have psychogenic as well as neurological characteristics, e.g. behaviour problems. Behavioural disorders take into account dysfunctions where the subject, in most cases a child, has difficulty with maintaining alertness, communicating, social skills, physical contact and so forth. Research into the use of massage therapy for these patients is limited but does indicate that massage can lead to some positive changes.

Emotional dynamics

In addition to the familiar stressed person, the massage therapist may be treating someone who is going through a complex and emotionally sensitive situation. It is therefore important that the therapist can recognize signs that point to emotional disturbances such as anxiety and depression (Box 4.4). While massage can be of benefit in such circumstances, it does not address the underlying factors. These are best worked through with a counsellor. Furthermore, the massage practitioner has to define his or her exact role in the overall treatment programme to avoid being overwhelmed by the emotional situation.

Box 4.4 Signs and symptoms of underlying emotional states

- Fatigue
- Inability to concentrate
- Disturbed or lack of sleep
- Headaches
- Muscle pain and stiffness
- Digestive signs such as upset stomach, diarrhoea and constipation
- Weight loss or gain
- Palpitations
- Breathing difficulty

If the massage sessions are continued over a period of time, a good rapport invariably builds up between clients and the therapist. This is significant in the healing process, because it indicates that clients are able to trust and 'open up' to another person. Building up a relationship with the therapist gives clients a feeling of being accepted and cared for; it also increases their self-esteem. They may feel secure enough to start talking about their feelings, perhaps for the first time. This is doubtless a good development; expressing feelings is much better than suppressing them or turning them against oneself. Emotions such as anger and resentment may be hidden and begin to show up as clients heal. As already discussed, however, the massage therapist must be aware of how much he or she can or should handle, and may need to encourage clients to talk to a trained counsellor or psychotherapist.

Massage is of immense benefit in several 'emotional' situations provided that its goals and limitations are well defined, both to the therapist and the patient. It can be applied in general mental–emotional states such as postnatal depression, bereavement, anxiety, withdrawal from drugs, anorexia, sexual abuse and panic attacks. While these emotional traumas have different aetiologies, the goal of the massage is more or less common to all of them. People under any form of mental–emotional stress can benefit from touch, support and relaxation. Some are likely to gain more than others; the extent and quality of the response depends on the character of the individual and the circumstances.

Touch

Touch in itself is of tremendous value, and conveys an immediate message of caring, acceptance, nurturing and support. It is an essential factor in establishing a feeling of self-worth in recipients. Accepting touch is a big step in the process of emotional healing, demonstrating that subjects are beginning to like themselves and to trust another person. It also helps to heal their psyche, and enables them to cope better with their problems or circumstances. Touch is also valuable in forming a bond between mother and baby; this closeness can be missing in some mental–emotional situations such as postnatal depression. Another benefit of touch is that it lessens the fear of imminent events, for instance in preoperative patients. Anxiety has been found to be similarly reduced in intensive care units by the touch of massage.

Relaxation

Relaxation is essential in counteracting many of the mental–emotional states, and massage is one of the best methods that can be used for this purpose. Its soothing effects can be enhanced with the addition of essential oils; however, these do not necessarily suit every individual and should only be used by a trained therapist. It is noteworthy that, while relaxation is of great value, it may not be appropriate in certain situations. Clinically depressed people are very lethargic and unmotivated; further sedation can therefore be counterproductive, and massage is only carried out with the approval of the patient's counsellor. A similar precaution is needed in postnatal depression. The mother may not want to be touched at all, in which case massage cannot be carried out. The anorexic person, however, may find difficulty in relaxing and the massage is consequently of great benefit.

Massage application

- Effleurage and other massage movements can be carried out in a soothing manner and with relaxation in mind. The choice of strokes is dependent on the therapist and, in many ways, the recipient. As a general rule, light effleurage stroking is applied with alternating hands and in a continuous fashion: that is, as one hand finishes a stroke the other hand starts to massage. On the neck and back the movements are carried out in a caudal direction, which is more relaxing for the nervous system. Techniques such as vibrations and gentle kneading movements can also induce tranquillity.
- The cranial hold (see Chapter 10) is an extremely relaxing technique that is carried out with the patient supine.
- Another very effective procedure falls into the realm of bodywork. It is the simple 'rocking' movement, which is as instinctive as the

stroking of effleurage. As the recipient lies supine or prone, the whole body is gently rocked from side to side. The manoeuvre is carried out by placing one hand on the pelvis and the other on the ipsilateral shoulder. A gentle push is applied with one or both hands; this action rocks the body towards the contralateral side, and the hands are immediately partially lifted off to allow the body to recoil. This is repeated, and in this manner the body is rocked from side to side, the movement and the resultant relaxation being synonymous with that of a baby rocking in a cradle.

- Massage to the hands and feet is very soothing, and can be of enormous value when the patient is unable or unwilling to receive any other massage movements on other regions of the body; for example, patients in intensive care and those suffering from very advanced cancer or who are terminally ill.
- One movement that is often neglected for its relaxing effect is massage to the head. This simple technique is extremely relaxing, and has the advantage of easy application with the recipient in the sitting position. It should be included in all massage strokes for insomnia, anxiety and so forth.

Mind–body connection

Tension in the muscles is frequently evident in anxiety. In some cases, the tightness is subconsciously used as a form of 'body armouring' or 'guarding' against the outside world. With a recurrent or prolonged anxiety state, the muscle tightness can become chronic and characteristic of the posture. Such a postural change can influence the whole body and be difficult to reverse. Tension in the muscles can also exacerbate other symptoms such as headaches, pain, difficulty in breathing and panic attacks. Massage is applied to ease the muscle tension and reverse the 'holding on' of rigid postural patterns.

Breathing

Difficulty in breathing can be a feature of stress and, even more so, of anxiety attacks. The experience in itself can be frightening, and thus causes further stress. During an attack, massage to the back can be applied to help calm the person and restore a relaxed breathing pattern. A convenient and comfortable arrangement is for the recipient to be sitting and leaning forward, resting the arms on a table. Massage is carried out on a regular basis in between anxiety attacks. The continued relaxation promotes a more comfortable breathing pattern and helps the subject to become more at ease.

Insomnia

Another symptom of stress is insomnia, which is both distressing and leads to fatigue. The relaxation that massage induces in the recipient is often followed by deep and uninterrupted sleep. Essential oils can increase the efficacy of the massage treatment. Lavender oil, for example, has been found to increase alpha brain-wave activity, which is an indication of a restful mental state (Tisserand, 1992). Promoting sleep in this natural way reduces the need for sedation with medication. Sleep is important to recover from fatigue and to enable the person to cope with stress; it also speeds up the healing process.

Massage for promoting sleep is ideally carried out before the patient retires to bed, although this is not always a feasible option for the massage therapist. However, some basic movements can be carried out by a family member or friend. The massage therapist can offer some basic instruction in carrying out simple effleurage strokes on the neck and shoulders. At other times the massage is performed by the massage therapist, using a number of techniques. Effleurage is essential; the strokes are continuous and are applied at a steady rhythm, not necessarily slowly. Gentle vibration movements are also included, and can even be combined with the continuous effleurage stroke. If the patient is in the sitting position, the strokes are carried out from the occiput or neck area towards the shoulders. Other massage techniques are also applied to the head, face and hands. The same routine can be carried out with the patient lying down. Rocking movements complete the massage treatment for insomnia.

Connecting with the body

The continual thinking processes that are so much a part of anxiety mean that, in some mental–emotional states, subjects may be living not so much in their bodies as in their heads. As a result, the body is 'ignored' or rejected; this is even more so if the aetiology of the condition was related to some form of physical trauma such as sexual abuse. By appreciating the physical movements of massage, clients are able to 'make contact' with their bodies once more. One such situation arises when a client is undergoing a drug withdrawal programme. In addition to making contact with the body, massage brings the person to a point where the mind can heal. By accepting the massage, clients are also accepting their own body and themselves. Such a step is essential in situations where surgery has been performed, as in mastectomy.

Changing the body image

A step on from connecting with the body is that of changing the body image. Anorexia provides a good example. This very complicated and delicate condition is not truly an eating disorder, but rather one of deep-rooted insecurity about the self and the outside world. In an attempt to gain some control, the anorexic person exercises restraints on food intake. The internal turmoil is deepened by a distorted body image, which is created through self-doubt and lack of self-worth. Agreeing to massage indicates that subjects are accepting themselves and, in turn, are changing their own body image. This transition is a vital aspect of recovery. It also applies in many situations, such as cancer and bone marrow transplant, where subjects wrongly see themselves as having a 'debilitated' body. Accepting the body and its image is likewise a vital step to recovery in cases of sexual abuse. In all these situations, massage helps subjects to build up a new body image and, in so doing, to restart the process of loving themselves.

Autism

Among the characteristics of autism are disinclination to make physical contact, unwillingness to relate socially with others, inability to maintain concentration, atypical responses to sensory stimuli such as sound, and irregular behaviour patterns. The outcomes of one study that was carried out with a group of preschool autistic children (average age 4.5 years) indicated that massage therapy can have some very positive benefits for these children (Field, 2000). Following the massage therapy programme, the study showed that the physical contact of massage was accepted, the social interaction had improved, the level of attentiveness had increased, the typical autistic behaviour such as sensitivity to sounds was also reduced, and the irregular behaviour patterns had changed. One explanation for the improvements is based on other studies which showed that massage therapy can stimulate vagal activity (Field, 1990) and that alertness and maths performances are improved following massage therapy (Field et al., 1996b).

Depression

A study on the effects of back massage carried out daily for a 5-day period was carried out on hospitalized children and adolescents suffering from depression and adjustment disorders (i.e. behavioural problems). Symptoms associated with these conditions include anxiety, muscle tension, increases in cortisol levels and sleep disturbances. In addition to their confinement, exacerbation of stress in these children was considered to be related to touch deprivation. Assessment criteria included self-reports on anxiety and depression, behavioural observations, activity levels, heart rate, saliva samples for cortisol, urine samples for cortisol and catecholamines (norepinephrine, epinephrine and dopamine), and time lapse videotaping of sleep patterns. The study revealed a decrease in anxiety, deeper sleeping sessions and improved cooperative behaviour following the 5-day period of daily massage treatments. Saliva cortisol was reduced but only during the massage, whereas urinary cortisol levels were reduced over the 5-day period, especially in the depressed group. Levels of urine norepinephrine were also reduced over the 5-day period in the depressed group. No changes in epinephrine and dopamine were recorded (Field et al., 1992).

Post-traumatic stress

Post-traumatic stress disorder following natural disasters or human-induced disasters is common in adults as well as in children. Symptoms including stress, anxiety and behavioural misconduct often result from the trauma and can last for months. A study on 60 school children (average age 7.5 years) who were suffering from post-traumatic stress (in this case following a hurricane) was carried out at the Touch Research Institute. The purpose of the study was to determine whether massage therapy might reduce the anxiety and depression levels of the children as measured by a number of factors, including behavioural observations, the children's drawings and their cortisol levels. A 30-min massage treatment which consisted of moderate pressure and smooth stroking on the neck and back, was carried out twice a week over a period of 1 month. The study showed that the children had less anxiety and depression after the massage, and that there were also reduced saliva cortisol levels. Their self-drawings and behavioural conduct were also more positive and their relaxation level ratings were higher than before the massage. A very noteworthy observation was made that the children may have benefited considerably from the physical contact of massage because they may have been deprived of physical contact by their parents who themselves may have been suffering from post-traumatic disorder. It is not clear whether the benefit of the massage diminishes once the massage treatment is discontinued, but very positive immediate effects emerged after the treatment (Field, 2000).

TOXICITY

Toxins

Toxins are noxious or poisonous substances which can be harmful to the body. They are mostly made up of plant or animal matter but can also include inorganic elements or compounds, some of which are essential and form the mineral constituents of cells. These compounds or trace elements include aluminium, calcium, phosphorus, potassium, sulphur, sodium, chlorine, magnesium, iron, fluorine, iodine, copper, manganese and zinc. Although they largely exist in a harmonious stability, an excess of one element, such as aluminium, can be harmful to the body.

The most common group of toxins to occur are those produced by bacteria. These are either released by micro-organisms (referred to as exotoxins) or occur as a result of the bacteria being destroyed (known as endotoxins). Toxins can be located within the tissue cells or in the interstitial spaces. They can also be transported in the blood. For instance, poisonous substances that are produced by bacteria growing in a local or focal site can be distributed throughout the body via the circulatory system, leading to the condition of toxaemia. The generalized symptoms of toxaemia include fever, diarrhoea, vomiting, and changes in the pulse rate and in respiration.

A distinction can be made between toxins that are endogenic, i.e. generated within the body as a result of infection or during the normal process of metabolism, and those that are exogenic, introduced into the body. Exogenic toxins can enter the body through the skin as in the case of a bee sting, a snake bite or an open wound. They can also be taken in through the mouth in the form of fluids, e.g. alcohol (intoxication), foods, drugs, chemicals, preservatives, additives and so forth. It is noteworthy that even a high protein diet can result in highly toxic products, including ammonia, phenols and hydrogen sulphate. Furthermore, toxins can also result from poor digestion of proteins. It is one belief that some toxic materials are released into the body by certain procedures in dentistry and, to an extent, conventional medicine. Typical examples are metals such as mercury, palladium and nickel, as are chemicals such as formaldehyde (a colourless poisonous gas, made by the oxidation of methanol). Allergic materials such as pollens are also poisonous and invariably cause a hypersensitive reaction that is either transient or cumulative in nature. Environmental pollution is one certain way of introducing airborne poisons into the body; the insecticide organophosphate is one such primary suspect.

The extent of toxic poisoning can be assessed by the severity and number of symptoms that accompany the condition (Box 4.5). Laboratory tests, especially those for investigating metals such as mercury, are used to provide more specific evidence. Investigations include blood tests such as the memory lymphocyte stimulation assay test and the saliva IgA test for immune function, as well as a urine test for liver function (Hall and Winkvist, 1996). The immune function can often be linked to stress, and it is generally accepted that continual stress weakens the body's immune system and consequently exacerbates the effects of toxins. Other conditions that can be associated with toxicity are numerous; some of these, however, go undiagnosed as their symptoms are often attributed to other disorders.

Treatment of toxicity

Toxins that are circulating in the blood are normally eliminated through the colon, kidneys, lungs, liver (via the bile), mucous membranes and sweat glands in the skin. Other toxins, including bacteria and minute particles such as coal dust, are transported and neutralized by the lymphatic system. Toxic substances can also bind to proteins in the interstitial tissues, where they are broken down by the action of phagocytes.

Box 4.5 Conditions that may be caused by toxicity

- Autoimmune diseases
- Multiple sclerosis
- Chronic fatigue syndrome
- Lethargy and muscle fatigue
- Psychogenic states, e.g. anxiety, depression, claustrophobia
- Cancer
- Colds
- Joint pain
- Arthritic changes
- Fevers
- Skin eruptions
- Digestive disturbances

In treating toxicity it is first necessary to identify all the substances that have caused or are causing the accumulation in the first place. While it is imperative to avoid such harmful products it is not always feasible to remove them entirely from the diet or from the environment. A bigger problem concerns medication for an illness; this cannot and indeed must not be stopped without the approval of a doctor or without appropriate substitute or treatment. Some diet changes are easy to implement, albeit that they are best carried out under the guidance of a naturopath or clinical dietitian. Fasting is one of the best methods of eliminating toxins, but this too requires similar supervision when it is undertaken for more than a day or two. Supplementation with minerals, especially sodium ascorbate (Vitamin C), and with herbs is also effective. All these factors must be taken into consideration before, or alongside, the massage treatment.

Effects and application of massage

Massage is beneficial in the treatment of toxicity as it helps to relieve some toxic symptoms, such as headaches, myalgia and fatigue. It also improves the function of the organ or system affected. The use of massage for detoxification dates back to the origins of Swedish massage when the 'Movement Cure', a treatment regime that included exercise and massage, was advocated for general health. The 'Movement Cure', as Swedish massage was then called, proposed that great benefits were to be gained from detoxification of the systems and therefore from good circulation, good oxygenation, drainage of the colon, reduction of oedema, and stimulation of organs such as the liver and kidneys.

Improving the digestion

Regular emptying of the bowels is an all-important element in the treatment of toxicity and for this reason it is essential that the digestive system functions well and that good peristaltic action is maintained. Diet changes may be necessary to improve the function of the bowel while massage to the abdomen and colon may also be needed to reduce constipation. Digestion is also improved with massage and, with this, the metabolism of nutrients and antioxidants which is needed to neutralize the toxicity. Further assistance is provided by the transportation of lymphocytes and phagocytes that takes place with the enhanced blood circulation and lymph flow.

Improving the circulation

- Massage is first applied to improve the circulation systemically to secure a good nutritional supply to all tissues. It is also used to enhance the venous return, which is essential for the removal of toxins.
- Toxic substances that may be circulating in the body can also affect muscle tissue and may lead to inflammation and pain. Muscles also produce their own toxic by-products, including lactic acid, carbon dioxide and water. Elimination of these products is more rapid when the circulation through the muscles is improved and, to this end, techniques such as effleurage and petrissage are indicated.
- Circulation to the visceral organs can be enhanced using petrissage and effleurage movements to the abdomen. Specific visceral methods such as compression massage for the liver and kidneys are also of use (see Chapter 7).
- Toxins can infiltrate the periarticular structures of joints and may create inflammation and pain. Gout is one example, albeit an extreme one, where there is a toxic build-up in the periarticular soft tissues such as the ligaments and tendons. A 'gouty-joint' is too painful to massage, but in most other conditions effleurage is used to increase the venous return and the arterial flow to and around the joint. Transverse friction movements are also suitable for improving the circulation to the periarticular structures.

Enhancing the lymph flow

The lymphatic system is given considerable attention in the treatment of toxicity. Massage movements for the vascular and lymph circula-tion are applied to reduce oedema and improve the flow in the lymphatic vessels. A primary goal therefore is to reduce congestion in the interstitial tissues, where the formation of oedema is most likely. In the presence of congestion, the circulation to the tissue cells is diminished, and this in turn slows down their nutritional supply and metabolism. The congestion has the additional effect of preventing the removal of toxic wastes from the interstitial spaces. Increasing the lymph flow, on the other hand, has the benefit of delivering nutrients to the tissue cells, transporting lymphocytes to combat bacteria, neutralizing toxins and improving drainage. It is important to bear in mind that, if a viral or bacterial infection has caused severe inflammation, lymph massage is contraindicated until the acuteness has abated, to avoid spreading the pathogen.

Improving kidney function

The nephrons of the kidneys are the physiological filters that remove toxins from the blood. Among these toxins are uric acid (which is a naturally occurring product of catabolism), nucleic acids (which are derived from food or cellular destruction), and benzoic acid (which is a toxic substance in fruits and vegetables and is believed to be eliminated from the body in the form of hippuric acid). Massage, applied systemically and also locally to the kidney area, increases the circulation to and from the kidney, thereby improving the filtration and elimination processes. As noted above, systemic lymph massage has a similar function.

Improving the liver function

A major function of the liver is to destroy worn-out blood cells, bacteria and toxic substances. It also removes drugs like penicillin, ampicillin, erythromycin and sulphonamides. The liver is said to be a semi-solid organ that is encased by a fibrous capsule and, as it is largely protected by the rib cage, direct manipulation is limited to its lower borders. The organ is, however, influenced by external pressures such as those exerted by the diaphragm from above, an adjoining viscus or, indeed, that of palpation. Compressive massage movements as described in Chapter 7 exert sufficient pressure through the tissues to influence its circulation. Massage can also assist the portal circulation to the liver through the hepatic portal vein. It increases the oxygenated blood supply to the liver via the hepatic artery. Circulation is enhanced along the lobes of the liver, along the central and hepatic veins, and to the superior vena cava. Secretion of bile is augmented to some extent by the advanced blood flow and by the mechanical pressure of the technique.

Assisting respiration

Full movement of the rib cage and deep breathing are both necessary for the unrestricted uptake of oxygen and the elimination of gaseous toxins. To this end massage movements are carried out on the muscles of respiration, in particular to the intercostals, the pectoralis minor, the sternocleidomastoid, the scalene group (scalenus anterior, medium and posterior), the rectus abdominis, the serratus posterior inferior and superior, and the levator scapulae.

Elimination of toxins through the skin

The skin is an organ of elimination and consequently skin eruptions are an indication of toxic-

ity and the body's attempt to eliminate them. This process can be assisted by the massage movements that increase the circulation to the skin and decongest the pores. Effleurage movements are of particular use. The skin rolling technique is another effective method as it involves a compression and upward stretch of the superficial tissues, primarily the skin and subcutaneous fascia (Fig. 4.7).

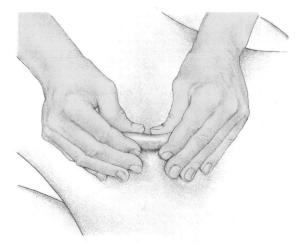

Figure 4.7 Skin rolling—the tissues are lifted off the underlying structures and rolled between the fingers and thumb.

5

Massage for body regions—the back

OBSERVATIONS AND CONSIDERATIONS

The general condition of the back is assessed before any massage. This procedure applies in particular if the patient is presenting with pain in the back. While the discomfort may be superficial, involving only the soft tissues, it may also be symptomatic of an underlying condition, possibly even one that contraindicates massage. The patient's posture is first considered during the taking of the case history; it can also be observed when they are moving about, getting on to the treatment table and lying down. Movements that the patient finds difficult to carry out or that cause obvious pain are noted and recorded. Observation of the spine may reveal changes such as scoliosis, which is related to changes in the muscles. Imbalances or malfunctions that can be addressed with massage may also be observed in the musculature of the back. Some of the more common considerations associated with the back are discussed in this section.

Spinal curvatures

Lordosis in the lumbar area may be observed when the patient is lying prone; the spine can be lordotic without the corresponding lumbar muscles being in a tense state.

Congenital scoliosis is acquired at birth or during the early years. It is generally noticeable in both the upright and lying down postures. If the scoliosis is functional, it can change with the posture; consequently it may be prominent in the standing position but less so when the person is lying prone.

Kyphosis of the thoracic spine may likewise be more noticeable in the upright posture, especially if it is caused by problems in the lumbar spine. When the person is lying prone, the curvature may be reduced.

Hypertrophied muscles

The musculature of the back may show differences between the muscle groups. Muscles on one side of the spine may be hypertrophied when compared to the corresponding group on the opposite side. Over-developed muscles can result from repetitive physical activity, and can also be indicative of overuse. Subconscious contractions of the muscles can occur; for instance, if the body is attempting to correct imbalances in the posture. Rotation of the spine or irregularities of the rib cage can give a false impression of hypertrophied muscles on one side of the spine.

Muscle atrophy

Atrophy of the muscles can be a sign of insufficient nerve supply. This in turn can be associated with musculoskeletal problems, or with pathology that affects the nervous system. Atrophied muscles will not respond to techniques such as percussive strokes if an underlying nerve impairment is present; they can, however, benefit from the improved circulation and stimulation.

Psoriasis

This condition, of unknown cause, shows itself as dry and itchy patches on the skin; it may also be accompanied by chronic back pain. Plenty of oil or cream is first applied to the back if massage is to be carried out. The treatment may be contraindicated in cases where there is bleeding of the blemishes.

Back pain

In describing back pain, it is necessary also to enlarge upon its various forms and causes. Discomfort in the region can range from a dull ache to a sharp pain. It can be localized to one area, or can radiate to other regions such as the groin or the leg. Movements can exacerbate the pain or, indeed, alleviate it. Some of these problems fall into the realm of the more specialized musculoskeletal therapies; however, a number of the causes can be discussed within the scope of massage treatment.

Lumbago

Lumbago is synonymous with chronic back pain, and describes a non-specific dull ache across the loin area. At times, lumbago is persistent with no apparent cause; however, the most likely factor is the formation of nodules and adhesions, which impinge on nearby nerves. Massage is used to increase the local circulation and to relax the muscles. Deep effleurage and cross-friction techniques are of particular use for the reduction of nodules. The tissues can also be manipulated and lifted off the underlying structures; this helps to reduce the adhesions and to stretch the muscles and fascia.

Muscle tension and fatigue

Tightness of the muscles and fascia is the primary cause of back pain, generally a 'dull ache'. Muscle tightness that is felt on palpation may be caused by extensive physical activity; for instance, a sporting pursuit. This is invariably accompanied by muscle fatigue. A similar situation may arise after a period of gardening or decorating, or from long periods of travelling. Allowing for such factors, there should still be a certain amount of 'yield' when the muscles are palpated. Muscles which are 'held rigid' are indicative of anxiety, muscle strain or a disc problem.

Psychogenic factors causing back pain

Anxiety and depression are frequently associated with acute or chronic back pain; other regions may also be involved. Headaches and lethargy are also common symptoms of anxiety and depression.

Muscle strain

A strain of the lumbar muscles is a common occurrence, and results in acute and severe pain when the sufferer attempts to carry out certain movements. Bending forward is perhaps the most frequent movement, involving mostly the extensor muscles of the back; twisting or rotating the trunk is a similar manoeuvre, which causes the rotator muscles to stretch and contract at the same time—this also occurs when the sufferer is turning over while lying down. Pain is also elicited when the subject attempts to get into and out of a car. If the rupture is severe, the pain is elicited on palpation of the muscle and as the patient attempts to move or turn over on the treatment table. Complications such as spinal misalignments and a herniated disc may also be present in addition to the strain.

Widespread muscle spasm is likely to spread across the back. This occurs as a spontaneous and subconscious protective mechanism, and acts like a splint. Massage to relax the muscles is therefore counterproductive. The sufferer may manage to get onto the treatment table for the massage treatment; however, on attempting to move or get up again all of the back muscles may go into sudden spasm. The patient may end up being 'stuck' in one position. If this unfortunate situation arises, heat is applied to relax the muscles as the patient is assisted into a standing position; he or she is then advised to rest for a few days and to seek advice from a doctor. In the acute stage cold packs can be applied on the area of injury to reduce the pain and oedema. The muscle can be treated after the acute stage to prevent adhesions and excessive scar tissue formation.

Misalignments of the spine

In some cases of back pain, two or more adjoining vertebrae may be misaligned. The misalignment or loss of mobility in these segments can lead to irritation of the nerve root(s) emerging from between the vertebrae. Corresponding muscles respond by contracting in an attempt to correct the abnormal posture. Back pain occurs as a result of the nerve root inflammation and the sustained contraction of the muscles. Misalign-ment of the spinal column can be genetic and fixed, but more often it is episodic and results from bad posture or from scoliosis, bad lifting or strenuous activities. The condition can be moderate or even asymptomatic; on the other hand, it may be sufficiently painful to require treatment. Palpation of the spinous processes can be used as a simple indicator of misalignments and immobility. A gentle pressure applied to the lateral side of the spinous process is likely to elicit pain if that segment of the spinal column is misaligned or malfunctioning; the more severe the discomfort, the more acute the condition is likely to be (Fig. 5.1). Massage is indicated to deal with the associated muscle tightness but not as a means of correcting the deviations; however, spontaneous corrections of the spinal alignments can often follow the muscle relaxation. The treatment is contraindicated on areas of considerable pain or if there is very severe radiating pain to the limbs.

Sciatica

A nerve root emerges through the intervertebral foramen, i.e. the aperture between two adjoining vertebrae. Dysfunction of the vertebral column can alter the integrity of the foramen, causing nerve root irritation and sciatica (see also Chapter 4). Occipital neuralgia and radiating pain down the arm are of a similar nature.

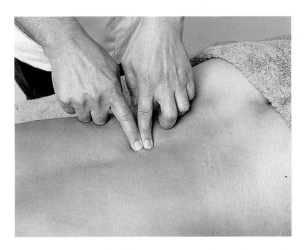

Figure 5.1 Palpation of the spinous processes. Pressure is applied to the lateral side, towards the midline.

Hypersensitivity in the superficial tissues, usually the dermatomes near the spine, is another common consequence of the nerve root irritation. Massage is contraindicated along a nerve route if it is inflamed (as occurs in sciatica). It is also carried out with great care or omitted altogether on hypersensitive areas close to the spine.

Intervertebral discs

Herniated or prolapsed discs present with severe pain, mostly in the lumbar area, which can make even the tiniest movement extremely difficult (see also Herniated disc in Chapter 4, p. 135). Pronounced tenderness is found in the region of the dysfunction and along the dermatomes. All of these symptoms are severe and should immediately prompt the massage therapist to refer the patient to a doctor. Massage is therefore contraindicated, particularly on the area of the lumbar spine involved and along the path of nerve pain. Cold packs may be beneficial until the patient receives the appropriate treatment.

Osteoporosis

Osteoporosis refers to a loss of bone substance, leading to brittle and weakened bones. These changes can affect any bone, but the vertebral bodies are most susceptible and can undergo compression and collapse. In mild forms of osteoporosis the subject is able to move without discomfort; in more advanced stages there is pain on movement, and in severe cases the patient is unable to lie down. Palpation of the spinous processes can bring on the pain; this may be difficult to differentiate from the pain associated with misalignments of the spine or that of nerve root problems. However, the muscle spasms that accompany misalignments are not always present in osteoporosis. Massage to the back is none the less contraindicated in severe cases of osteoporosis.

Osteoarthritis of the spine

A frequent cause of back pain, especially in those who have reached middle age, is osteoarthritis of the vertebral column. The lumbar and cervical areas are the worst affected segments. While inflammation is not always present, the pain of osteoarthritis can be chronic and is exacerbated by activity. The patient is likely to be pain-free while lying down, but experiences great discomfort on attempting to rise and move about. Massage is indicated for this condition, as it does not involve movements of the spine. Effleurage techniques are used to increase the circulation to the muscles as well as to the joints; they also help to reduce any muscle tightness that may develop as a protective mechanism to the arthritic changes. Congestion may be prominent around the spinal column; this is treated with deep thumb effleurage. Cross-friction movements are applied across the fibres to reduce the adhesions of the soft tissues that can also develop close to and around the joints. In more advanced stages, and in some sufferers, the muscles may show signs of weakness. These tissues are more sensitive to pressure because of the reduction in bulk, and all massage movements are therefore carried out with this in mind. Spondylitis (arthritis) of the cervical area is a very painful condition, in which most movements can cause great discomfort, and massage is best avoided or applied only lightly owing to the fragility of the bony structures and vascular vessels. Rotation, side bending or flexion movements of the neck are to be avoided.

Rheumatoid arthritis

Rheumatoid arthritis is a systemic inflammatory condition affecting the joints and other tissues. The spine is not always affected at the onset of the condition; if there is involvement, however, palpation of the spinous processes will elicit pain. In the early stages of the disease the patient may still be able to lie down on the treatment table, although with some discomfort. As the condition progresses, this position becomes less comfortable, and the massage is carried out with the patient in the sitting position. Systemic atrophy of the muscles occurs because of the reduced mobility; massage is therefore applied with minimal pressure, and only during the non-inflammatory periods. The benefits of the massage are to increase the circulation, reduce pain, relax the patient (stress can bring on an attack) and maintain some tonicity in the musculature. Treatment is contraindicated during periods of inflammation.

Ankylosing (rheumatoid) spondylitis

This is a progressive disease similar to rheumatoid arthritis. It affects mostly the costovertebral and sacroiliac joints, which are tender on palpation. Ankylosing (immobility and fixation) of the back gives rise to the 'poker back', and sclerosis or fusing of the sacroiliac joints leads to immobility and low back pain. Muscle stiffness and shortening are likely to occur alongside the spinal column. Massage is indicated to improve the circulation, decongest the area and facilitate stretching. However, if the condition is chronic, massage may be ineffective and may even cause discomfort; in this case it is contraindicated.

Circulatory conditions

Heart problems can refer pain to the shoulder, chest, arm and back. The pain of angina, for instance, is felt in the midline of the back or in the area of either scapula. Tissue changes, for example tension relating to heart function, can extend to the whole left side of the thoracic region. The lower border of the rib cage is likely to be tight, as well as the area between the left scapula and the second and third thoracic vertebrae. If the circulation is systemically impaired, the tissues of the back will feel cold and dry. Conversely, an elevated blood pressure, the intake of alcohol or a fever can cause the tissues to redden and feel hot. Another circulatory condition that can cause back pain is an aneurysm of the aortic arch, which refers pain to the mid-back; an aneurysm of the abdominal aorta can refer pain to the lower back. Myocardial infarction, however, is rarely a cause of back pain. Massage is indicated to increase the venous return and assist the function of the heart. Unless it proves uncomfortable, massage on areas of referred pain and tissue changes can help improve heart function via reflex pathways. Hot packs have the effect of increasing local circulation as well as relaxing the muscles.

Oedema

Oedema can often be observed and palpated in the lower back and the sacral region. The fluid build-up may be hormonally influenced in women (for example, premenstrual tension and pregnancy); it may also be associated with obesity, which can cause disturbances in the circulation and fluid retention. Inflammation is another cause, whether it is of the soft tissues, nerves or joints. Hodgkin's disease is a condition that can result in back pain because of the disturbances in lymph flow as well as the enlargement of the lymph nodes, spleen and liver. Right heart failure leads to fluid retention in the sacral area and, more significantly, in the legs and elsewhere. In this condition the muscle contractions on the right side of the heart may be too weak to pump the blood through to the lungs, and a back pressure in the veins builds up, which then causes fluid retention. Massage is indicated to the sacral area to enhance the lymph drainage, and gentle effleurage movements can be carried out on the back to assist the venous return. The treatment is contraindicated if there is persistent oedema, or if there is severe heat or tenderness on palpation; these symptoms could indicate an underlying condition that may require further investigation.

Visceral organs

Pathology or severe malfunctioning of a visceral organ can cause referred pain, and frequently muscle spasms, in distant regions. Examples affecting the back include the following.

1. Problems in the liver and gallbladder can cause:

- Referred pain in the right side of the neck.
- Referred pain in the right scapula at the inferior part of its medial border.
- Tissue changes in the right thoracic region; at the lower border of the rib cage on the right side; and in the area between the scapula and the spine on the right side at the level of the fifth and sixth vertebrae.
- Congestion at the level of the seventh cervical vertebra.

2. Stomach malfunction can refer pain to the upper thoracic area of the back. The tissues involved are those of the central region, between the fourth and ninth vertebrae. Changes in the tissues may also extend to the whole of the thoracic back, on the left side; for example, gastric ulcers and gastritis can cause tissues changes in the left scapula region.

3. Constipation can cause tightness and tenderness in the region of the piriformis muscle. While massage to this area can be applied to encourage bowel movement, the changes in the tissues must not be mistaken for a malfunction of the piriformis muscle.

4. Other visceral organ malfunctions or conditions that can refer pain or cause tissue changes to the back include obesity, ulcerative colitis and pancreatitis.

Massage is indicated to reduce the referred pain and enhance the function of the associated organ via a reflex pathway. It is, however, contraindicated if palpation of these referred pain areas causes very severe discomfort. A local malfunction of the musculoskeletal tissues may also be present; this would need further assessment and treatment.

Headaches

Aches and pains in the head can cause tissue changes in some regions of the back. The changes are mostly tight zones in the midline tissues, which can also be tender to palpation. Massage is applied to these tissue zones for its reflex effect on the head area. Changes occur in the following tissue zones:

1. The middle thoracic area, in between the two scapulae—this area is often related to headaches and insomnia.
2. The central area of the spine at the level of the lower rib cage.
3. The lower region of the sacrum, which can be related to headaches arising from disorders of the digestive system.
4. The occipital border, which is often related to tension headaches.

Respiratory conditions

Conditions of the respiratory system that can cause back pain include carcinoma of the bronchioles. The left lung (and possibly the right) as well as the diaphragm can also refer tenderness and pain to the back. Carcinoma of the oesophagus can have a similar effect. The regions involved are the left side of the upper thoracic area and the upper side of the left shoulder. Massage applied to these regions helps to improve the function of the related organs.

Kidney malfunction and pelvic conditions

Infection of the kidneys can lead to pain in the lower back and trunk, extending also to the lateral borders of the buttocks and upper thighs. The pain can resemble that arising from spinal misalignments, nerve root irritation or lumbago; the difference, of course, is that these disorders are not accompanied by the proteinuria and haematuria of kidney infection. The ureters descend from the kidneys and pass deep to the transverse processes of the lumbar spine, and tenderness on palpation of the paravertebral muscles may therefore be that of ureteralgia and not of muscular origin.

Kidney infections are generally accompanied by heat in the lumbar region. Oedema is another characteristic; it can be local, systemic or in the lower limbs. There may also be systemic toxicity, which can intensify the pain; as a result, the hypersensitivity can extend to the upper back. Massage to the kidney area on the back is contraindicated if there is a known kidney condition or if the area is very tender to palpation. It can otherwise be carried out for its reflex effect. General massage can be applied as it enhances the systemic circulation; it also stimulates kidney function. Massage to the abdomen has the same effect and is likewise indicated.

Kidney disorders can also cause renal colic, with spasm in the region of the kidneys and towards the thigh. The passage of a calculus is accompanied by pain radiating from the kidney region and over the abdomen into the groin. In renal colic, massage on any of the referred pain areas (maybe extending to the anterior abdominal wall) is likely to be uncomfortable and is therefore contraindicated.

Some of the other conditions involving the urinary and reproductive systems that can cause back pain include:

1. Cystitis
2. Pregnancy
3. Malfunctioning ovaries
4. Dysmenorrhoea
5. Pelvic abscess
6. Chronic cervicitis
7. Carcinoma of the kidney
8. Pyelonephritis
9. Infection or new growth of the prostate.

Cancer

Chronic back pain can result from a primary or secondary tumour of the spinal canal and nerve roots, often associated with Hodgkin's disease or myeloma. Massage, both local and systemic, is contraindicated.

MASSAGE TECHNIQUES FOR THE WHOLE BACK REGION

Introduction

For all of the massage movements on the back, unless otherwise indicated, the patient lies prone, with the head turned to one side or resting in the face hole. If the treatment table is not fitted with this opening, support the patient's forehead on a folded towel. Place a cushion under the patient's abdomen to avoid excessive extension of the lumbar spine, and a second cushion underneath the chest. Use a bolster cushion or a rolled up towel to raise the ankles and support the feet. The arms can rest on the treatment table or hang comfortably over the edge.

Soft tissue stretching

Effects and application

- Palpation of the superficial tissues (skin, subcutaneous fascia, deep fascia and musculature)

can reveal tightness, restrictions and hypersensitivity.
- Tightness can be palpated as taut tissues, which are unyielding to longitudinal or transverse stretching.
- Restrictions can be felt as reduced or absent 'gliding' between two layers, mostly in between the superficial and the deep fascia.
- Hypersensitivity may be present in the same areas of restriction and tightness. All of these tissue changes may result from one or more stressors (e.g. organ malfunction, mechanical stress). Stretching techniques are applied as a way of assessing for these tissue changes. The same movements are also used to help normalize the tissue dysfunction. Skin rolling can also be used to assess tightness and sensitivity. These movements are best carried out without the use of lubricants. Some of the effleurage strokes, especially those with the forearms, have a similar stretching component to them when carried out with minimal lubrication.

Practitioner's posture

Forearm stretch. Stand in the upright posture, with the feet slightly apart and the body weight equally distributed on both feet. Lean forward to reach over to the contralateral side of the back. Lean slightly so that you can apply pressure, at the same time avoiding any strain on your own back.

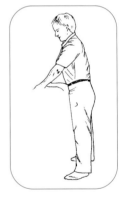

Procedure

Position the forearms on the contralateral side of the back, one forearm on the lumbar region and the other in the region of the scapula (Fig. 5.2). Exert a gentle pressure on the tissues by leaning forward slightly. Without any sliding of the forearms, apply a slight stretch to take the 'slack'

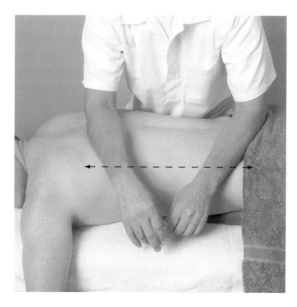

Figure 5.2 A longitudinal stretch is applied with the forearms on the contralateral side of the spine.

out. The stretching is achieved by pushing the forearm on the scapula level toward the head, and the forearm on the lumbar area toward the pelvis. Assess the 'give' in the tissues and hold the position for a few seconds to increase the stretch. Release the tissues and repeat the procedure a few times. Move round the treatment couch to repeat the stretching technique on the opposite side of the back.

Light stroking technique

Longitudinal effleurage

Effects and applications

- Light stroking effleurage is implemented to induce relaxation in the patient.
- It enhances the systemic flow of blood and that of lymph.
- Circulation is improved in the musculature of the back.
- The light stroking effleurage can be repeated several times. It can be applied as a warm up to other massage techniques or carried

out as a finishing manoeuvre.

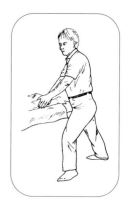

Practitioner's posture

Stand in the lunging posture, with one foot slightly behind but in line with the other; this position allows you to shift your body weight backwards and forwards. In order to effleurage the back in this posture, you will also need to rotate your upper body. Bear in mind that over-rotating your trunk can easily put your own back under stress.

Procedure

Position the hands on the lower back, one hand on either side of the spine (Fig. 5.3). Make contact with the palm and fingers of each hand. Keep the hands relaxed throughout the movement; this helps you to palpate and assess the tissues as well as monitoring the patient's response. Effleurage with both hands in a cephalad direction (towards the head). Apply pressure by shifting your body weight to the front leg (you will also need to flex the knee) and adding a force through your arms. Move the hands at a steady rhythm, taking about 5 seconds to reach the upper back, then separate the hands and slide them laterally towards the shoulders. Cup each hand and massage round the shoulder, maintaining the pressure. Trace the hands down the left and right borders of the trunk, while shifting your body weight onto the back leg to release the pressure. Continue the stroke to the iliac crest and then finish on the central region of the lower back. Repeat the whole routine several times. Massage the muscles close to the spine and then position the hands further laterally away from the centre to massage the outer group of muscles. Use a very light pressure to begin with, particularly if you want to emphasize the relaxation aspect of the movement. Light pressure also benefits the superficial circulation (vascular and

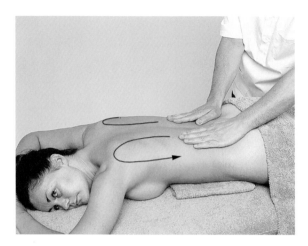

Figure 5.3 Longitudinal effleurage to the lower and upper regions of the back.

lymph). Apply a heavier pressure to increase the deeper circulation and to reduce tightness in the musculature.

Light stroking technique

Criss-cross effleurage

Effects and applications

- This technique, applied with very little pressure, is particularly relaxing.
- It is effective in increasing the circulation to the whole of the back region.
- The movement can also be applied with a heavier stroking action, and can therefore be carried out as a kneading-type stroke to all the muscles of the back.

Practitioner's posture

Stand on one side of the patient. Start in the upright posture with the feet slightly apart and the body weight equally distributed on both legs. You can also use the t'ai chi posture as

an alternative position, or interchange this with the upright posture.

Procedure

Place the hands on the lower back, one on the ipsilateral side and the other on the opposite side of the spine (Fig. 5.4). Apply the effleurage across the back, guiding the hands past each other as you move them to opposite sides, then repeat the stroke in a reverse direction. Carry out the criss-cross effleurage slightly further up the back, overlapping the previous stroke, and continue with this pattern all the way up the back. At the top of the back, extend the effleurage stroke to the shoulders and the upper arms. Repeat the series of strokes all the way down the back.

Shift your body weight slightly onto your cephalad leg (nearest to the head) as you effleurage up the back. You may also want to flex the knee slightly if you are in the upright posture. As you effleurage down the back, shift your body weight onto the other leg. The rhythm of the criss-cross effleurage is fairly slow and relaxing, taking about 3–4 seconds to travel from one side to the other; a faster speed will have a stimulating rather than a relaxing effect.

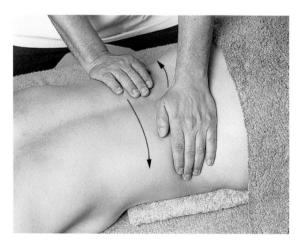

Figure 5.4 Criss-cross effleurage to the lower and upper back.

Deep stroking technique

Effleurage with reinforced hands

Effects and application

- The benefits of these movements are akin to those of other effleurage methods; however, a heavier pressure can be applied with this method. This is invariably needed for the deep muscles of the back, to ease any tightness and improve the circulation.
- This heavy pressure is also used to stretch tight fascia and to reduce any nodules (knotted areas).
- The muscles that benefit most from this technique are those close to the spine, i.e. the paravertebral muscle group as well as the rhomboids and the trapezius on either side.

Practitioner's posture

Position yourself to the side of the treatment table, standing in the upright posture and with the feet slightly apart. Massage the ipsilateral side of the spine and then move round the treatment table to work on the opposite side. For this movement, the patient's head is turned away from the side you are massaging (i.e. towards the contralateral side).

Procedure

Place your more medial hand on the ipsilateral side of the spine, with the ulnar border of the hand beside the spinous processes (Fig. 5.5). Palpate and assess the tissues with this hand as you apply the effleurage. Exert pressure with the more lateral hand by placing it across the more medial one. Effleurage with both hands in this position, starting from the lumbar region and moving towards the head. Adjust the pressure to suit the state of tension of the tissues, increasing

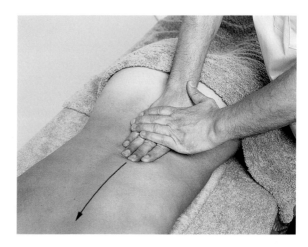

Figure 5.5 Deep effleurage to the lower and upper back using reinforced hands.

the pressure on tight areas and reducing it where there is less resistance.

Start with the body weight equally distributed on both legs. Shift your body weight onto the cephalad foot as you effleurage in the same direction. Bend the knee of the same leg as you shift your body weight forward, to achieve an easier movement and to exert a perpendicular force through the cephalad arm and hand. When you reach the upper back, cup your underneath hand slightly to massage around the shoulder, still maintaining the pressure. Having massaged the shoulder ease off the pressure and, with the hands still on top of each other, effleurage lightly down the lateral region of the trunk. During this manoeuvre, shift your body weight equally onto both feet. Return the hands to the lower back and repeat the routine.

Deep stroking technique

Effleurage using the forearm

Effects and applications

- Effleurage with the forearm can be used when heavy pressure is required to increase the local circulation. It is particularly useful when the muscles are well developed, as in the athlete or mesomorphic person. The pressure of this movement is also of benefit where the muscles are very tense or rigid. All the muscles of the back can benefit from forearm effleurage, in particular the paravertebral group. The forearm can be very effectively substituted for the hands when carrying out effleurage stroking. While this method can be used to avoid a strain on the hands it does not provide the same precise contact with the tissues that the fingers and palms can offer; sensory receptors in the palmar surface of the hands far outnumber the ones on the forearms. For the assessment of tissue dysfunction therefore the hands are better tools. Forearm effleurage is best applied to increase the circulation and for the relaxation of muscles. The manner of application is dictated by what is most suitable to the subject.

Practitioner's posture

Ipsilateral stroking. Stand in the lunging posture, with your feet slightly apart. Rotate your back foot laterally so that it is almost at right angles to the front one, and rotate your trunk so that you are facing towards the patient's head. Start this movement with

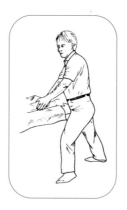

your body weight equally balanced on both feet and position yourself in line with the patient's pelvis.

Procedure

Position the forearm of the more lateral arm on the subject's lower back, on the ipsilateral paravertebral muscles (Fig. 5.6A). Hold the forearm at the wrist with your other hand. Apply the effleurage with the anterior region of the forearm (the muscle mass of the flexor digitorum superficialis). Effleurage with the forearm towards the head as you shift your body weight onto the front leg, and flex the knee at the same time; this manoeuvre helps you to increase the pressure. You can also add pressure by pushing harder with the hand that is holding the wrist. Adjust the pressure as you palpate the tissues for tension. Avoid any unnecessary heaviness or jabbing with the elbow on the ribs, and take care not to press with the ulnar side of the forearm. At the level of the inferior border of the scapula, rotate the humerus medially so that the massaging forearm lies parallel to the spine (Fig. 5.6B). Continue to effleurage towards the head, along the area between the spine and scapula. You may need to shift your weight further onto the front leg and raise the heel of the back leg to carry out this manoeuvre. Ease off the pressure as you

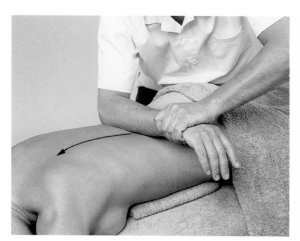
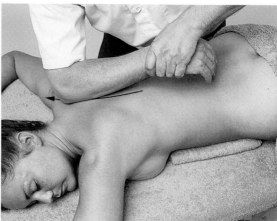

Figure 5.6 A and B   Effleurage with the forearm over the whole back region.

move round the upper shoulder, then effleurage lightly down to the lower back. Set the forearm on the lower back again and repeat the routine. Massage the ipsilateral side of the spine only, then move round to the other side of the treatment table to effleurage the opposite side.

Alternative or additional strokes

Contralateral stroking. Stand in the upright posture and on one side of the treatment couch. Lean forward towards the contralateral side of the back. Adjust the pressure as you lean onto the subject's back, at the same time protecting your own back from any overstretching or strain. If reaching over to the contralateral side proves to be awkward, carry out this movement on the ipsilateral side.

Cephalad stroking. Place the more cephalad forearm on the lumbar region, and position it so that it is roughly at right angles to the spine. Rest the other forearm on the pelvic area; exert some weight with this forearm to stabilize the pelvis. Apply some pressure as you lean onto the back, and maintain the pressure as you effleurage in a cephalad direction i.e. towards the shoulder region. Continue the stroke as far up the back as is comfortable and then lift the forearm and return to the starting position. Repeat the movement as necessary.

Caudal stroking. A similar movement is carried out with the cephalad forearm, only this time it is directed in a caudal direction and therefore towards the pelvis. The forearm is positioned on the upper region of the back, and at a right angle to the spine. Place the other forearm or hand on the ipsilateral side of the back. Apply some pressure by leaning forward and carry out the stroke towards the pelvis. If the patient is suitably undressed and if it is ethically agreeable the stroke can be continued over the gluteal region. Repeat the movement as necessary. As with the previous movement, should it prove uncomfortable to reach the contralateral side of the back, carry out this movement on the ipsilateral side.

Effleurage from the head end. Using the same part of the forearm, the effleurage can be applied from the head end of the treatment table. Position yourself so that you can lean to reach the upper thoracic region of the back. Make contact with the fleshy part of the flexor muscles of the forearm and position it so that the pressure is directed on the muscles to the side of the spine. Hold the wrist with the other hand to help you direct the movement of the forearm. Lean forward slightly to apply pressure, and effleurage the upper region of the back in a caudad direction (Fig. 5.6C). Do not attempt too much forward bending or to reach far down the back, as this may cause you to strain your own back. Having carried out some strokes on the one side of the spine, place the forearm on the other side and repeat the procedure.

Light stroking technique

Reverse stroke effleurage

Effects and applications

- The primary benefit of this effleurage is relaxation. It can therefore be applied at any time during the massage routine to the back. In some cases it may be most appropriate at the

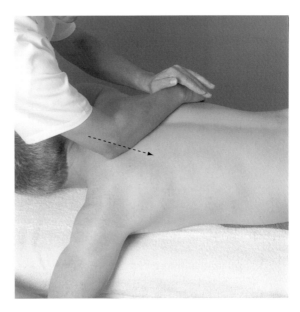

Figure 5.6 C Forearm effleurage from the head end of the treatment table.

beginning; however, at most times it is carried out at the end of the massage sequence to the back or in between other movements.

- Part of the massage stroke is applied in the opposite direction to the venous return. This is not, however, detrimental to the circulation, which is only temporarily neglected for the benefit of relaxation.

Practitioner's posture

Stand at the head end of the treatment table; you can use either the to-and-fro or the leaning posture for this movement. Select the one that allows you to bend forward and reach down the back without putting a strain on your own muscles. The patient's head is not rotated for this movement, and the face is resting in the face hole or, if this is not available, on a folded towel. However, should both these positions prove uncomfortable, the patient can turn the head to the side.

Procedure

Start with your hands at the top of the back, one on either side of the spine. Keep the fingers and thumb closed together, and the fingers pointing away from you. Make contact with the palm and the fingers, and apply an even pressure with the whole of the hand. Effleurage in a caudal direction (towards the feet). Move slowly, and reach down the back without putting any strain on your own muscles. When you reach your furthest point, slide the hands towards the lateral border of the trunk, one hand on either side (Fig. 5.7A).

Continue the massage by sliding your hands along the outer trunk towards the shoulders, with the fingers still pointing in a caudal direction but the thumb opened out away from the fingers. Move the hands over the shoulder and

then down the upper arm, the thumbs sliding on the lateral border of the upper arm (Fig. 5.7B). Rotate the hands and effleurage up the upper arm towards the shoulders, with the thumbs now sliding over the medial border of the upper arm and the fingers on the outer side (Fig. 5.7C). Continue the movement over each shoulder and onto the neck. Apply a gentle compression of the tissues between the two hands, then gently slide and lift them off (Fig. 5.7D). Place the hands on the upper back again and repeat the routine.

MASSAGE TECHNIQUES FOR THE GLUTEAL REGION

Massage to the gluteal region does not have to be omitted, provided that it is ethically acceptable to the patient. In some cases, palpation of the gluteal muscles can result in a spontaneous tensing of the same muscle group. While this could be a reaction to some disorder, such as inflammation of the sciatic nerve, it is more often a natural guarding mechanism which will only subside if and when the subject loses any feeling of vulnerability. Tension can also result from anxiety states, some of which may have sexual implications. Massage to the gluteal region is therefore carried out with these factors in mind and, consequently, with the utmost consideration for the patient.

Light stroking technique

Criss-cross effleurage

Effects and applications

- The effleurage is particularly useful to enhance the circulation of the gluteal region.
- It can be used for relaxation, and combined with criss-cross effleurage to the back.

Practitioner's posture

Stand in the t'ai chi posture, with the body weight equally distributed on both legs. Maintain this position during the movement, but rotate the trunk to apply pressure. As you twist

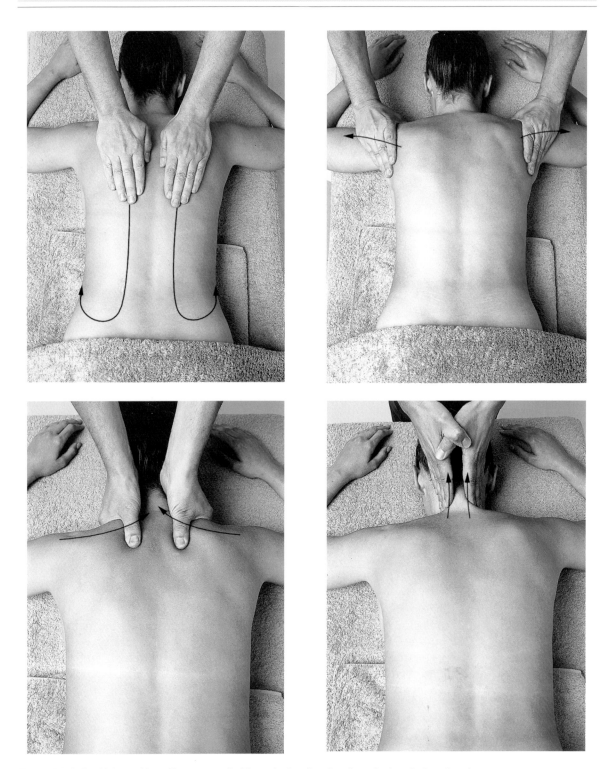

Figure 5.7 A–D Light stroking effleurage applied from the head end and used primarily for relaxation.

the trunk, push slightly towards the contralateral side with one hand and pull the other hand towards you. The patient lies prone, as for the other techniques for the back. Tactfully uncover the area being massaged and drape all other areas with a towel.

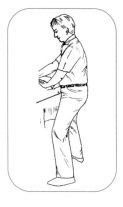

Procedure

Place one hand on the contralateral gluteal area and the other hand on the ipsilateral side (Fig. 5.8). Apply the effleurage across the buttocks, guiding the hands past each other as you move them to opposite sides, then repeat the stroke in a reverse direction. Add some pressure through the arm as you effleurage from the ipsilateral side towards the centre, then reduce it completely as you move the same hand beyond the midline and towards the contralateral side. Apply a gentle pull through the other arm as you slide the hand from the contralateral side towards the midline; then reduce the pressure completely as you move the hand beyond the midline and towards the ipsilateral side. In this

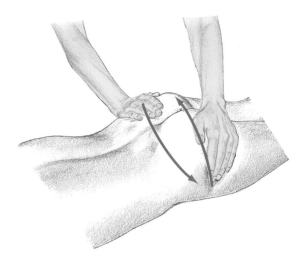

Figure 5.8 Effleurage to the gluteal region with the hands exerting pressure as they travel towards the midline.

manner, you compress the buttocks slightly towards the midline as you apply the effleurage in the same direction. Then reduce the pressure as you cross the hands and slide them from the midline towards the lateral borders, this avoids any separation of the buttocks. Reverse the action so the hands travel in opposite directions, repeating the effleurage of each buttock from the lateral border towards the midline.

Deep stroking technique

Effleurage *du poing* on the iliac crest

Effects and applications

- This deep effleurage is used to ease tightness in the muscles of the lower lumbar area and the upper gluteal region.
- It can also be employed to apply a transverse stretch to the muscles and fascia.
- Considerable pressure can be exerted with this technique; it is therefore useful when treating well-developed muscles such as those of the sports person.

Practitioner's posture

Stand in the upright posture, with your feet slightly apart and your body weight equally distributed. Position yourself close enough to the treatment table so that you can keep your back fairly straight and comfortably reach the ipsilateral side of the pelvis.

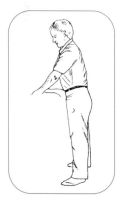

Procedure

Make a fist with each hand. Close the fingers and align them on the thenar and hypothenar eminences, thereby making a fist (Fig. 5.9). Keep the distal interphalangeal joints straight so that the fingers are straight and the fist does not assume

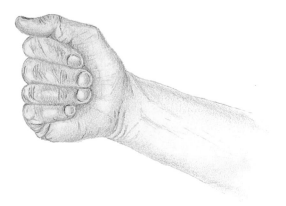

Figure 5.9 Position of the closed fingers for effleurage *du poing*.

the shape of a 'boxing' fist. Use the proximal phalanges of the fist to effleurage, avoiding any pressure with the knuckles of the metacarpophalangeal joints or those of the interphalangeal joints.

Place the cephalad fist on the superior border of the iliac crest, close to the sacrum. Position the caudal fist on the inferior border. Interlock the hands by placing one thumb inside the second fisted hand. Keep the fists flat to the surface of the tissues, and apply pressure through your arms (Fig. 5.10). Effleurage along the iliac crest, with the cephalad fist running along the superior

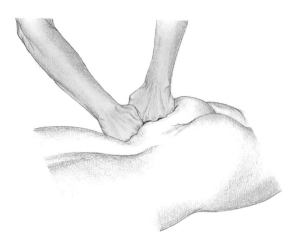

Figure 5.10 Effleurage *du poing* to lower lumbar and upper gluteal tissues.

border of the iliac crest and the caudal one along the inferior border. Apply the stroke from the central area in a lateral direction, across the muscles and fascia. As you move over the lateral tissues, adjust each wrist so that the fist remains flat to the skin surface; it is vital that you do not dig the knuckles into the tissues. When you reach the outer borders of the pelvis, reduce the pressure and return the hands to the central area to repeat the movement. Carry out this treatment on the ipsilateral side of the spine only, then move round to the other side of the treatment table to repeat the stroke on the opposite side.

Compression technique

Kneading

Effects and applications

- This compression movement reduces tightness and contractions in the gluteal muscles.
- It is also used to stretch the muscles and fascia.
- A fair degree of pressure can be exerted with this method; it may therefore be applied as an alternative technique to the petrissage movement.

Practitioner's posture

Stand to the side of the treatment table, in the upright posture. Lean against the treatment table and reach to the buttock on the contralateral side. Keep your back more or less straight, and do not bend forward too much.

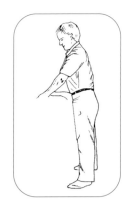

Procedure

Place the thenar and hypothenar eminences of the cephalad hand (nearest to the head) on the ipsilateral buttock, near to the midline. Set the fingers of the same hand on the contralateral side; use this arrangement to approximate the buttocks together (Fig. 5.11). Use the caudal hand

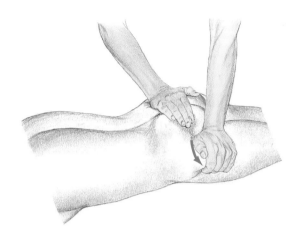

Figure 5.11 Kneading of the gluteal muscles.

(nearest to the head) to apply the kneading movement, which is carried out in two actions. First lift the tissues with the fingers, then apply a kneading pressure with the heel of the hand. Add pressure through the arm by leaning forward. The kneading action is achieved by compressing the tissues between the heel of the hand and the fingers, and rolling them laterally. When this is complete, release the tissues and repeat the lifting and kneading.

Compression technique

Petrissage

Effects and applications

- Adipose tissue is invariably present, to some degree, in the gluteal region. Petrissage is used to help break up and disperse the fat globules.
- The circulation to the muscles is also enhanced with this movement.
- Muscles of the gluteal region are encouraged to relax with this technique. As noted earlier, this may be a difficult task due to the 'holding of tension' in the same muscles.

Practitioner's posture

You can petrissage the contralateral gluteal region while standing in the upright posture.

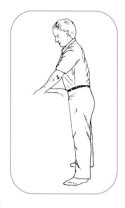

Lean against the treatment table to support your weight, and maintain a straight back as you reach over to the other side.

Procedure

For this technique, use the thumb and thenar eminence of one hand against the palm and fingers of the other hand. Lift and compress the muscles on the contralateral side with the hands close together and pressing against each other in this manner (Fig. 5.12). An alternative hold is to substitute the thenar and hypothenar eminences for the thumb; this may be a better hold when the muscles are well developed.

Maintain the compression and gently twist the tissues in a clockwise direction, avoiding pinching of the skin, then release the grip and allow the hands to slide over the tissues. Repeat the petrissage by reversing the position of the hands, i.e. substitute the fingers for the thumb in one hand and vice versa with the other. Maintain the compression as before, and apply a gentle twist in an anticlockwise direction. Then release the

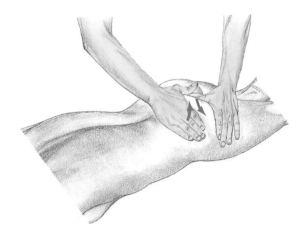

Figure 5.12 Petrissage to the gluteal region. Compression is applied with the fingers of one hand and the thumb and thenar eminence of the other.

grip and let the hands slide over the tissues. Continue to alternate the position of the hands as you repeat the petrissage technique a few more times.

MASSAGE TECHNIQUES FOR THE LOWER BACK

Deep stroking technique

Thumb effleurage

Effects and applications

- Thumb effleurage increases the circulation of the lumbar muscles.
- Increasing the circulation has the additional effect of reducing tightness and nodules or 'knotted areas'.
- The deep pressure of the technique has a stretching effect on the superficial lumbar fascia and, to some extent, the deeper fascia.
- It also helps to break up adhesions (fibrous congestion) which can be present in conditions such as osteoarthritis and lumbago.
- Muscles that benefit from thumb effleurage on the lower back include the iliocostalis lumborum, the longissimus thoracis, the spinalis thoracis and, if the pressure is deep enough, the multifidus. As the technique is applied further up the back towards the head, other muscles are also included (see also Effleurage *du poing*).
- Particular attention is drawn to areas of hypersensitivity. The sacral area is prone to oedema (mainly in women), which renders it sensitive to palpation and pressure. The lower back can also be very sensitive, especially near the spinous processes. This can be caused by misalignments of the spinal column, soft tissue strains, nerve root compression, osteoarthritis or osteoporosis. Pressure should be applied gradually and removed immediately if excessive pain is experienced by the patient.

Practitioner's posture

Stand in the to-and-fro posture, with one foot slightly behind the other, but facing towards the

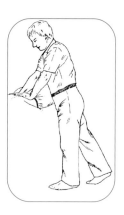

head. Adjust your stance further by rotating your trunk slightly to a comfortable angle. Position yourself at the level of the patient's pelvis and keep your arms locked at the elbow; this enables you to use your body weight behind the movement. If this posture is uncomfortable, you may prefer to sit on the edge of the treatment table.

Procedure

Place the hands on the lumbar region so that the thumbs are on each side of the spine (Fig. 5.13). Apply the effleurage stroke with both thumbs simultaneously moving together along the paravertebral muscles on each side of the spine, and exerting an equal pressure. The length of each stroke is about 5 cm (2 inches) and the direction is cephalad with a slight lateral curve. You can also slide the hands forward along with the thumbs. This avoids excessive stress on the metacarpal/phalangeal joints of the thumbs. The pressure, however, is still applied primarily with the ball of each thumb.

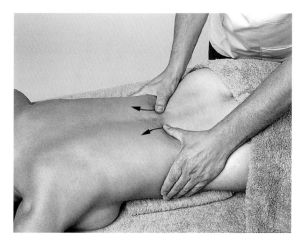

Figure 5.13 Deep stroking effleurage with the thumbs to the paravertebral muscles.

Use your body weight to increase the pressure. Keep your elbows fairly straight and lean forward slightly, without necessarily flexing the front knee. Apply the pressure gradually and adjust it to the rigidity and resistance of the tissues. Monitor also the response of the tissues to the effleurage stroke. For instance, tension in the muscle tissue can increase if the pressure is applied too quickly and deeply. Overtreating an area can cause hypersensitivity. An indicator that the tissues are treated sufficiently is a feeling of 'sinking in' with the thumbs. This 'giving' of the tissues, however, is not quickly accomplished, sometimes not at all. Allow about 2 seconds for each stroke and repeat the thumb effleurage several times before treating another section of the muscle group. Use this technique on the muscles of the lower back; you can also extend it to the thoracic region as far as the lower border of the scapula.

Alternative hand position

An alternative method for thumb effleurage is to use only one thumb on the ipsilateral side. Place the palm and fingers of the more lateral hand on the lateral border of the trunk, and rest the thumb close to the spine. Apply pressure with the thumb as you slide the whole hand cephalad. Use short strokes, and repeat these several times over one area before moving the hand further along the back. Shift your body weight forward with each thumb stroke to add pressure behind the movement. This technique is demonstrated in Chapter 2 (Fig. 2.10).

Deep stroking technique

Effleurage *du poing*

Effects and applications

- Effleurage *du poing* is used on well-developed or very tight muscles, such as those of the lumbar area. The technique can be carried out in this region as an alternative method to thumb effleurage, or in addition to it.

- The circulation of the deeper muscles and fascia is enhanced with the movement.
- As the effleurage *du poing* movement exerts considerable pressure, particular caution is needed on the kidney area—this should be avoided. Atrophied or small musculature are also contraindications to this movement.
- Contracted fascia and fibrotic tissue are stretched with this technique. These include the following structures:

a. Superficial layer

- Thoracolumbar fascia, posterior layer
- Lower fibres of the latissimus dorsi muscle
- Lower fibres of the trapezius muscle

b. Second superficial layer

- Serratus posterior inferior muscle

c. Middle layer

- Erector spinae muscle and common tendon
- Iliocostalis lumborum muscle (lateral border of paravertebral muscle group)
- Longissimus thoracis muscle (middle)
- Spinalis thoracis muscle (medial muscle of paravertebral muscle group)

d. Deep layer

- Fascia of transversus abdominis muscle
- Multifidus and rotators (not easily palpated).

Practitioner's posture

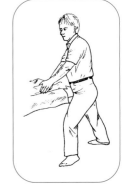

Stand in the lunging posture, with the feet well apart and the front knee flexed. In this position, you can easily shift your body weight onto the front leg as you apply the stroke. Rotate the trunk slightly so that you can place your hands on the ipsilateral side of the spine. Lean slightly towards the centre of the treatment table, and position yourself approximately 'behind' the movement.

Procedure

Close the fingers of the cephalad hand (the one nearest to the patient's head). Align the fingertips on the thenar and hypothenar eminences, thereby making a fist (Fig. 5.14). Keep the distal interphalangeal joints straight, so that the fingers remain straight. Use the proximal phalanges of the fist to effleurage, avoiding any pressure with the knuckles of the metacarpophalangeal joints or interphalangeal joints.

Position the fist on the ipsilateral side of the spine (Fig. 5.15). Rest the thumb of the same hand on the contralateral side, provided you can extend it that far. The thumb acts as a guide as you slide it along the opposite side of the spinous processes. Grip the wrist of the massaging hand with the more caudal hand; this hold allows you to lock the wrist of the massaging hand and push the fist along the musculature. Apply the pressure in two directions; in a perpendicular direction through the cephalad hand and in a forward direction through the more caudal arm.

Effleurage from the lumbar area in a cephalad direction (towards the head). Extend the stroke

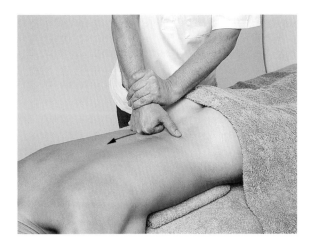

Figure 5.15 Effleurage *du poing* to the paravertebral muscles on the right.

to the inferior medial border of the scapula, and shift the body weight onto the front leg to increase the forward pressure. When you reach the level of the scapula, lift the hands off and shift the body weight onto the back foot. Place the fist on the lumbar area again, and repeat the stroke. Use a medium rhythm, taking about 5 seconds to effleurage from the lumbar area to the scapula.

Increase the pressure slightly on muscles that feel tight, provided this is still comfortable to the subject, then reduce it as the tissues relax and yield. Reduce the pressure if the muscles react to the movement by 'guarding' and tensing, which may be caused by nerve irritation, spinal misalignment or other disorders.

Alternative stroke

Instead of applying a continuous stroke from the lumbar region to the scapula, you can use a series of shorter strokes. The technique is the same; apply the pressure as you shift your body weight forward and then return the weight onto the back leg once you finish the stroke. If you opt for this method, repeat the stroke a few times over one area and then move the hands further up the back and repeat the procedure. Continue in this manner until you have covered the area to the scapula.

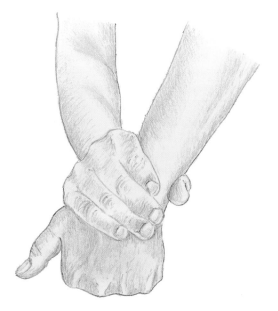

Figure 5.14 Hands position for massaging the left side of the back.

Compression massage

Petrissage on the lateral border

Effects and applications

- The circulation is improved in the local muscles and fascia, primarily the quadratus lumborum, the transversus abdominus and the lumbar fascia. Along with the circulation, the lymph drainage of the muscles and that of the superficial tissues is enhanced.
- Muscle and fascia fibres are stretched. The technique also reduces adhesions between the tissue layers.
- The action of petrissage helps to break up and disperse the fat globules of adipose tissue.
- Although it is generally carried out with a firm pressure, this technique is also relaxing. It may not be suitable, however, if the subject is in a very tense state.

Practitioner's posture

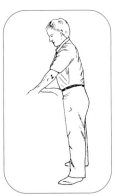

Stand in the upright posture, with the feet slightly apart. Lean against the treatment table and reach over to the contralateral side. Maintain a straight back to avoid any strain.

Procedure

In this method, the tissues are compressed and manipulated between the fingers of one hand and the thumb of the other (Fig. 5.16). Place the fingers of the cephalad hand on the very outer border of the loin area. Set the thumb of the caudal hand on the same tissue, but more medially and therefore closer to the spine. Use the whole length of the thumb and thenar eminence; this allows for a better grip and avoids any uncomfortable digging into the tissues. With the same fingers and thumb, compress and lift the muscle group from the underlying tissues, applying an equal pressure between the two hands.

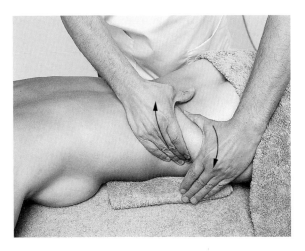

Figure 5.16   Petrissage to the outer region of the trunk.

Maintaining this hold, twist the tissues in a clockwise direction while avoiding any pinching of the skin and then release the grip and allow the hands to relax and to travel in opposite directions, so that the caudal fingers are placed furthest away and the cephalad thumb is more medial. Repeat the compression in a reverse direction and apply an anticlockwise twisting action. Relax the hands once more, and return them to the original position. Repeat the movement several times. The technique can also be carried out further along the outer border of the trunk. It is particularly indicated when there is a considerable accumulation of fat or if the muscles are well developed. It may also be extended in a caudal direction to include the gluteal region.

Compression movement

Kneading the lateral region

Effects and applications

- Kneading is an additional or alternative method to petrissage, and is used similarly to loosen the muscles. The heavy pressure exerted by this movement makes it suitable where the muscles are well developed.
- The primary effect of the technique is to apply a lateral stretch to the paravertebral muscles and those of the outer region of the lumbar

area. Muscles that are chronically contracted, such as those found in lumbago, can benefit a great deal from this kneading movement.

- Little or no lubrication is used to avoid any accidental slipping of the hand over the tissues; this also allows a good grip and, therefore, a better stretch.

Practitioner's posture

Stand in the upright posture and at the side of the treatment table. Reach over to the contralateral loin area. Apply the body weight by leaning forwards slightly, with minimal bending of the back. An alternative arrangement is to stand in the to-and-fro posture. This stance enables you to use a heavier pressure by shifting your body weight forwards and raising the heel of the back foot.

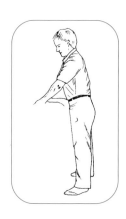

Procedure

Place the caudal hand on the contralateral side, close to the spine (Fig. 5.17). Avoid any pressure

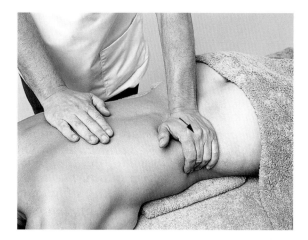

Figure 5.17 Kneading the lateral border of the lower back. The tissues are pulled medially with the fingers and then compressed and rolled forward with the heel of the hand.

on the spine itself. Position the cephalad hand further up the back, and use this to stabilize your posture. The kneading action is performed in two stages. Using the fingers, lift the tissues and pull them medially towards the spine. Then apply a kneading pressure with the heel of the hand to compress and roll the tissues forward; emphasize the lateral stretching action of the movement. Apply pressure through the arm by leaning forward or by shifting the body weight, then release the grip on the tissues as you lean backward. Repeat the routine a few times in the same region.

Deep fingertip friction

Transverse friction on the paravertebral muscles

Effects and applications

- As well as being tight, the paravertebral muscles often adhere to surrounding structures. Friction is used to reduce the adhesions between tissue layers such as fascia and muscle, fascia and bone, and adjacent muscle bundles.
- The deep and localized pressure of the movement has the effect of exerting a transverse stretch to fibrotic tissue, improving its pliability.
- It is useful to note that, as well as the hyperaemia this movement may cause, there is the possibility of some micro-inflammation as the adhesions are 'broken up'. In the unlikely event that the tissues become tender, they are easily treated with a cool pack for about 5 min; the irritation will gradually reduce over a day or two.

Practitioner's posture

Stand in the upright posture and to the side of the treatment table. Position yourself at a slight distance from the edge, so that you can shift your body weight forward and backward with the movement. Maintain a comfortable stance with the back fairly straight.

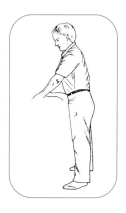

Procedure

Place the fingertips of both hands on the ipsilateral side of the spine; have the fingers more or less straight and close together (Fig. 5.18). No lubrication is needed for this movement. Apply a considerable pressure with the fingertips, and move the tissues backward and forward without sliding over them. The aim of the technique is to 'grip' the muscles or tissues by compressing them, and to move them over the underlying structures. Lean forward slightly to exert additional pressure. Continue with this action for about 10 seconds, then move to another segment of the lumbar area and repeat the movement.

Bodywork technique

Neuromuscular technique to the paravertebral muscles

Effects and applications

- Neuromuscular movements are used to treat the deep paravertebral muscles of the lumbar region. The position of the thumbs can be adjusted to address particular muscles; for example, when the thumbs are close to the spinous processes the technique is applied on muscles like the spinalis thoracis, the multi-

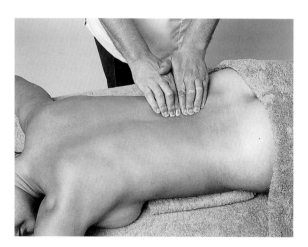

Figure 5.18 Deep fingertip friction. The fingertips are used to compress the tissues and to move them over the underlying structures.

fidus, the deep rotators and even the interspinalis. As the thumbs are moved further away from the spinous processes, the iliocostalis lumborum and longissimus thoracis are addressed, together with the more superficial latissimus dorsi.
- The neuromuscular technique (NMT) is of particular benefit for lumbago-type backache, and can be used in addition to other techniques already described. The movement can also be extended to the tissues of the middle back.
- If the lumbar muscles are very rigid or well developed, effleurage *du poing* may be used in conjunction with or in place of the NMT.
- The main contraindications to the NMT are pain in the lumbar region that radiates to other areas, and any tenderness that leads to spontaneous muscle contraction on palpation.

Practitioner's posture

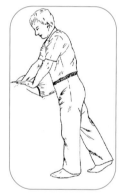

Take up the to-and-fro posture and position yourself in line with the subject's pelvis. Rotate your body slightly so that you can comfortably place your hands on the subject's lower back. Lean against the treatment table and move your body towards the midline, so as to apply pressure in line and behind the movement.

Procedure

Place the hands on either side of the spine. While keeping the fingers on the outer borders of the back, rest both thumbs on the ipsilateral side of the spinous processes. Set the thumbs next to each other but pointing in opposite directions, the lateral thumb pointing medially and vice versa (Fig. 5.19). Line up the tips of the thumbs one behind the other. Allow the thumbs to flex slightly at the interphalangeal joints and lock them in this position to prevent any backward extension at these joints. Carry out a short stroke

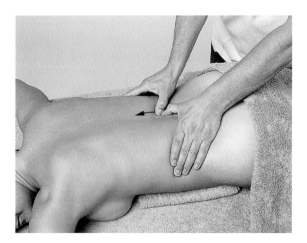

Figure 5.19   The neuromuscular technique to the lumbar muscles.

with both thumbs together, each stroke covering an area of about 5–7 cm (2–3 inches).

Apply pressure through the forearms, and increase it by adding body weight. Flex the front knee and raise the heel of the back foot, shifting your body forwards and adding weight behind the movement. Apply pressure equally with both thumbs, increase it on the hardened nodular zones and reduce it as you feel the tissues yield. Adjust the pressure according to the resistance and 'give' in the tissues. By using this method, you can assess the tissues for any tightness and treat them simultaneously. Once you complete the forward stroke, ease the pressure completely and return the thumbs to the more distal point before repeating the movement. Having carried out the stroke a few times, position the hands further up the back and repeat the routine on another section; continue with this method until you reach the thoracic area.

Applying neuromuscular technique with the fisted hand

An alternative method of applying the NMT is to use the 'fisted' hand. This method helps you to reduce unnecessary strain on the thumbs and allows some extra pressure. The position of the fisted hand is similar to that used for effleurage *du poing*, and the practitioner's posture is also

comparable. Pressure is, however, applied differently, mostly with the bony (knuckles) of the metacarpophalangeal joints. When this technique is applied very close to the spine the knuckles of the first and second fingers are mostly used. When you use it over a wider area to take in the width of the erector spinea muscles, then you can add the third and fourth knuckles (the thumb is not used in this technique). As you maintain contact with the skin, press into the tissues with the knuckles and swivel your wrist so that you perform an arced stroking movement, more or less like a scooping action. Assess the tissues as you take the knuckles through the arc so that you start with little pressure at one end of the arc, apply pressure as you dig into the tissues and then finish by easing off the pressure at the end of the movement (Fig. 5.20A). Throughout this action, keep the wrist in one area and avoid any sliding forward of the hand. The scooping action therefore covers no more than 5–7 cm (2–3 inches) as for the usual NMT with the thumb. Repeat the movement as necessary and then continue with the technique further along the back.

Applying neuromuscular technique with the elbow

The elbow is also a useful tool to use for the NMT. It must be stressed at this point that the aim of using the elbow is not to exert extreme or painful pressure but to avoid unnecessary strain on your thumbs or knuckles. The method does allow for some additional pressure, however, and can therefore be used to reduce tightness in the muscles that are very hypertoned or fibrotic. It is not applied when dealing with hypersensitive zones or some of the nodules as the thumbs or the fisted hand can provide sufficient weight for the movement.

Place the elbow on the ipsilateral side of the spine, close to the spinous processes and on the paravertebral muscles (Fig. 5.20B). Keep the forearm as close to the horizontal as possible; the more flexed the elbow is the more 'digging' there is with it. Hold the wrist of the massaging forearm with the other hand, so that you can control the position of the elbow much more efficiently.

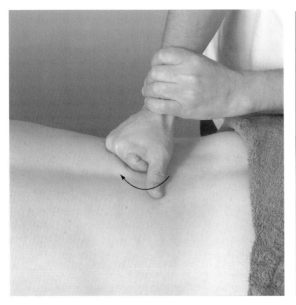

Figure 5.20 A   Neuromuscular technique on the lumbar region—using the fisted hand.

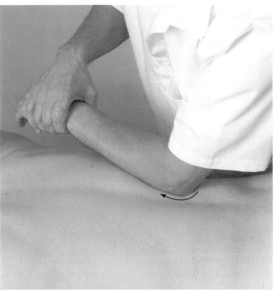

Figure 5.20 B   Neuromuscular technique on the lumbar region—using the elbow.

Position the forearm at about 45° to the spine, on the horizontal plane, and maintain this angle as you carry out the technique. Use your body weight to exert some pressure, while still maintaining control over the overall force being applied. Carry out the stroke by sliding the elbow a few inches, assessing and treating the tissues. Repeat as necessary before moving on to another segment of the back.

MASSAGE TECHNIQUES FOR THE UPPER BACK AND NECK

Deep stroking technique

Thumb effleurage on the scapula

Effects and applications

- The deep stroking massage is well suited to the muscles on the inferior region of the scapula, namely the infraspinatus, the teres minor and the teres major. The technique enhances the circulation of the muscles and, in so doing, helps to remove any build-up of metabolites; this also encourages the muscles to relax.
- This movement also stretches the muscle fibres as well as their associated fasciae, and reduces adhesions between these structures.

Practitioner's posture

Position yourself in the upright posture with the feet slightly apart. Lean against the treatment table, and extend your arms to reach the scapula on the contralateral side. While your body weight is mostly supported by the treatment table in this position, you can also apply some weight through your arms. For this movement the patient's head is turned towards you; alternatively, it can be rested in the face hole or, if this is uncomfortable, away from you.

Procedure

Place the hands on the contralateral scapula. Rest the cephalad hand (nearest to the patient's head) on the superior region of the scapula, with the fingers curved round the upper shoulder. Place the caudal hand on the lower region, with the palm and fingers curved round the posterolateral border of the rib cage (Fig. 5.21). Apply thumb effleurage to the posterior muscles of the scapula, inferior to the spine. Use alternating thumb strokes, each stroke being about 5 cm (2 inches). Starting from the more medial side of the scapula, move each thumb in a slight curve and in a lateral direction. You may find it easier to move the whole hand forward as you slide the thumb over the scapula; in this case follow a straighter line while exerting the pressure predominantly with the thumb. Repeat the strokes a few times, then reposition the hands to massage the outer border area of the scapula, which includes the teres major and minor.

Compression technique

Kneading the upper side of the shoulder

Effects and applications

- While performing a deep massage, this kneading technique is also very relaxing. A suitable

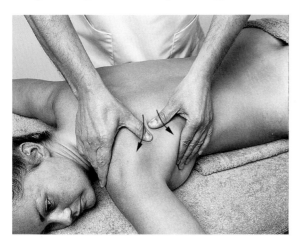

Figure 5.21 Thumb effleurage to the posterior muscles of the scapula.

application is therefore for stress headaches or tension. These states, however, can cause the tissues in this area of the back to be very tight or hypersensitive. Pressure is therefore introduced gradually and with regard to the responses of the muscles and the recipient. Should the reaction to the movement be one of increased tightness, then relaxing effleurage techniques are used instead. These can replace the kneading, or be used until the tissues begin to show signs of easing; at this time, the kneading technique can be resumed. Apart from emotional factors, tenderness and tightness on palpation may result from disorders involving the nerve roots and the spinal column. If these reactions to the massage persist, a referral would be advisable.

- The main groups of muscles treated with this technique are the upper fibres of the trapezius, levator scapulae, medial fibres of the supraspinatus, and upper fibres of the rhomboids.

Practitioner's posture

Stand in the to-and-fro posture, with one foot slightly behind the other. Extend your cephalad arm (the one nearest to the patient's head) to the shoulder on the contralateral side. Hold your elbow locked in extension, to transfer your weight through your arm. Add body weight by leaning forward and raising the heel of the back foot slightly. For this movement, the patient lies with the head resting in the face hole of the table; alternatively, the head can be turned away from the side being treated.

Procedure

Use the cephalad hand (the one closest to the head) to massage the contralateral side of the upper back, and rest the caudal hand on the middle or lower region. Place the fingers of the cephalad hand on the anterior region of the trapezius. Set the thenar/hypothenar eminences of the same hand between the scapula and spine, or as near to this level as you can comfortably reach.

Lift the tissues gently with the fingers, avoiding any excessive pressure that may cause discomfort; then compress the tissues with the thenar and hypothenar eminences while applying a simultaneous counterforce with the fingers (Fig. 5.22). With minimal sliding of the hand, push the tissues forward to stretch them gently transversely; synchronize this action with that of shifting your body weight onto the front foot. Release the grip with your thenar and hypothenar eminences while maintaining contact with the fingers. Position the heel of your hand between the scapula and the spine again. Lift the tissues with the fingers once more, and repeat the routine. Increase the pressure gradually with each stroke, and repeat the technique several times until the muscles feel sufficiently relaxed.

Deep stroking technique

Thumb effleurage on the upper back

Effects and applications

- The deep stroking effleurage is effective in reducing nodules and stretching tight muscles,

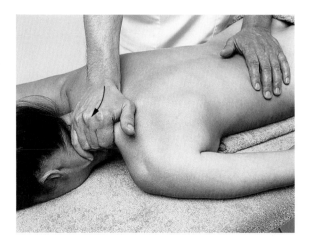

Figure 5.22 Kneading the upper side of the shoulder. The muscles are compressed and stretched across their fibres.

fascia or fibrotic tissue. In addition, it enhances the circulation and promotes relaxation. Consequently the movement can be used to alleviate pain in the cervical area, particularly when this is associated with muscular spasms and contractures in the upper regions of the back.

- The muscles that are treated with this movement include the middle fibres of the trapezius and the rhomboids (mostly across their fibres). When the pressure is sufficiently deep, the following muscles are also treated: the semispinalis cervicis (along its lower fibres); the iliocostalis cervicis (along its fibres); the longissimus cervicis (along its fibres); and the upper fibres of the longissimus thoracis.
- Massage on this region can have reflex benefits for heart function, the stomach, insomnia and headaches.

Practitioner's posture

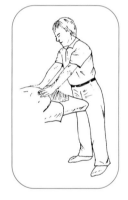

Stand at the head end of the treatment table in the leaning posture, with the feet apart and parallel to each other. Lean forward to transfer your body weight through your arms. Alternatively, adopt the to-and-fro posture with one leg placed slightly behind the other. In this arrangement you can apply the pressure by raising the heel of the back foot and leaning forward. The patient lies with the head resting in the face hole of the table, or the head can be turned to one side.

Procedure

Place the hands on the upper back so that the thumbs rest on each side of the spine (Fig. 5.23). To prevent stressing the thumbs hold them flat to the surface and therefore without any extension at the interphalangeal joints. Apply the effleurage stroke with both thumbs simultaneously or alternating with each other. Starting from the upper region of the back, slide each thumb in a

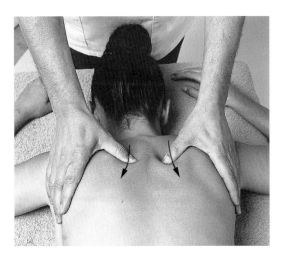

Figure 5.23 Thumb effleurage to the upper back muscles exerts a deep pressure, which is increased in gentle stages.

curved line and in a caudal direction (towards the feet); each stroke is about 5 cm (2 inches). You may find it easier to slide the whole hand along with the thumb. In this case move the hand in the same direction while applying the pressure primarily with the thumb. Lean forward to add body weight to the movement; introduce the force gradually and in balance with the rigidity and state of the tissues. Nodules, for example, can be quite tender on palpation and respond best to pressure which is increased in gentle stages. Repeat the effleurage strokes a few times before repositioning the hands to massage another section of the paravertebral muscles. Continue the thumb effleurage stroking along the thoracic region, only reaching forward to a comfortable point and without straining your back.

Deep stroking technique

Effleurage *du poing* on the upper back

Effects and applications

- Effleurage *du poing* is used when a heavier pressure than that exerted by the thumbs is required. Such a situation arises when the muscles are well developed, or if they are very

tight. This state is common in the muscles of the upper back and neck, owing to their use in maintaining the upright posture and their susceptibility to tension. The technique has the effect of stretching those tissues that are fibrotic, especially those of the paravertebral muscles (for example, the spinalis and semispinalis thoracis). Despite its heaviness, the effleurage is also very relaxing.

- The muscles treated with this technique include the middle fibres of the trapezius, rhomboids (across their fibres), lower fibres of the splenius capitis, lower fibres of the splenius cervicis, spinalis thoracis, semispinalis thoracis, and lower fibres of the iliocostalis cervicis.

Practitioner's posture

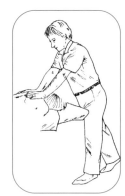

Position yourself at the head end of the treatment table and take up the leaning posture or the to-and-fro stance. Stand a short distance away from the edge of the treatment table so that you can lean forward and exert pressure behind the movement. For this movement, the patient lies with the head resting in the face hole of the table.

Procedure

Make a fist of each hand by closing the palms and placing the fingertips on the thenar and hypothenar eminences (Fig. 5.24). Place the hands on each side of the spine, at the upper thoracic area (Fig. 5.25). Use only the 'flat' part of the fist, i.e. the proximal phalangeal bones, and avoid any pressure with the metacarpophalangeal joints (knuckles). An additional adjustment to the position of the hands is made by placing one thumb inside the closed fist of the other hand. This arrangement enables you to keep the hands close together but on either side of the spine.

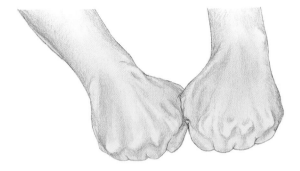

Figure 5.24   Both hands in a fist and interlocked.

Starting at the upper end of the back, effleurage in a caudal direction (towards the feet) to the level of the inferior border of the scapula or to the nearest comfortable point. Adjust the pressure by leaning forwards, keeping the fists flat to the tissues. Having completed the stroke, lift the hands and return them to the upper thoracic area. Repeat the same procedure several times.

Alternative method

The effleurage *du poing* stroke can be applied with one rather than both fists. With this option, the movement is slightly easier to apply and requires less body weight. Carry out the stroke with the fist on one side of the spine. Keep the other hand open, and use it as an effleuraging 'guide' on the other side of the spine. Interlink the two hands by placing the thumb of the open hand inside the fist (Fig. 5.26). Effleurage one side a few times before reversing the position of the hands and massaging the other side of the upper back.

Deep stroking technique

Effleurage *du poing* on the neck and shoulder

Effects and applications

- The effects of this technique are synonymous with those already described in the previous

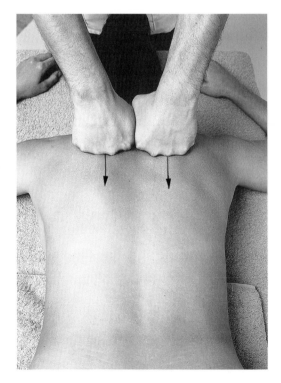

Figure 5.25   Effleurage *du poing* on the upper back, using both hands.

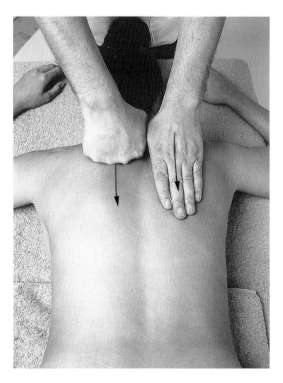

Figure 5.26   Effleurage *du poing* carried out using only one fisted hand.

section. Effleurage *du poing* exerts a heavy pressure, and is therefore indicated on muscles that are highly developed or very tight.

- The effleurage assists the circulation, reduces tightness and applies a stretch to the tissues.
- It is also relaxing.
- This technique is not applicable when the muscles are flaccid or atrophied. It is also replaced with lighter movements when there is tension related to psychogenic factors.
- Muscles treated with this technique include the levator scapulae, medial fibres of supraspinatus, upper fibres of the trapezius, splenius capitis, splenius cervicis, lower fibres of the longissimus capitis, upper fibres of the longissimus cervicis, and upper fibres of the iliocostalis cervicis.

Practitioner's posture

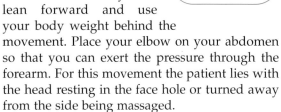

Stand at the head end of the treatment table. The to-and-fro posture is the most suitable for this technique; an alternative is the leaning posture. Take up a position at a slight distance away from the edge of the treatment table; this clearance is needed for you to lean forward and use your body weight behind the movement. Place your elbow on your abdomen so that you can exert the pressure through the forearm. For this movement the patient lies with the head resting in the face hole or turned away from the side being massaged.

Procedure

Massage the side of the shoulder that is nearest to your hand; that is, use the right hand to massage the left shoulder and vice versa. Make a fist of the hand and place it at the base of the neck, at the level of the lower three or four cervical vertebrae. At this stage you may need to flex the wrist slightly to position it flat on the tissues. Use only the flat part of the fist to massage with; avoid any pressure with the interphalangeal or metacarpophalangeal joints (knuckles). Avoid also any pressure on the spine. Rest the non-massaging hand on the upper back, and use it to stabilize your posture and to counterbalance the pressure applied with the fisted hand.

Effleurage from the base of the neck in a lateral direction towards the acromioclavicular joint (Fig. 5.27). Adjust the pressure to suit the tightness and bulk of the muscles and, as you move the hand over the tissues, keep it flat to the surface. When you reach the lateral part of the shoulder, ease off the pressure; guard against going over the prominence of the acromion of the scapula. Lift the hand and return it to the base of the neck. Repeat the stroke several times. Continue to adjust the pressure to the response and 'give' of the tissues to avoid any discomfort, in particular as you effleurage across the fibres of

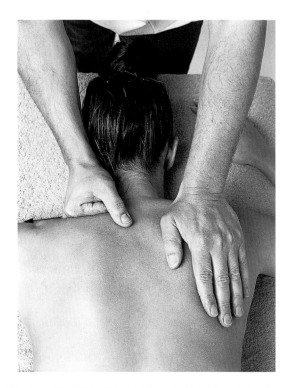

Figure 5.27 Effleurage *du poing* on the neck and shoulder.

the iliocostalis cervicis and longissimus cervicis, which are often tense.

Compression technique

Kneading the lateral/posterior muscles of the neck

Effects and applications

- With this kneading movement, the muscles and tissues are gently compressed and stretched. The circulation to all the tissues of the neck is also enhanced.
- The technique can be applied to help alleviate headaches associated with muscle tension. It can also be included in the general relaxation massage routine.
- Although not contraindicated, the movement is applied with caution if there is degeneration of the cervical vertebrae. This is common in elderly patients.
- The muscles treated with this movement include the levator scapulae, upper fibres of the trapezius, semispinalis capitis, longissimus thoracis, upper fibres of the scalenus medius, and upper fibres of the sternocleidomastoid.

Practitioner's posture

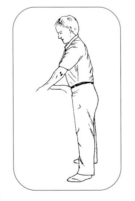

Position yourself to the side of the treatment table at the level of the patient's shoulder. Stand in the upright posture, with the feet parallel and slightly apart. You can also lean against the treatment table, provided this does not disturb the patient. Apply the movements while you are on this side of the patient; there is no need to repeat it from the other side. If you stand on the right side use the left hand to carry out this stroke, and vice versa. The patient's head should be straight and resting in the face hole. Another option is for the patient's forehead to rest either on the hands, which are placed on top of each other, or on a rolled up towel.

Procedure

As you stand facing the side of the treatment table, use your caudal hand to apply the massage. Rest your cephalad hand on the patient's head; use this hand if necessary to lift the patient's hair gently out of the way. Place the fingers of the caudal hand on the contralateral side of the neck. Set the thumb of the same hand on the ipsilateral side. At this stage, rest the palm on the back of the neck. Keeping the fingers and thumb fairly straight, apply a gentle compression to the lateral/posterior muscles of the neck (Fig. 5.28A).

Maintain the compression as you slowly lift and stretch the tissues upward, allowing the hand to slide a little at the same time (Fig. 5.28B). You can lean backward slightly to help you with this move. Alternatively, use the hypothenar eminence as a fulcrum and extend your wrist to create an upward lift, bearing in mind that this action can stress your wrist joints. As you reach the upper tissues of the neck with your thumb and fingers, gradually reduce the grip to prevent any pinching of the skin. Then resume the initial hand position and repeat the movement.

Alternative hand position (1)

An alternative method for this movement is to use both hands, placed next to each other. In this case, both thumbs are placed on the ipsilateral side of the neck and the fingers of both hands are on the contralateral side. Compress the tissues with the hands in this position and with very little sliding, simultaneously adding a gentle stretch upwards.

Alternative hand position (2)

The kneading technique can be applied while you stand at the head end of the treatment table, still in the upright posture. Use only the fingers for this movement, and avoid any pressure with the thenar or hypothenar eminences. Compress the tissues with the fingers of both hands, placed one on either side of the neck. Hold the hands in this position as you simultaneously apply a

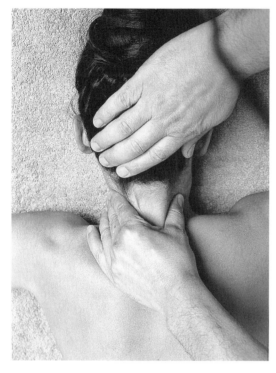
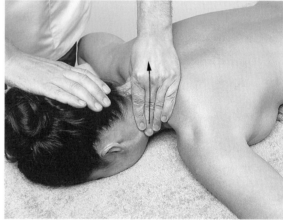

Figure 5.28 A and B Kneading the lateral/posterior muscles of the neck from the side.

gentle stretch upward (Fig. 5.29). Lean backward slightly to help you exert a gentle pull on the tissues. Allow the fingers to slide upward slightly without pinching the tissues. Release the compression and place the fingers further down the sides of the neck once again. Repeat the stroke a few times.

Bodywork technique

Neuromuscular technique on the occipital border

Effects and applications

- The fascia at the base of the occiput is a common insertion for the posterior and lateral muscles of the neck and for those of the posterior cranium. As a result of physical, chemical or emotional stressors, the tissues at the occipital border are frequently tender to palpation

and the seat of tension headaches. The NMT is carried out in this region to help alleviate tension and improve the state of the tissues.
- The technique lessens the intensity of the discomfort by reducing any irritation of the nerves and, in turn, the hypersensitivity. It also promotes relaxation of the associated muscles and, accordingly, their circulation. Improving the blood flow reverses the ischaemic state of the tissues.
- A common condition that benefits from this technique is tension headache. In some instances, pain may be referred to the ear and eyes from these sensitive tissue areas. Normalizing these tissues can therefore alleviate the pain.
- Muscles and fasciae treated with the NMT include the trapezius, sternocleidomastoid, splenius capitis, semispinalis capitis, occipitalis, deep superior oblique and deep rectus capitis posterior minor.

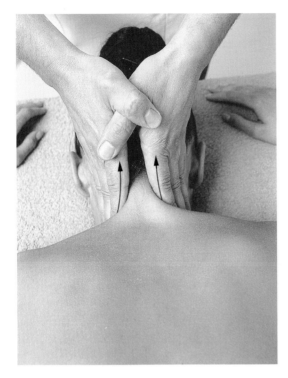

Figure 5.29 Kneading the lateral/posterior muscles of the neck from the head end of the treatment table.

Practitioner's posture

Position yourself to the side of the treatment table. Align yourself with the patient's shoulder, and stand in the upright posture with your feet apart and parallel to each other. The to-and-fro position is an alternative, and enables you to lean forwards and apply pressure behind the movement. In both cases the pressure is minimal. The patient lies prone with the head resting in the face hole.

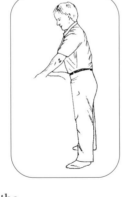

Procedure

As you stand to the side of the patient, use the caudal hand (the one nearest to the feet) for massage. Rest the cephalad hand on the patient's ipsilateral shoulder or head; if necessary, use this hand to push the subject's hair out of the way. Set the thumb of the caudal hand under the mastoid process of the occipital bone, and the fingers on the contralateral side of the neck (Fig. 5.30). Apply pressure with the thumb as you move it medially along the facial insertions at the occipital base. Keep the fingers stationary, and use them as a counterforce. Adjust the pressure according to the condition of the tissues, i.e. the tightness and degree of tenderness. When you reach the midline area of the occiput, ease off the pressure completely and then lift the thumb and return it to the mastoid process. Repeat the stroke a few times. Move round the treatment table to massage the other side of the occipital border.

Bodywork technique

Neuromuscular technique on the upper back

Effects and applications

- As noted earlier, the NMT reduces congestion in the fascia by increasing the local blood circulation. This occurs via a reflex mechanism that has the effect of relaxing the involuntary muscles of the blood vessels.

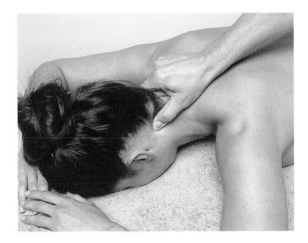

Figure 5.30 The neuromuscular technique is carried out on the fascial insertions along the occipital border.

- The mechanical pressure of the technique, together with the improved local circulation, has the additional effect of reducing nodules (hard and indurated areas) within the muscles or fascia.
- Fibrous infiltrations (adhesions), which can occur between the tissue layers and within the muscle, are separated by the mechanical effect of the movement.
- A further benefit of the technique is to decrease chronic muscular contractions. By improving muscle function, it also increases the mobility of associated joints, in this case those of the spine.
- Treatment of the superficial tissues with the NMT has a normalizing and beneficial effect (reflex) on related organs, in this case the heart and lungs.
- Muscles and fascia treated with this technique include the medial insertion of the rhomboids into the scapula, facial insertion of the trapezius into the thoracic vertebrae, iliocostalis thoracis (with deep pressure), spinalis thoracis (with deep pressure), longissimus thoracis (with deep pressure), and thoracic superficial and deep fascia.
- As well as the upper back, the NMT is applied to other areas such as the rhomboids, trapezius and the medial border of the scapula. The effects and applications are common to all these regions.

Practitioner's posture

Stand at the head end of the treatment table and take up the to-and-fro posture. Position yourself a short distance from the edge of the treatment table so that you can lean forward and exert body weight behind the movement. Raise the heel of the back foot to add body weight from a more perpendicular angle. For this movement, the patient lies prone with the head resting in the face hole.

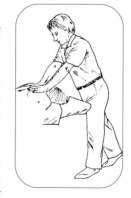

Procedure

Position both thumbs on one side of the upper back, and arrange the thumbs one behind the other and close together (Fig. 5.31). Apply equal pressure with the lateral border of the ball of each thumb. Lean forward to add body weight behind the movement. Allow about 4 seconds to cover an area of about 5 cm with each stroke. Use the thumbs to search for nodules, and treat these by increasing the pressure of the stroke. Reduce the intensity if an area of 'give' is encountered within the same stroke, or once the nodules themselves yield to the pressure. Repeat the technique several times, until the tissues lose their tightness and the hypersensitivity is reduced. Carry out the treatment on one area before moving the hands to a new position to repeat the procedure. Treat both sides of the spine.

Apply the NMT in the following directions:

1. Close to the spinous processes in a caudal direction (towards the feet), starting at the upper thoracic area and working down to the middle region.

2. Along two or three similar lines in a caudal direction, but working between the scapula and the spine.

3. Along the medial border of the scapula, from the superior medial angle to the inferior angle. This movement can also be applied while standing to the side of the treatment table (described below).

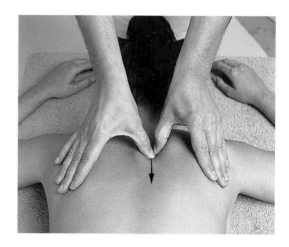

Figure 5.31 The neuromuscular technique to the muscles and fascia of the upper back.

Bodywork technique

Neuromuscular technique along the rhomboids and lower trapezius

Practitioner's posture

Stand in the upright posture and to the side of the treatment table. Maintain a position in line with the patient's shoulder.

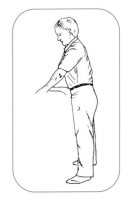

Procedure

Place the thumbs on the medial border of the scapula. Arrange the fingers of the more cephalad hand over the supraspinatus and clavicle, and those of the more caudal hand on the lateral border of the scapula (Fig. 5.32). Starting from their insertion into the scapula, trace the rhomboids' fibres towards the upper thoracic vertebrae. Use both thumbs simultaneously and close to each other. Apply an equal and even pressure with both thumbs as you assess and treat the tissues. Carry out the technique using only short strokes, and repeat them several times on each section. As you move in a cephalad direction, be aware of the deeper iliocostalis

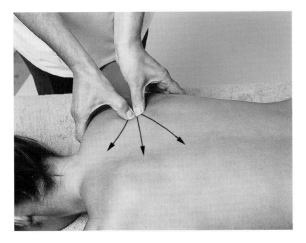

Figure 5.32   The neuromuscular technique along the rhomboids and trapezius.

cervicis; if these fibres are in a tense or fibrotic state, they can be tender on palpation. Having addressed the rhomboids, carry out the same procedure on the lower fibres of the trapezius. Start at its insertion in the spine of the scapula and continue the strokes towards the middle and lower thoracic vertebrae. In this region you transverse some fibres of the iliocostalis thoracis; these can also be painful if they are tense or fibrotic. Repeat the technique along the middle fibres of the trapezius.

Bodywork technique

Neuromuscular technique along the medial border of the scapula

Practitioner's posture

Stand in the upright posture and to the side of the treatment table. Maintain a straight back as you extend your arms to the scapula on the contralateral side of the trunk.

Procedure

Hold and stabilize the scapula at its upper border, using your cephalad hand (the one closest to the patient's head). Raise the scapula gently while holding it in this manner, or by inserting a folded towel under the same shoulder. This upward manoeuvre shortens and relaxes the rhomboids and the middle fibres of the trapezius. Place the thumb of the more caudal hand on the medial border, and the fingers on the lateral border of the scapula (Fig. 5.33). Trace and palpate the insertions of the rhomboids into the scapula as you move the thumb along the medial border. Apply a counterforce with the fingers as you exert pressure with the thumb. Use short strokes, and repeat them several times over one section before moving to another area. Treat the whole medial border of the scapula while you are in this position.

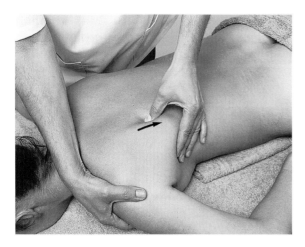

Figure 5.33 The neuromuscular technique along the medial border of the scapula.

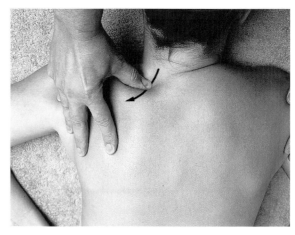

Figure 5.34 The neuromuscular technique to the levator scapulae, trapezius and supraspinatus.

Bodywork technique

Neuromuscular technique to the levator scapulae, trapezius and supraspinatus

Practitioner's posture

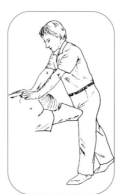

Stand in the to-and-fro posture at the head end of the treatment table. Minimal body weight is employed for this technique; you can therefore be in a position fairly close to the treatment table.

Procedure

Apply the technique to one side of the neck. Place one hand on the shoulder to be treated, and the other hand on the upper back or on the opposite shoulder. Spread and extend the fingers of the hand applying the treatment, and rest the fingertips on the scapula and the shoulder muscles. Place the thumb on the lateral–posterior region of the neck, close to the cervical spine (Fig. 5.34). With the tip of the thumb, trace the fibres of the trapezius and levator scapulae. Continue the stroke over the

supraspinatus muscle, stopping before you reach the acromioclavicular joint. Throughout the movement, stabilize the hand by keeping the fingers extended. Allow them to slide over the scapula and the shoulder as your thumb travels over the supraspinatus. Repeat the stroke several times.

Bodywork technique

Treatment of trigger points

Effects and applications

- A nodular formation can develop into a chronic and hypersensitive zone. When this happens, the area can act as a trigger point and refers a sensation, usually of pain, to a distant region. The sensation is exacerbated by palpation of the trigger point area. Reducing the irritability of this hypersensitive zone helps to alleviate the referred perception. In addition, the treatment helps to normalize the underlying stressor (mechanical imbalances, organic malfunction, etc.) that is associated with the nodule formation.
- Trigger points and their target areas tend to have the same pathway in every person; for example, if the target area is the lateral parietal

area of the head, the trigger point will be in the splenius capitis muscle, below the mastoid process.

Practitioner's posture

Stand in the to-and-fro posture; alternatively, choose the standing or leaning stances. This technique requires very little body weight; consequently, you can position yourself to the side of the treatment table or at the head end.

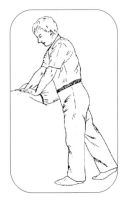

Procedure

Place the thumb or the middle finger on the trigger point zone, e.g. the levator scapulae insertion (Fig. 5.35). Apply sufficient pressure to create the sensation in the target area, and maintain the pressure for 6–10 seconds. Reduce the pressure slightly for a few seconds, then apply it again for a few more seconds. Continue with this on-and-off procedure until the patient experiences a reduction in the sensation, or for a maximum of 2 min.

Follow the pressure treatment with passive stretching of the tissues, preferably having cooled

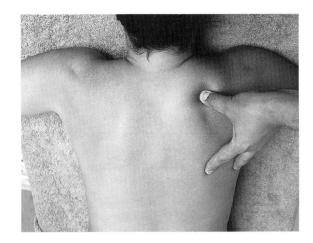

Figure 5.35 Treatment of trigger points on the insertion of the levator scapulae muscle.

the area first with ice, spray or cold towels. Trigger points require the tissues to be passively stretched following their treatment, and this can involve procedures that fall into the scope of bodywork rather than massage. However, a simple stretching effect is achieved by lifting the tissues off the underlying structures. An additional or alternative method is to apply a passive stretch across or along the fibres of the muscle being treated. Mobilization of the scapula, as described further on, illustrates a method of passively stretching the muscles (see Figs 5.36 and 5.44).

Bodywork technique

Mobilization of the scapula

Effects and applications

- The technique stretches the muscles that insert into the scapula, primarily the rhomboids and middle fibres of the trapezius. The fascial connections of the scapular–costal (soft tissue) joint are also stretched with this movement.
- The rotational action of the technique helps to mobilize the whole shoulder girdle.

Practitioner's posture

Stand in the upright posture and to the side of the treatment table. Position yourself in line with the patient's shoulder and extend your arms to the contralateral side.

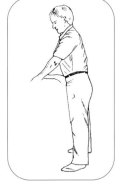

Procedure

Place the fingers of the cephalad hand on the shoulder, and those of the caudal hand on the lateral border of the scapula. Grip the scapula with both hands in this position and lift it gently. Press both thumbs on the medial border (Fig. 5.36). Maintain this hold with the fingers and thumbs,

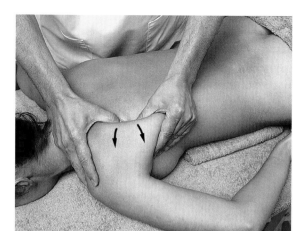

Figure 5.36 Mobilization of the scapula.

and push the scapula in a lateral direction. It is important to bear in mind that this manoeuvre is only possible if the muscles (and naturally the patient) are relaxed; therefore, apply pressure gradually and only if the tissues are responding by yielding to it. Hold the stretch for a few seconds before allowing the tissues to recoil to their normal resting state. Repeat the stretch technique once or twice.

A rotational movement can also be applied to the scapula. Maintain the grip with the fingers in the same position and reduce the pressure with the thumbs. Move the scapula in a clockwise direction, and hold this position for a few seconds before carrying out the same action in an anticlockwise direction. Repeat the procedure once or twice.

SUPPLEMENTARY TECHNIQUES FOR THE BACK: SUBJECT SIDE-LYING

The patient may be unable to lie prone for reasons such as injury, pregnancy, obesity or old age. In such a situation, you can massage the back while the subject is in a side-lying posture (the recovery position). Comfort and safety are important; therefore, support patients with cushions where necessary. Place a pillow of the right height underneath the head, and perhaps another at the front of the abdomen; this may be required in pregnancy or if the patient is overweight or eld-

erly. While lying on the side, the patient can keep the uppermost knee, which extends forward over the lower one, resting on a cushion. This arrangement is not only comfortable, but also checks any rolling forward. An alternative set-up is for both knees to be flexed and resting on the massage table, one on top of the other. Some padding can be placed between the knees. The side-lying patient may also require support underneath the trunk to prevent the spine from bending into a scoliotic curve. Although twisting of the spine is best avoided, the patient may find it comfortable to rotate the trunk forwards towards the lying prone position rather than maintaining a more vertical side-lying posture. A slight rotation is appropriate provided it does not cause any pain or misalignments of the spine. Some additional support under the chest may also be needed. Whatever posture is chosen, it must not cause the back muscles to tense. Furthermore, it is vital that you stabilize the subject in a secure position with the non-massaging hand.

Effects and applications

- Most of the massage movements described with the patient lying on the side are similar to those carried out when the patient is prone. Furthermore, the effects and applications are common to both sets of techniques. As these have already been described in earlier sections, they are not repeated here unless additional information is appropriate.

Stroking technique

Effleurage to the whole back

Practitioner's posture

Stand in the lunging posture, with one foot in front of the other. Position yourself at the level of the patient's pelvis, and twist your trunk slightly so that you are facing towards the patient's head. Guard against straining your back by keeping any forward bending to a minimum. Carry out the massage on the uppermost side of the spine. Once the patient has turned onto the other side, you can repeat the strokes. If the patient is unable to turn over, apply the massage to both sides of the spine simultaneously.

An alternative arrangement is to carry out this effleurage technique while sitting on the edge of the massage plinth. This is ethically correct, provided that it is acceptable to the recipient. If you opt for this posture, keep one foot resting on the floor to support your body weight.

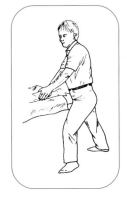

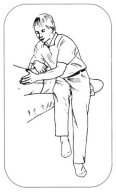

Procedure

Place the forearm or hand that is closest to the patient on the iliac crest (Fig. 5.37). Use this hold to stabilize and limit the movements of the trunk and legs. Effleurage the uppermost side of the spine, using the palm and fingers of the outer hand. Apply the stroke from the sacral area in a cephalad direction (towards the head). Increase the pressure slightly, with the thenar and hypothenar eminences, on the lumbar area. Guard against straining or overextending your wrist. Flex your front knee, and move your whole body forward to

apply weight behind the stroke. When you reach the upper back, cup your hand and continue the stroke over the shoulder. Then proceed with a light effleurage towards the feet (caudal direction), as far as the lateral pelvis. Starting once more at the sacral area, repeat the routine several times. Use only a slow rhythm, taking about 5 seconds to reach the upper back.

Deep stroking technique

Effleurage *du poing*

Practitioner's posture

Stand in the lunging posture with the front knee slightly flexed. Rotate the trunk and the front foot towards the head end of the plinth. Place the elbow of the massaging arm on your abdomen or pelvis. Rest the non-massaging hand on the patient's pelvis and use it to steady and support the body.

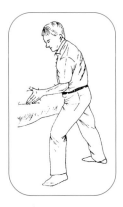

Procedure

Make a fist with the massaging hand, by closing the fingers and resting the distal phalanges on the thenar and hypothenar eminences. Hold the wrist straight or with minimal flexion or extension.

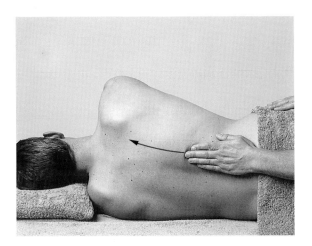

Figure 5.37 Effleurage on the upper side of the spine.

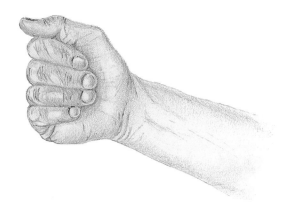

Avoid applying any pressure with the knuckles (metacarpophalangeal and interphalangeal joints). Place the elbow of the same massaging arm on your abdomen or pelvis; this position enables you to lean towards the side of the plinth and exert pressure through your forearm. Effleurage with the flat fist, using the proximal phalanges only, in a cephalad direction (towards the head). From the lumbar area, massage upwards to the mid-thoracic region or to a point that can be reached comfortably (Fig. 5.38). Flex the front knee further so that you can move your whole body towards the patient's head. Simultaneously, apply pressure to the tissues by leaning forward towards the plinth and thereby transferring body weight through the forearm. When you reach the middle of the back, reduce the pressure by leaning backward slightly. Then return the hand to the lumbar area. Repeat the movement several times. To effleurage the upper thoracic area, rearrange your body position so that you stand at the level of the patient's lower ribs.

Effleurage du poing on the sacral region

When it is applied in a caudal direction, the effleurage *du poing* movement has the effect of stretching the lumbar and sacral fascia.

Additional pressure can also be exerted over the apex of the sacrum, which helps to reduce any lordosis in the lumbar spine.

Practitioner's posture

To carry out this technique, reverse your stance so that you face towards the pelvis. The position of the hands is also changed; stabilize the trunk with the more medial hand while applying the massage with the outer one. Place the elbow of your massaging arm on your abdomen or pelvis as you carry out the stroke with the fisted hand. Using the non-massaging hand, apply a simultaneous stretch to the fascia by pushing the pelvis in a caudal direction.

Procedure

Make a fist of the massaging hand and apply the effleurage from the lumbar area towards and over the sacrum and coccyx (Fig. 5.39). Add body weight by leaning towards the plinth. Flex the front knee and move the whole body in the direction of the stroke. Carry out the stroke very slowly, allowing 4 seconds for the hands to effleurage from the lumbar area to the apex of the sacrum. Repeat the stroke several times.

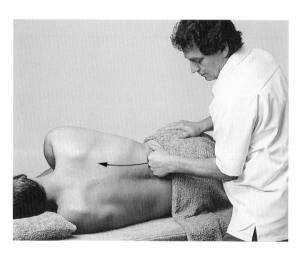

Figure 5.38 Effleurage *du poing* to the lower and middle back.

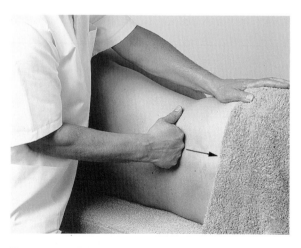

Figure 5.39 Effleurage *du poing* to the sacral area stretches the fascia and encourages a reversal of lumbar lordosis.

Deep stroking technique

Thumb effleurage on the paravertebral muscles

Practitioner's posture

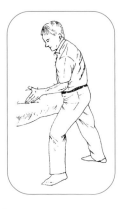

Stand in the lunging posture. Rotate your upper body slightly so that you are facing towards the head end of the treatment table, and point the front foot in the same direction. Rest the elbow of the massaging hand on your abdomen or pelvis; this position allows you to apply body weight behind the movement.

Procedure

Place the more lateral hand on the lumbar region, with the palm and fingers pointing towards the treatment table and curving round the lateral border of the trunk. Position the thumb on the uppermost side of the spine and pointing towards the head (Fig. 5.40). Flex the thumb slightly at the interphalangeal joint. Maintain this position throughout the movement, and avoid extending the interphalangeal and metacarpophalangeal joints. Rest the other hand on the patient's pelvis and use it to stabilize the torso. Effleurage the paravertebral muscles with the pad of the thumb, using a short stroke of about 5 cm (2 inches). Add pressure behind the movement by flexing the front knee and shifting your whole body weight forward. To facilitate an easier movement, slide the whole hand while directing the pressure with the thumb. Apply sufficient force to compress the thumb into the tissues as you slide it forward, then release it again at the end of the stroke. Once you have carried out a few strokes, or when the tissues have eased, move your hand to another position and repeat the series of strokes. Continue with the routine along the side of the spine and to the level of the scapula.

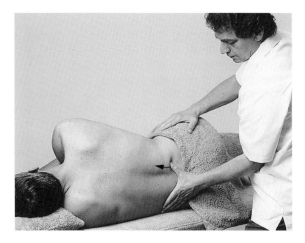

Figure 5.40   Thumb effleurage on the paravertebral muscles.

Bodywork technique

Neuromuscular technique on the paravertebral muscles

Practitioner's posture

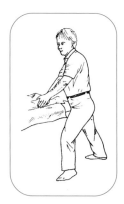

Stand in the lunging posture. Rotate your body so that you face towards the head end of the massage plinth, and point the front foot in the same direction. Position yourself at the level of the patient's pelvis or lumbar area, whichever is more comfortable.

Procedure

Position the thumbs on the uppermost side of the spine, one behind the other and very close together (Fig. 5.41). Flex the interphalangeal joint of both thumbs and lock them in this position as you carry out the neuromuscular stroking. Carry out a series of short strokes with both thumbs moving together and maintaining their proximity. Press into the tissues with the very tip of each distal phalanx, and with both thumbs applying an equal pressure. This force on the paravertebral muscles is deeper than that of the thumb effleurage. As you move your hands in a

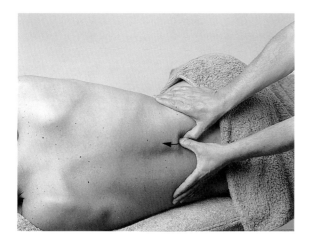

Figure 5.41 The neuromuscular technique is applied with both thumbs exerting an equal pressure.

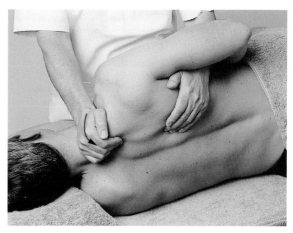

Figure 5.42 Kneading the upper shoulder muscles.

cephalad direction flex the front knee and shift your body forward, thereby adding body weight behind the movement. Increase the pressure on any hardened nodular zones, and reduce it as the tissues yield. Repeat each stroke a few times before moving on to another section. Carry out the neuromuscular stroking on the lower lumbar area, extending it gradually to the thoracic region.

Compression technique

Kneading the upper side of the shoulder

Practitioner's posture

Stand in the upright posture, facing the patient. Position yourself in line with the patient's shoulders and close to the treatment table. Lean forward slightly to add weight behind the movement.

Procedure

Set the cephalad hand on the upper shoulder muscles. Place the thenar and hypothenar eminences on the anterior region, and the fingers on the posterior side. Use the thenar and hypothenar eminences (heel of hand) to compress the muscles

against the fingers (Fig. 5.42). Maintain this gentle grip as you stretch the tissues away from you, without sliding your hand. Lean forward slightly to apply some pressure behind the movement, while avoiding any excessive compression with the heel of the hand on the supraclavicular area (between the sternocleidomastoid muscle and the anterior border of the trapezius). Release the pressure and, keeping the fingers in the same position, lift the heel of your hand and return it to the more anterior region of the shoulder. Repeat the procedure and the routine several times. Place the other hand on the scapula or the shoulder. Use this hold to control the movement of the shoulder and to add a degree of counterforce as you apply the stretch.

Compression technique

Kneading the lateral/posterior muscles of the neck

Practitioner's posture

Stand in the upright posture and close to the treatment table. Keeping the back straight, lean forward slightly to facilitate an easier movement.

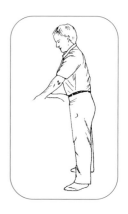

Procedure

Carry out the kneading movement on the lateral/posterior muscles of the neck with the cephalad hand. Set the fingers on the contralateral or underside of the neck, and the hypothenar and thenar eminences (heel of hand) on the ipsilateral or upperside. Apply compression between the fingers and heel of the hand, guarding against any excessive force (Fig. 5.43). Maintain this grip as you stretch the tissues backward, i.e. away from you. Allow your body weight to facilitate the stretch by leaning forward slightly. Having applied the stretch, slide the fingers and the heel of the hand (in an effleuraging fashion) away from you. Reduce the pressure altogether as you complete the stroke, and adjust the hand position to start again. Repeat the procedure a few times. Throughout the movement keep the caudal hand on the shoulder or the scapula, and use this hold to create a slight counterforce to the kneading stroke.

Bodywork technique

Mobilization of the scapula

Effects and applications

- The mobility of the scapula is restricted when the surrounding muscles are contracted and

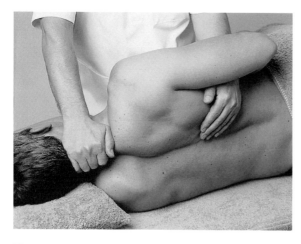

Figure 5.43 Kneading the lateral and posterior muscles of the neck.

shortened. This technique applies a passive stretch to these muscles and, in so doing, increases the range of movement of the scapula. The muscles that benefit most from this movement include the serratus anterior, levator scapulae, all fibres of the trapezius, and the rhomboids.

Practitioner's posture

Stand in the upright posture, leaning against the massage table and facing the patient. No body weight is required for this movement. Some leaning forward is involved, but this should be only minimal.

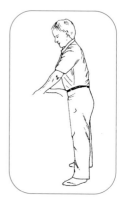

Procedure

Hold the shoulder with your cephalad hand, placing the fingers on the upper regions of the scapula, the palm over the acromioclavicular joint and the thumb over the anterior region. Grip the lower border of the scapula with your caudal hand, using the fingertips on the medial border and the hypothenar and thenar eminences on the lateral border (Fig. 5.44A).

Encourage a rotational movement of the scapula whilst maintaining a firm grip. The axis of rotation is in the centre of the scapula. Lift the lower border whilst pressing down the upper region. Hold the position at the end of the movement to apply a passive stretch to the muscles. Those mostly affected are the rhomboids and the lower fibres of the trapezius.

Having mobilized the scapula in one direction, reverse the action by lifting the upper region while pressing down on the lower border (Fig. 5.44B). Use a similar passive stretch to the muscles, primarily to the upper fibres of the trapezius, the serratus anterior and the levator scapulae. The subscapularis, teres major and minor and infraspinatus are also stretched to a lesser extent. Once this stretch is complete, repeat the whole procedure, mobilizing the scapula in both directions.

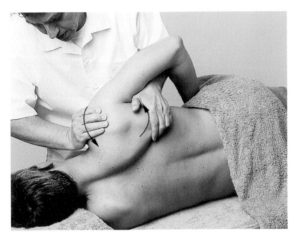

Figure 5.44A The scapula is mobilized with a rotational movement in one direction.

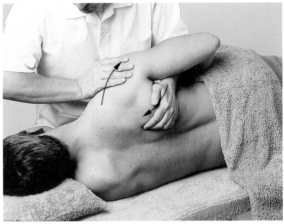

Figure 5.44B The rotational movement is reversed and carried out in the opposite direction.

Deep stroking technique

Effleurage *du poing* on the neck and shoulder

Practitioner's posture

Stand at the head end of the treatment table in the to-and-fro posture, with one foot slightly behind the other. As you stand facing in a caudal direction (towards the feet) use the medial hand, which is closer to the centre of the treatment table, to apply the massage. Stabilize the shoulder with the more lateral hand, the one closer to the outer edge of the treatment table. For this movement the patient's head needs to be in a flat position; therefore, use only a small cushion for support.

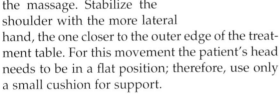

Procedure

Make a fist with the massaging hand by closing the fingers and aligning the fingertips on the thenar and hypothenar eminences.

Use the proximal phalanges of the fist to effleurage and avoid exerting any pressure with

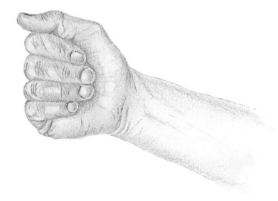

the knuckles of the metacarpophalangeal or interphalangeal joints. Place the fist on the upper fibres of the trapezius, near to the mastoid process. Arrange the hand so that the dorsum of the fist is towards the anterior region of the neck (Fig. 5.45). Effleurage, with the fist in this position, along the muscles of the posterior border of the neck and towards the shoulder. Continue the stroke over the upper side of the shoulder, in the region of the supraspinatus. The weight of the fisted hand is generally sufficient for this stroke; therefore, avoid applying any heavy pressure. You can, however, add some pressure by leaning forward or shifting your body weight to the front foot. Release the pressure when you reach the clavicle, and return the fist to the upper region of the neck. Repeat the routine several times. It is

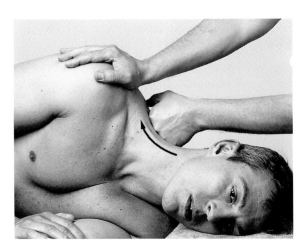

Figure 5.45 Effleurage *du poing* on the posterior muscles of the neck.

vital that you carry out this technique only on muscles on the posterior region of the neck, i.e. the upper fibres of the trapezius, and the levator scapulae, and the more central structures such as the scalene muscles are therefore avoided.

Bodywork technique

Neuromuscular technique on the neck and shoulder

Effects and applications

- The NMT is used to reduce nodules and chronic contractions in the muscles of the neck and upper side of the shoulder. It also applies a passive stretch to the tissues and assists in reducing adhesions.
- The muscles that benefit most from this technique include the upper fibres of the trapezius, levator scapulae, splenius capitis, splenius cervicis, lower fibres of the longissimus capitis, upper fibres of the longissimus cervicis and iliocostalis cervicis, and the medial and upper fibres of the supraspinatus.

Practitioner's posture

Stand in the upright posture and at the side of the treatment table. Align your position close to the patient's shoulder. Rotate your body so that you are facing in a cephalad direction (towards the head). Another option is to sit on the edge of the treatment table; this arrangement is very practical, although it does involve a degree of forward bending of the trunk.

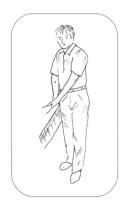

Procedure for the neuromuscular technique (1)

Hold and stabilize the shoulder with the more medial hand, i.e. the one nearest to the centre of the treatment table. Maintain this grip as you apply a gentle pull on the shoulder during the movement. Place the thumb of the more lateral hand on the upper side of the shoulder, in the region of the supraspinatus. Rest the palm and fingers of the same hand on the upper back region (Fig. 5.46). Apply a series of short strokes with the tip of the thumb flat to the tissues. You may want to flex the distal interphalangeal joint of the thumb to apply some extra pressure. Repeat the stroke over the same area until the tissues relax or, in the case of nodules, until the sensitivity is reduced. Bear in mind that too long a treatment on one area can cause bruising.

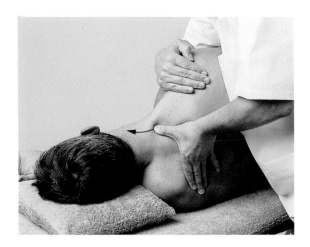

Figure 5.46 The neuromuscular technique to the muscles of the neck and shoulder.

Carry out the NMT on the upper side of the shoulder, and proceed along the lateral and posterior regions of the neck until you reach the occiput. As you stretch the tissues in a cephalad direction with each stroke, apply a counter-stretch with the hand holding the shoulder (in a caudal direction).

Procedure for the neuromuscular technique (2)

The NMT can be carried out using this alternative method. Sit on the edge of the treatment table, or stand in the same upright posture. Place the fingers of both hands close together on the posterior/lateral muscles of the neck, close to the occiput and the mastoid process. Position the hands so that both sets of fingers are in contact with each other (Fig. 5.47).

Flex the distal interphalangeal joints of all the fingers, and press the fingertips into the tissues. Apply the neuromuscular stroke with both hands simultaneously, maintaining the proximity of the fingers. Carry out one continuous stroking action, from the occipital region to the upper side of the shoulder. Lean back slightly to increase the pressure and to stretch the tissues. When you reach the lateral border of the shoulder, ease the pressure, return the hands to the upper cervical region and repeat the routine.

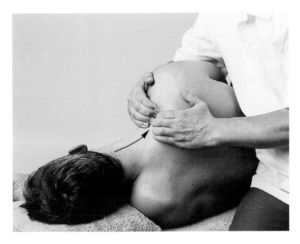

Figure 5.47 The neuromuscular technique is applied from the cervical region to the upper side of the shoulder.

SUPPLEMENTARY TECHNIQUES FOR THE BACK: SUBJECT SITTING ON THE TREATMENT TABLE

The patient may be unable to lie down on the treatment table owing to some condition such as emphysema. In this situation, you can carry out the massage movements to the back with the patient sitting on the treatment table. Other movements can be applied with the patient sitting on a chair or stool; these are described further on.

The patient can sit at one end of the treatment table while you take up a position to the side. Stand very close to the patient, in the upright posture, and place one arm across the patient's upper chest. Reach across to hold and stabilize the contralateral shoulder. Support the patient's weight by allowing him or her to lean against your torso (Fig. 5.48). Continue to adjust this posture until the patient is fully relaxed, particularly the muscles of the back. You may want to insert a cushion between your chest and the patient for a more comfortable support. In addition, you can place a cushion or folded towel on your shoulder to support the patient's head, which should be kept more or less vertical, as too much side bending of the neck can be painful and dangerous in conditions such as spondylosis. When massaging the patient sitting on the treatment table, the table has to be low enough for you to reach the upper back comfortably. If the treatment table is not adjustable or too high you may prefer to carry out this massage with the patient sitting on a chair, with you sitting next to them, applying the same method to hold and support them. This would also be a better option if the patient is not comfortable sitting on the treatment table.

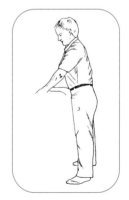

Effects and applications

- Most of the massage movements in this section are similar to those carried out when the patient is lying prone. Both sets of techniques also share the same effects and applications. As these have already been described in earlier sections, they are not repeated here unless additional information is appropriate.

Stroking technique

Effleurage to the whole back

Procedure

While holding and supporting the patient with one hand, as already described, effleurage the back with the other hand (Fig. 5.48). Carry out the stroking in any one of the following directions: across the back, in a circular fashion, or in a cephalad direction (towards the head). Introduce a slight rocking action with each effleurage stroke by shifting your body weight from one foot to the other or by leaning backwards and forwards. This enhances the soothing

and relaxing effect of the effleurage, especially if it is carried out with a slow rhythm. The most likely recipient of this technique is an elderly person; if this is the case, use only minimal pressure. Otherwise, adjust the pressure depending on the condition and size of the tissues.

It is not necessary to repeat the stroke from the other side of the trunk.

Compression technique

Kneading the paravertebral muscles

Procedure

Follow the same holding position as for the previous movement, and carry out the kneading technique to the contralateral side of the spine. Use the thenar and hypothenar eminences (heel of hand) to exert pressure on the paravertebral muscles, just lateral to the spinous processes (Fig. 5.49). With the hand in this position, apply a stretch to the tissues in the same contralateral direction (i.e. away from the spine). Lean forward slightly to increase the pressure through your arm; avoid any slipping of the hand over the tissues. Start at the lower back and gradually proceed with the strokes upwards to the upper thoracic region. Massage the contralateral side only, then move round the treatment table and repeat the procedure.

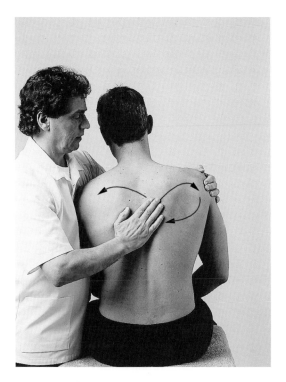

Figure 5.48 Effleurage to the back is carried out across the back, in a circular fashion or in a cephalad direction.

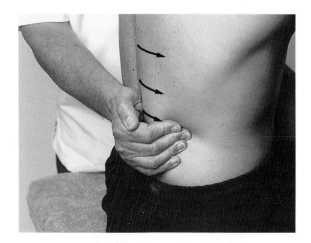

Figure 5.49 Kneading the paravertebral muscles on the contralateral side of the spine.

Compression technique

Kneading the upper side of the shoulder

Procedure

Maintain the holding and standing position as for the previous movements, and massage the contralateral upper side of the shoulder. Check that the patient's head is not bending sideways towards you excessively, as this will tighten the muscles on the contralateral side. Place the fingers of the massaging hand on the anterior region of the trapezius, and the thenar/hypothenar eminences (heel of hand) on the posterior region of the upper back (Fig. 5.50).

Compress the tissues between the heel of the hand, which applies most of the pressure, and the fingers. Simultaneously roll and stretch the tissues forward in an anterior direction. Guard against too much sliding of the heel of the hand and any pinching of the skin. Once you have compressed the tissues in this manner, release the pressure altogether and return the heel of the hand to the upper back. Repeat the routine several times. Massage the contralateral side only, then move round the treatment table and carry out the same procedure to the other side.

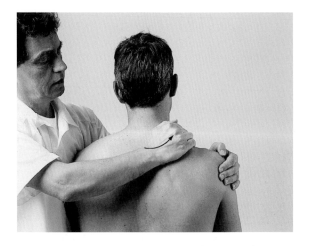

Figure 5.50 Kneading the upper side of the shoulder.

SUPPLEMENTARY TECHNIQUES FOR THE BACK: SUBJECT SITTING ON A CHAIR

If the patient is unable to lie down, some massage techniques to the back can be carried out with the patient sitting on a stool or a chair. In this position, they can lean forward and rest the forearms and head on the treatment table or any similar item of furniture. Use cushions for support as necessary. Encourage the patient to adjust his or her position for comfort, and so that the muscles of the back are relaxed. Choose your own posture to carry out the massage; kneel on the floor, sit on a chair next to the patient, or stand. Alter this posture if necessary, and massage for short periods only to avoid any back strain.

Effects and applications

- Most of the massage movements in this section are similar to those carried out when the patient is lying prone. Both sets of techniques also share the same effects and applications. As these have already been described in earlier sections, they are not repeated here unless additional information is appropriate.

Stroking technique

Effleurage to the whole back

Practitioner's posture

One of the positions for applying the effleurage is to kneel down on one leg. Having the other knee flexed with the foot resting on the floor enables you to shift your body weight forward during the movement. You can also kneel on both legs.

Procedure for the effleurage to the back (1)

Support the subject by placing one hand on their pelvis. Effleurage the back, on one side of the spine only, with the other hand (Fig. 5.51). Start at the lower lumbar region, or as far down as you can comfortably reach, and proceed in a cepha-

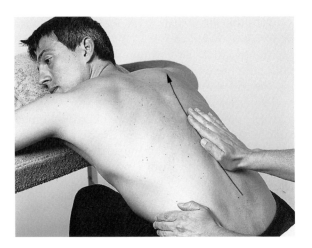

Figure 5.51 Effleurage to the back is carried out with the patient sitting and the therapist in a kneeling position.

lad direction (towards the head). As you effleurage upward, lean forward to apply some body weight. Continue the stroking over the shoulder and then trace your hand along the outer border of the torso. Repeat the stroke several times. Reverse your position so that you rest on the opposite knee and, having also changed hands, massage the other side of the spine.

An alternative stroking action is to massage both sides of the spine simultaneously, using one hand on either side of the spine. This manoeuvre is more practical if you are kneeling down on both legs.

Procedure for the effleurage to the back (2)

An alternative to the kneeling posture is to sit on a chair next to the patient. Support the patient by holding the shoulder with one hand, and carry out the effleurage with the other hand (Fig. 5.52). Trace your hand in a cephalad direction, in a circular fashion, or across the back, applying a series of strokes over the whole region of the back.

Deep stroking technique

Effleurage with the thumb on the paravertebral muscles

Practitioner's posture

The kneeling down position is perhaps the most practical position in which to perform this effleurage with the thumb. Sitting on a stool or on a chair is another option.

Procedure

Place the thumbs one on each side of the spine, on the paravertebral muscles (Fig. 5.53). Effleurage with both thumbs simultaneously, applying a series of short strokes. Massaging with one thumb only can sometimes be more comfortable than using both thumbs at the same time. Hold

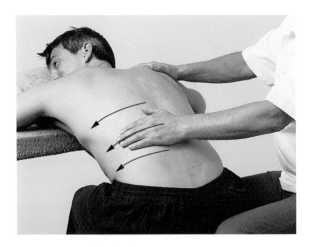

Figure 5.52 Effleurage to the back is applied with the therapist sitting next to the patient.

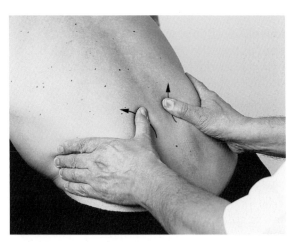

Figure 5.53 Thumb effleurage on the paravertebral muscles.

each thumb fairly straight, or flex it slightly at the distal interphalangeal joint. Apply pressure by leaning forward slightly. Repeat the strokes over one area a few times, or until the tightness is reduced, and then move the thumb(s) further cephalad and repeat the procedure. Continue with the massage to the level of the scapula.

Deep stroking technique

Effleurage *du poing*

Effects and applications

- The primary effect of this technique is to apply deep pressure to the lumbar muscles when these are very contracted. In addition to easing the muscles, the effleurage *du poing* technique has the effect of stretching the lumbar fascia, which is invariably tight.

Practitioner's posture

Stand behind the patient and lean forward to reach the lumbar area. The to-and-fro posture may be the most suitable for this movement, as it enables you to shift your body weight backward and forward. As the effleurage *du poing* involves a degree of body weight, it is impractical to carry it out while sitting on a chair.

Procedure for effleurage du poing *(1)*

Make fists of both hands, by closing the fingers and resting the fingertips on the thenar and hypothenar eminences.

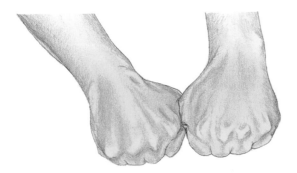

Place the fisted hands on the upper lumbar region, one on either side of the spine (Fig. 5.54). Maintain a flat fist position as you effleurage with both hands simultaneously over the lumbar region and the sacrum. Massage the paravertebral muscles and the fascia close to the spine; guard against exerting pressure over the kidney area or prodding the tissues with the interphalangeal or metacarpophalangeal joints. Increase the weight of your stroke by leaning forward

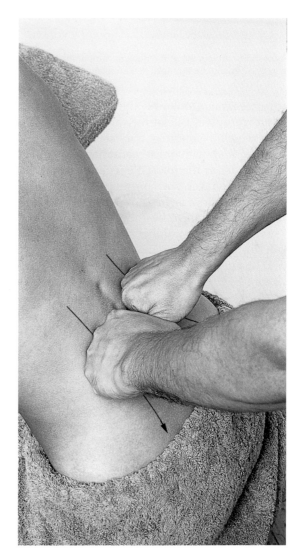

Figure 5.54 Effleurage *du poing* is applied over the lumbar region and the sacrum.

slightly. Complete the stroke at the lower end of the sacrum, then ease the pressure and return the fisted hands to the upper lumbar region. Repeat the procedure a few times.

Note that this technique is contraindicated if the patient suffers from severe back pain, sciatica, a herniated disc or other such disorders.

Procedure for effleurage du poing (2)

A second method for applying the deep effleurage is to stand next to the patient and administer the massage on the ipsilateral side of the spine. In this standing mode you can also start the massage further up the back and proceed in a caudal direction.

Use one fisted hand as already described to apply the effleurage. Hold it flat to the tissues, and avoid exerting pressure with the knuckles (Fig. 5.55). Carry out the effleurage *du poing* with the fist in this position, tracing the paravertebral muscles and the lumbar fascia. Repeat the long stroke over the whole lumbar region several times. Support and stabilize the back with the non-massaging hand. Note that, instead of using the fisted hand, you can also carry out the effleurage with the flat palm and fingers. While you exert less pressure with the flat hand, it is a better 'tool' for palpating the tissues.

Compression technique

Kneading the upper side of the shoulder

Practitioner's posture

Stand in the upright posture and behind the patient. Massage the left and right sides of the upper back simultaneously. A second option is to stand to one side of the patient and massage the contralateral side.

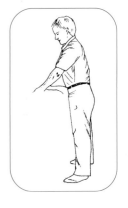

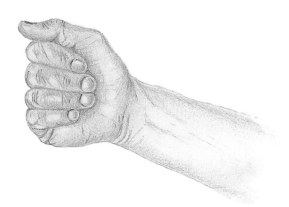

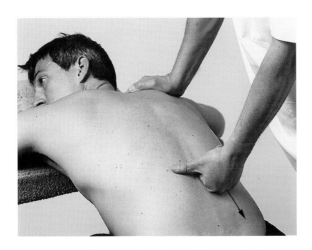

Figure 5.55   Effleurage *du poing* carried out with only one fisted hand.

Procedure

To massage both sides of the upper back simultaneously, place the fingers on the anterior aspect of the upper side of the shoulders, in the region of the clavicles. Extend the thumbs to the posterior aspect, and place them between the spine and the scapulae. Apply pressure with both thumbs and compress the tissues against the fingers on the anterior side (Fig. 5.56). Maintain this grip, and roll the tissues forward with the thumbs to stretch the fibres transversely. Then release the grip and set the thumbs in the more posterior position. Repeat the routine several times. If you choose to stand to one side of the patient and

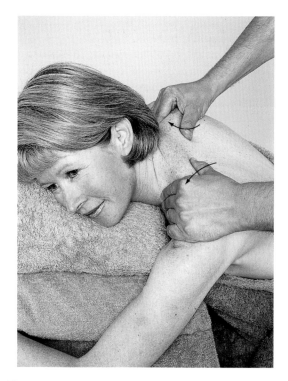

Figure 5.56 Kneading the upper side of the shoulder with both thumbs simultaneously.

treat the contralateral side, substitute the thenar and the hypothenar eminences (heel of hand) for the thumb. Carry out the same manoeuvre, compressing the tissues and rolling them forward.

6

Massage for body regions—the lower limb

OBSERVATIONS AND CONSIDERATIONS

Observation and palpation of the tissues of the lower limb is carried out with patients lying both prone and supine. It is worth noting that some of the visual signs that can be observed when subjects are standing may alter when they are recumbent, and these changes are mostly caused by the pull of gravity. The state of the musculature and the bony alignments may therefore differ in the two positions; for instance, muscles that contract excessively to maintain the upright posture may relax when the subject is lying down. Oedema in the lower limb is also subject to modification; it can become less obvious when the person is lying down.

Skeletal disorders

Lateral rotation of lower limb

Observation of the feet when the patient is lying supine may show that one or both feet are 'turned out'. This deviation indicates a lateral rotation of the whole lower limb, which in turn is associated with tightness in the muscles on the ipsilateral side. The primary lateral rotator muscles involved are the piriformis, gluteus medius and sartorius.

Flexion of the hip and knee joints

When the subject is supine, one or both knees can be in a slightly flexed position. In the absence of bony deformities or arthritic changes, such flexion can be caused by tightness in the quadriceps muscle group. Should the rectus femoris be involved, then hip flexion may also be observed. Spasm of the psoas muscle will likewise cause flexion at the hip joint.

Joint pain

Pain in the joints of the lower limbs is not infrequent, especially in older patients. It is not within the scope of massage to diagnose problems of the skeletal system and, when there is doubt as to the cause of acute or chronic pain in the joints, it is therefore always advisable to refer patients to their doctor. However, common conditions present with some obvious symptoms, and it is very helpful for the massage therapist to be aware of them and of any possible contraindications.

- Pain in the hip joint that is exacerbated with activity may indicate osteoarthritis. A common indication for this condition is limitation or pain in the hip joint when the femur is passively rotated or adducted.
- Osteoarthritis of the hip joint may refer pain down the anterior aspect of the thigh, as far as the knee. It can also result in weakness of the quadriceps muscle group. Hip joint disease will also refer pain to the medial aspect of the thigh.
- Arthritic knees are similarly painful on use. Crepitus (a grinding sound and feel) is a common feature of the condition and is experienced on passive movement of the joint.
- Arthritic degeneration may also affect the joints of the ankle and of the foot. Pain or crepitus are likewise elicited on passive movements of the joints.
- Rheumatoid arthritis presents not only with inflammation but also with bony deformations, as well as painful and restricted movements.

Referred pain

Misalignments or other disorders at the level of the second and third lumbar vertebrae may refer pain to the anterior aspect of the thigh; there may also be loss of sensation, and muscle weakness. The distribution of the pain may also extend to the anterior shin and the inner aspect of the foot; in this case, the origin of the problem is at the level of the fourth and fifth lumbar vertebrae, or the first sacral segment.

Tissue changes and referred pain

Malfunction or disorders of organs can lead to tightness, tension or hardening of the superficial tissues and muscles. For instance, the iliotibial band may be tight because of dysfunction of the bladder; disorders of the digestive system can be reflected in the tissues of the thigh; kidney problems can refer pain to the upper/lateral region of the thigh; and problems of the ureter and urinary bladder can refer pain or cause tissue changes in the upper/medial thigh area. Massage is applied on these reflex zones to normalize the tissues and improve the related disorder.

Sciatica

Sciatica is very often a cause of concern, and may be acute or chronic. It radiates from the buttock, down the posterior aspect of the thigh and along the posterior or lateral aspect of the calf to the foot. The ailment results from irritation of the nerve roots, lumbosacral plexus and sciatic nerve. The irritation in turn is a consequence of other disorders, such as intervertebral disc problems, vertebral dislocations, spondylosis, pressure on the lumbosacral plexus by the uterus during pregnancy, gluteal bursitis and tumours. In addition to the pain, other related symptoms can be present; these may include hypoaesthesia (decreased sensitivity), hyperaesthesia (increased sensitivity), or paraesthesia (numbness, prickling, etc.). Although not necessarily damaging, massage is not indicated for any of these malfunctions until their cause is diagnosed; referral is therefore the first step. Once approval has been granted by the patient's doctor, then techniques such as friction are used on each side of the sciatic nerve to release adjacent adhesions. This massage is, however, carried out without irritating the nerve. It is also applied frequently to increase its efficiency.

Massage techniques such as thumb effleurage can also be applied to the region of the greater trochanter and the ischial tuberosity. Extra attention should be given to the piriformis muscle, owing to its close proximity to the sciatic nerve; a spasm of this muscle can easily result in sciatica. The gluteus medius and maximus can likewise be involved if they are in a fibrotic state. Tissue changes may also be found in the upper end of the iliotibial band, the popliteal area and the upper end of the Achilles tendon. These zones may be tender or tight, and are treated with effleurage or the neuromuscular technique (NMT). Treatment for sciatica should also include massage to the anterior thigh and the calf muscles. Passive stretching of the whole limb is introduced gradually, and only when the acuteness of the pain has subsided.

Muscular malfunctions

- Tightness in the muscles is generally a consequence of overuse; however, in some cases the contractions are associated with anxiety.
- Atrophied muscles may result from lack of use. Another cause is an absence of motor impulses travelling from the brain or from the peripheral nerves. Toning up massage techniques can be used for underused muscles. However, treatment is contraindicated in the presence of any pathology of the nervous supply unless it is approved by the patient's doctor.
- A strained or ruptured muscle is generally tender to palpate. Loading (using isometric contractions) or stretching the muscle passively will also elicit pain. A compensatory mechanism to the strain often leads to spasm of associated muscles, or of bundles within the same muscle.

Oedema

To test for pitting oedema, apply gentle pressure with your thumb or fingers and maintain this for about 5 seconds. When assessing the knee for oedema, place a hand superior to the patella and compress the tissues. Palpate for oedema on top and around the patella, using the fingertips of the other hand (Fig. 6.1). If oedema is present the pressure will cause pitting; this is seen as a depression in the skin once the thumb or finger is removed. Common sites for testing are behind the malleolus, over the dorsum of the foot and over the shins. Oedema can be a consequence of a number of factors.

Oedema in one or both legs

- The most common causes for oedema in one or both legs are heart or kidney failure.
- Bursitis may affect one or both knees, and is frequently a consequence of overuse or injury. In severe cases, full flexion of the knee is limited and painful. A build-up of synovial fluid may also be present; this is generally contained within a cyst which extends into the back of the knee joint (Baker's cyst).
- Lymphoedema is caused by obstruction of the lymph vessels. Opinions differ as to whether pitting is always present in this condition, or whether it only occurs in the early stages; there is similar disagreement concerning whether the oedema is bilateral or asymmetrical. Skin thickening is present and, rarely, ulceration,

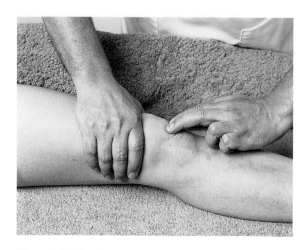

Figure 6.1 The tissues are palpated for oedema.

but there is no pigmentation. The distal leg is initially involved, and the feet will be swollen.

- Phlegmasia alba dolens refers to acute oedema from venous obstruction, usually a thrombosis, and is found mostly in women following childbirth.

Bilateral oedema

- Orthostatic oedema refers to bilateral oedema from prolonged standing or sitting. In this condition, pitting is often present on palpation.
- In lipoedema, there is fluid retention in both legs (the feet are spared) together with abnormal fatty deposits in the subcutaneous tissue. Fluid collects within the fat cells as well as in the interstitial spaces. One theory about the mechanism involved is that the pressure within the tissue is reduced and, consequently, there is free filtration of fluid into the interstitial spaces. However, this increase in fluid does not create sufficient force on the lymphatic system to drain it away. Lipoedema is almost exclusively found in women; it can be hereditary, and is unaffected by diet or elevation of the limbs. There is very little sign of pitting, and no ulcerations or pigmentation in the affected limbs, but there can be tenderness and pain as well as easy bruising. Shifting the fluid in this situation is not an easy task and the effect of massage may be limited, particularly if the condition is chronic and hereditary. The psychological support that massage offers to the sufferer is of great value; this can, however, be easily undermined by any inflated expectations of the treatment's outcome.

Unilateral oedema

- Blood in the urine and small haemorrhage spots on the skin can indicate obstruction in the kidneys. These signs can be accompanied by unilateral swelling of the calf and ankle. Discoloration can occur, particularly in the lower leg or foot, which is relieved by elevation.

- Oedema and puffiness in the foot may be indicative of an ovarian cyst.
- Venous obstruction or valvular incompetence are common causes of a pitting oedema that is generally unilateral and also involves the foot. Areas of ulceration and pigmentation are frequently present in the lower leg and ankle. Massage of the area and of the limb is contraindicated.

Circulatory malfunctions

Ulcerations

Ulcerations on the toes (and/or of the lower leg) could indicate insufficiency of the arterial supply. Massage, both on the area itself and distal to it, is contraindicated.

Varicose veins

In this disorder, the saphenous veins are prominent, swollen and distorted. Apart from the fact that palpation is painful, massage is contraindicated to avoid any clots becoming mobilized, particularly if the condition is chronic and severe.

Pain, heat and oedema in one or both legs

- Pain that affects the calf muscles and disappears with rest can be indicative of intermittent claudication. This is associated with insufficient blood supply to the muscles during activity. It may be due to a spasm of the arterial wall muscles, atherosclerosis, arteriosclerosis, or to occlusion (perhaps by a thrombus). In all of these situations, massage is only administered with the consent of the patient's doctor.
- The signs and symptoms of thrombosis can be present in isolation, or only in a mild form; however, certain changes do offer good indications. These include pain in the leg, redness, heat and unilateral oedema of the calf or ankle. Discoloration that is relieved by elevation can also occur, particularly in the lower leg or foot. Thrombosis itself is sometimes palpable as a tender cord within the affected vein. Massage

is contraindicated both for a known case of thrombosis and for potential sufferers.

- In iliofemoral thrombophlebitis the leg is swollen and painful, the veins are prominent and there is also heat. Massage is generally contraindicated.

Pain on palpation

- Pain on palpation may be due to thrombophlebitis in the calf. Although this is frequently asymptomatic, there may be tenderness in the area together with increased firmness and tension in the tissues when the calf muscles are squeezed. The tenderness on palpation must not be confused with the more obvious picture of muscle overuse or injury; massage is contraindicated for thrombophlebitis.
- The pain may be caused by superficial phlebitis. Redness and discoloration mark the thrombophlebitis along the saphenous veins, and it may be palpated as an indurated (hardened) cord in the subcutaneous tissue. Massage is contraindicated.
- The inguinal nodes may be enlarged and painful on palpation. This can be caused by a number of disorders, ranging from infection to carcinoma.

GENERAL MASSAGE TECHNIQUES FOR THE LOWER LIMB

When the patient is lying in the prone position, the feet should be supported with a cushion or rolled up towel. Place some padding under the abdomen to correct any lordosis in the lumbar region. Some patients may also need support under their knees when they are lying supine. Cover the body, and the leg that is not being massaged, with a towel, and use a second towel if necessary to keep the feet warm. As with all massage movements, apply any lubrication sparingly as manipulation of the tissues (e.g. the kneading technique) becomes difficult if the tissues are too slippery. The massage movements for the lower limb are demonstrated mostly on the posterior region; however, most of the movements can be repeated on the anterior region. It is important to add at this point that no set routine for leg massage is indicated in this section. The emphasis is on describing the techniques rather than putting them in any particular order.

Stroking technique

Effleurage on the leg (prone)

Effects and applications

- The circulation, in particular that of the venous return, is enhanced by this effleurage. Drainage of the lymph is likewise stimulated. The technique is therefore indicated when exercise or normal physical activity is limited or impossible—for instance, during confinement to bed for long periods; sitting down or standing for hours on end are similar examples.
- The movement is also used for its beneficial effect on all the muscles of the lower limb. Following sports activity, for example, the by-products of muscle activity are removed and the muscles supplied with oxygenated blood and nutrients.
- Massaging certain reflex zone areas of the superficial tissues has a stimulating effect on associated viscera, glands or organs. The lateral region of the thigh is considered to be one such zone, and relates to the digestive and urinary system.

Practitioner's posture

Stand in the lunging posture and to the side of the treatment table. Take up a position in line with the patient's feet, or beyond the foot end of the treatment table. Face towards the patient, with your front foot pointing in the same direction. Apply pressure behind the movement by shifting your body weight to the front leg.

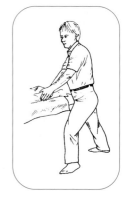

Procedure

Place both hands on the lower leg, just above the ankle (Fig. 6.2). Arrange them one behind the other as follows:

1. Set the more lateral hand in front of the more medial one. Rest the fingers of the lateral hand on the lateral region of the leg. Rest the fingers of the more medial hand on the medial side.
2. Line up the thumb of the lateral hand with the first finger of the medial one.
3. Complete the connection by lining up the thumb of the medial hand with the ulnar border of the lateral one.

Apply even compression all round the leg with the fingers and thumbs of both hands. Maintain this hold as you effleurage along the lower leg and the thigh, with both hands moving together as one unit. Add body weight by flexing the front knee and transferring your weight to the front foot. When you reach the upper thigh, separate the hands and move the lateral one to the outer region of the thigh, tracing the medial hand to the medial region. Then reduce the pressure altogether, and slide the hands towards the ankle to resume the movement. Shift your body weight to the back leg as you carry out this manoeuvre. Repeat the routine several times. Use a slow rhythm for this movement, taking about 5 seconds to effleurage in the cephalad direction. As you effleurage down the leg in a caudal direction, you can also apply a gentle compression with both hands. This has the effect of enhancing the arterial blood flow to the lower leg and the foot. Apply the same effleuraging method for the anterior region of the lower limb when the patient is lying supine.

Deep stroking technique

Thumb effleurage on the sole of the foot

Effects and applications

- Based on the theory of reflex zone therapy, massage to the sole of the foot stimulates reflex zones that relate to body systems and the various regions. It has an overall normalizing

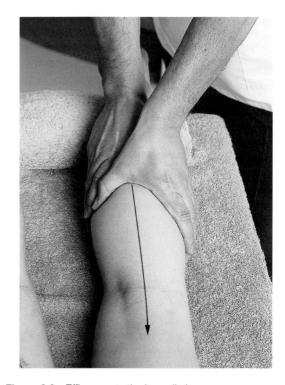

Figure 6.2 Effleurage to the lower limb.

effect on the body, and the technique is therefore applicable in many conditions as an adjunct to other treatments.
- Mechanically, thumb effleurage promotes circulation and stretches the plantar fascia.
- The majority of recipients generally find this technique very relaxing, provided the grip with the fingers is firm and the pressure of the thumbs is positive and deep. In some cases, however, the sole of the foot is too sensitive for thumb effleurage and the effleurage *du poing* method may be more relaxing (see Fig. 6.4).

Practitioner's posture

Stand in the upright posture, facing towards the foot end of the table. Another option is to sit on

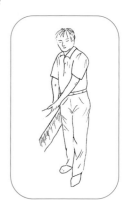

the treatment table, facing in the same direction. Maintain a comfortable upright posture, as there is no body weight involved in this movement.

Procedure

Raise the patient's lower leg and flex their knee. Support the foot with both hands and curve your fingers around the dorsum (Fig. 6.3). Effleurage using alternating thumb movements. Each stroke can be approximately 5 cm (2 inches), in a straight line or in a slightly curved direction. Repeat the strokes several times over one area before treating another zone. Adjust the position of your hands to maintain a comfortable hold as you proceed along the sole of the foot. Include the toes. In some cases, a degree of pain is elicited when you massage over a reflex zone; the quality of the pain is usually that of a 'needling' type. In the absence of any local trauma or inflammation, this tenderness may be referred from a malfunctioning organ or tissue in a distant region of the body. Provided the massage is bearable to the patient you can repeat the thumb effleurage stroke several times; invariably the intensity of the pain will reduce. An alternative method for this effleurage is to use only one thumb instead of two, and a further option is to carry out longer strokes, along the whole length of the sole of the foot.

Effleurage du poing *method*

Effleurage to the sole of the foot can be carried out with the fisted hand. Raise the lower leg as in the previous movement, and support the foot with the more medial hand. Carry out the effleurage stroke with the fisted hand, starting at the heel and continuing over the sole of the foot and the toes (Fig. 6.4). Apply an even stroke, avoiding excessive pressure with the knuckles (metacarpophalangeal and interphalangeal joints). Repeat the stroke a few times.

Stroking technique

Effleurage on the posterior lower leg

Effects and applications

- This effleurage to the lower leg assists the venous return and the lymphatic drainage.
- Muscles in this region benefit from an increased circulation, a reduction of metabolites and relaxation.
- The muscles addressed with this technique include the soleus, gastrocnemius, peroneus longus and brevis, tibialis posterior (located in the deep posterior compartment of the lower leg), and flexor digitorum longus (deep posterior compartment).

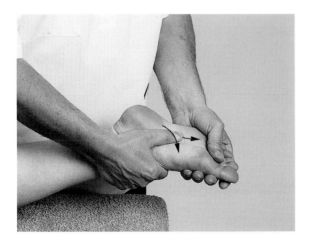

Figure 6.3 Effleurage on the sole of the foot, using alternating thumb strokes.

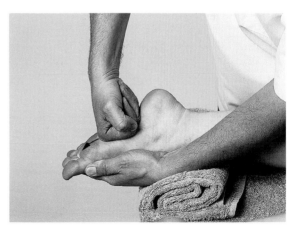

Figure 6.4 Effleurage *du poing* to the sole of the foot.

Practitioner's posture

Position yourself at the foot end of the massage treatment table, and stand in the to-and-fro posture. Apply pressure behind the movement by shifting the body weight from the back to the front foot. Alternatively, stand in the upright posture and apply weight by leaning forwards.

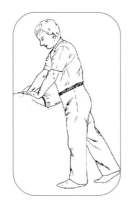

Procedure

Raise the patient's lower leg so that the knee is flexed and the foot is resting on one hand (Fig. 6.5). Perform the effleurage with the other hand, starting at the Achilles tendon area and extending the stroke to the popliteal fossa. Apply a gentle squeeze with the whole hand as you effleurage in a cephalad direction, while avoiding excessive pressure with the fingertips. If you can reach comfortably, continue the stroke over the popliteal fossa; however, pressure over this region needs to be considerably reduced. Return with a light effleurage to the distal end of the lower leg and repeat the procedure.

Effleurage to increase the arterial blood flow

Effleurage the lower leg and the foot to assist the arterial blood flow. Stand in the upright posture and support the foot with one hand, with the knee still in a flexed position (Fig. 6.6). Apply a gentle all-round pressure with the other hand, curving the fingers around the anterior region of the lower leg and keeping the thumb more or less on the posterior side. Effleurage from the middle of the lower leg to the foot; increase the compression over the foot and the toes. Lean backward slightly and use your body weight to exert pressure from in front of the movement. Carry out the same movement with the other hand, and repeat the alternating strokes several times.

Compression technique

Petrissage and kneading to the calf

Effects and applications

- Petrissage and kneading of the calf are included in the massage routine for general relaxation. They are also used more specifically for muscle tightness and congestion, which can result from long periods of standing, overuse of the muscles or periods of inactivity.
- As these particular methods of petrissage and kneading exert considerable pressure, they are additionally indicated when the muscles, pri-

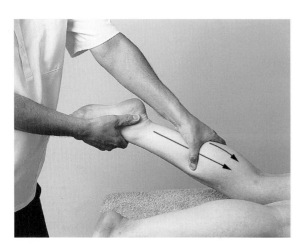

Figure 6.5 Effleurage along the venous return on the lower leg.

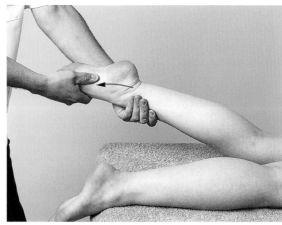

Figure 6.6 The effleurage is continued in a caudal direction to enhance the arterial supply.

marily the gastrocnemius and the soleus, are well developed or very tight. The sports person is therefore likely to benefit a great deal from these techniques.

Practitioner's posture

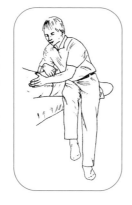

Sit on the edge of the treatment table. Flex the patient's knee and support the foot on your shoulder and the shin area on your chest (Fig. 6.7). If you need to lean forward to assume this position, guard against excessive bending of the trunk.

Procedure for petrissage to the calf muscles

This petrissage is applied with the fingers of both hands pressing against each other. The compression is then repeated with the hypothenar and thenar eminences of both hands, again pushing against one another. Curve the fingers of both hands, and place them on either side of the calf muscles (Fig. 6.7). Exert an even pressure with all the fingers as you compress the muscles and pull the tissues towards the midline. Maintain a steady grip during this manoeuvre and avoid sliding the fingers. Then release the pressure and substitute the fingers for the thenar and hypothenar eminences. Apply pressure as you compress the tissues and push them towards the midline. Follow this by easing the grip completely, then resume the compression with the fingers. Repeat the procedure a few times. Petrissage can also be applied with the patient's lower leg resting on the treatment table (see Fig. 2.14).

Procedure for kneading the calf muscles

Sit on the edge of the treatment table. Flex the patient's knee and hold the lower leg vertical. Grip the gastrocnemius muscle with both hands (Fig. 6.8). Place the thenar/hypothenar eminences of the medial hand on the medial region of the tibia. Keep the fingers of the same hand close together and set them on the midline, between the lateral and medial heads of the gastrocnemius. Place the more lateral hand, in a similar manner,

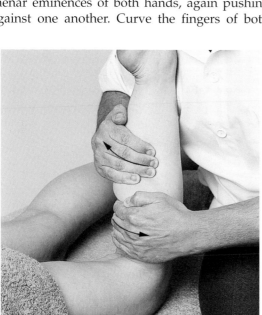

Figure 6.7 In this petrissage, the calf muscles are compressed towards the midline with the fingers or with the thenar/hypothenar eminences.

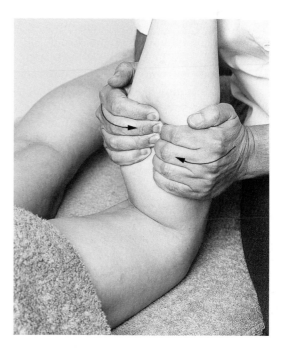

Figure 6.8 Kneading the calf muscles.

on the lateral side of the calf. Compress the gastrocnemius muscle between the fingers and the thenar/hypothenar eminences. Carry out this action with both hands simultaneously, then roll the muscle forward with the thenar/hypothenar eminences of both hands respectively, while keeping the fingers in a stationary position. Release the kneading compression and then repeat the procedure. Reposition the hands to massage another section of the muscle, and continue with the technique along the whole length of the calf.

Bodywork technique

Neuromuscular technique on the calf

Effects and applications

- Congestion in the fascial and fatty layers on the medial region of the lower leg can cause pain and create compression on vital structures such as the saphenous nerve. The NMT is used to help reduce congestion and improve the state of the tissues.
- While the saphenous vein is likewise affected, congestion may be present within the vein itself. This is generally reduced with effleurage movements, and is improved further with the NMT.
- The synovial bursa of the pes anserinus, in the more proximal region of the lower leg, is another structure that is susceptible to congestion and is treated with the NMT. The pes anserinus is the common tendon insertion of the sartorius, the gracilis and semitendinosus on the medial border of the tibia's tuberosity.
- Tightness of the fascial tissue that inserts along the medial border of the tibia is also common. Massage along this region of the tibia helps to lessen this irregularity.

Practitioner's posture

Stand in the to-and-fro or upright posture, at the foot end of the treatment table. Increase pressure from behind the movement by leaning forward.

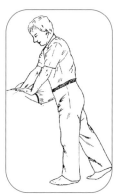

Procedure

Raise the patient's lower leg, with the knee flexed, and support the foot with the more lateral hand (Fig. 6.9). Position the more medial hand on the lower leg, curving the palm and fingers round the anterior region. Place the thumb, pointing towards the knee, on the medial/posterior border of the tibia. Flex the interphalangeal joint of the thumb and apply pressure using the thumb tip or pad. Start the technique at the distal end of the lower leg, proximal to the medial malleolus. Effleurage with the thumb along the medial border of the tibia in a cephalad direction (towards the head). Apply a very short stroke to assess and treat the tissues, and repeat it several times before moving on to another section. This whole region of the lower leg can be tender because of the congestion; therefore, adjust the pressure of the thumb according to the state of the tissues and the tenderness elicited. End the technique in the region just inferior to the medial condyle of the tibia. Add pressure behind the movement by leaning forward slightly. If you are standing in the to-and-fro posture, shift the body weight onto your front foot.

With the knee still flexed in this position, you can apply a similar movement on the lateral border of the tibia. In this case, massage the lower leg with the more lateral hand. Apply the stroke in between the lateral border of the tibia and the fibula, along the fibres of the tibialis anterior and the peroneus muscle group.

Deep stroking technique

Effleurage *du poing* on the posterior thigh

Effects and applications

- Effleurage *du poing* is a further technique that can be used when heavy pressure is indicated, generally when the muscles are over developed or very tight. A direct effect of the movement is to enhance the venous flow of the blood.
- The technique also eases contractures and tightness, which occur frequently in muscles like the hamstrings.

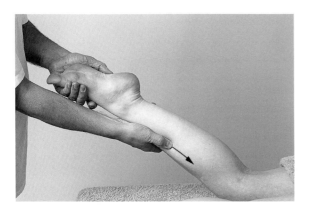

Figure 6.9 The neuromuscular technique is carried out with the tip of the thumb on the medial border of the tibia.

- The heavy pressure of the movement has the additional effect of stretching the superficial and the deep fascia. This manipulation of the tissues helps to reduce any fibrotic build-up and adhesions.
- This deep effleurage movement can be used in addition to the effleurage carried out with the palms of both hands (see Fig. 6.2).
- The effleurage is demonstrated on the posterior thigh. It can, however, be applied in a similar manner on the anterior thigh when the patient is lying supine.

Practitioner's posture

Position yourself in the lunging posture and to the side of the treatment table. Place both hands on the posterior region of the thigh, at the distal end. Keep the arms locked straight or slightly flexed at the elbow, to facilitate pressure behind the movement.

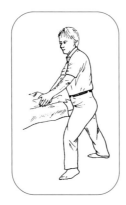

Procedure

Close the fingers and make a fist of each hand, aligning the fingertips on the thenar and hypothenar eminences. The technique is carried out with the proximal phalanges of each fist, and it is necessary to guard against applying pressure with the knuckles (metacarpophalangeal and interphalangeal joints).

Place one thumb inside the other fisted hand to interlock the hands. Apply the effleurage, with both fists simultaneously, on the posterior region of the thigh. Start the movement at the distal end, just above the knee, and effleurage in a cephalad direction (Fig. 6.10). Add pressure behind the movement by shifting your body forward onto the front foot and flexing the front knee at the same time. When you reach the more proximal end of the thigh, release the pressure and return the hands to the distal end. Repeat the stroke several times. If necessary, place both hands further medially or laterally to cover the whole width of the thigh.

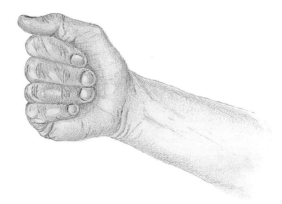

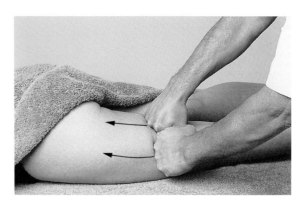

Figure 6.10 Effleurage *du poing* on the posterior lateral thigh.

Deep stroking technique

Effleurage *du poing* on the iliotibial band

Effects and applications

- The iliotibial band, running along the lateral region of the thigh, can be contracted owing to postural imbalances or heavy exercise. Tightness of the iliotibial band can lead to restricted movements of the limb and pelvis. Pain may also be elicited in the thigh, the knee or the back. The effleurage *du poing* movement helps to ease the rigidity and applies a stretch to the fascial band.
- Congestion and tenderness in the iliotibial band may be caused by its reflex connection to the digestive system and to the bladder. Massage to this region of the thigh is therefore very beneficial for normalizing the function of these associated organs.
- This technique can also be applied when the patient is lying supine.

Practitioner's posture

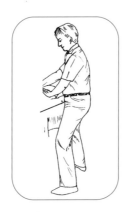

The basic stance for this movement is the t'ai chi posture, which allows for pressure to be applied sideways on to the thigh and the iliotibial band. Sliding of the hands along the thigh is facilitated by moving the whole body in a cephalad direction (towards the head).

Procedure

Close the more cephalad hand into a fist and place it on the lateral region of the thigh. Interlock the more caudal thumb inside the fisted hand, and spread the palm and fingers over the anterior and medial region of the thigh (Fig. 6.11). Apply some pressure with the fist and with the opposing hand to compress the tissues. Flex the more cephalad elbow, and rest it on your abdomen or pelvis. Keeping the hands interlocked and starting at the distal end of the thigh, effleurage in a cephalad direction. Exert pressure mostly with the fisted hand, leaning forward to transfer weight onto the same hand. Move your body forward with the movement by flexing the more cephalad knee and shifting your body weight onto the same leg. Continue the stroke as far as the buttock. Release the pressure and shift the body weight onto the more caudal foot again. Repeat the technique a few times.

Compression technique

Petrissage on the posterior thigh

Effects and applications

- Petrissage increases the circulation in the thigh muscles and furthers their relaxation. The muscles that benefit from this technique are the hamstrings group and the adductors. The technique is also effective in preventing and reducing muscle tightness, fibrotic tissue and fascial contractures. These disorders can occur due, for instance, to long periods of sitting and recurrent strains.
- This massage movement helps to break up and disperse the fat globules of adipose tissue, which are common in the thigh.
- Areas of varicosity are contraindications to this massage.

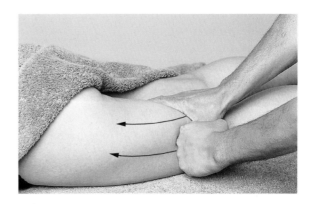

Figure 6.11 Effleurage *du poing* on the iliotibial band.

Practitioner's posture

Stand in the t'ai chi posture, and at a slight distance away from the edge of the treatment table. In this arrangement you can press forward through one arm and exert a pulling action with the other arm. Some twisting of the trunk may be involved in these actions.

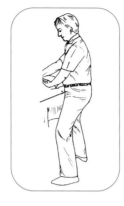

Procedure

Place the hands on the thigh, one on the medial and the other on the lateral region (Fig. 6.12). Compress the tissues by applying pressure with the fingers of one hand and the thumb of the other. The heel of the hand can be substituted for the thumb; using this allows for more pressure to be applied and lessens the risk of stressing the thumb. Maintain this hand position as you lift and twist the tissues in a clockwise or anticlockwise direction; at this stage do not slide the hands. Release the grip and relax the hands.

Allow the hands to slide to the outer and the medial borders of the thigh, respectively, then compress the tissues once more, having first swapped the hand positions (i.e. using the fingers of one hand instead of the thumb and vice versa). Maintain the compression as you lift and twist the tissues in an anticlockwise or clockwise direction

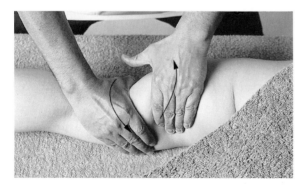

Figure 6.12 Petrissage to the thigh muscles is applied with the fingers of one hand pressing against the opposite thumb.

(whichever is practical). Release the grip and relax the hands before returning them to the outer borders of the thigh to resume the compression. Repeat the procedure a few times on one region and continue with the same routine along the length of the thigh. If your hands are not large enough to massage the whole width of the thigh, you may find it more practical to massage the posterior/medial region only; you can then move to the other side of the treatment table to apply the same movement to the posterior/lateral region.

Stroking technique

Effleurage on the leg (supine)

Effects and applications

- The technique increases the circulation in the lower limb, in particular the venous return. In addition, it has an influence on the lymphatic drainage, both locally and systemically.

Effleurage in the lunging posture

You can perform effleurage to the whole leg when you are in the lunging posture, using the palms of both hands. This technique is described for the posterior region of the leg (see Fig. 6.2). As an alternative, or in addition to this movement, you can apply the following technique while you stand at the side of the treatment table in the t'ai chi posture. It is more practical to keep your back straight while you are in the t'ai chi posture; however, you cannot apply as much pressure behind the movement as when you are standing in the lunging posture.

Effleurage in the t'ai chi posture

Stand in the t'ai chi posture and to the side of the treatment table. Adjust your position so that you can comfortably extend your hands to the foot as well as to the proximal end of the thigh.

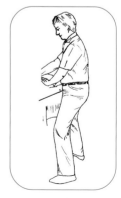

Procedure

Place the hands next to each other across the lower leg, with your fingers curved round the leg and pointing away from you (Fig. 6.13). Apply slight compression with both hands as you effleurage in a cephalad direction (towards the head). Bend your cephalad knee to shift your body in the same direction and therefore add weight behind the movement. Reduce the pressure as you reach the upper thigh, then trace the hands lightly back to the ankle. Repeat the routine several times.

Effleurage for the arterial blood flow

While you are in the t'ai chi posture, carry out an additional massage stroke to the lower leg to increase the arterial blood flow. Apply the effleurage with the caudal hand, placing the fingers on the medial region of the leg and the thumb on the lateral side (Fig. 6.14). Hold the wrist of the caudal hand with the other hand, and

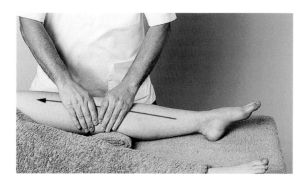

Figure 6.13 Effleurage to the leg while standing in the t'ai chi posture.

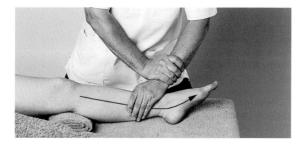

Figure 6.14 The effleurage is continued in a caudal direction to enhance the arterial supply.

maintain this position as you carry out the effleurage along the lower leg. Start at the knee and travel over the whole region of the lower leg, including the foot and toes, then return the hands to the knee area and repeat the stroke.

Stroking technique

Effleurage to the foot

Effects and applications

- This effleurage stroke is used to help increase the general circulation of the foot. As it is applied in the direction of the toes it has the additional benefit of aiding the blood supply to this area. As with other massage movements on the feet, this effleurage is also relaxing to most subjects.

Practitioner's posture

Stand in the to-and-fro posture at the foot end of the massage table. You will need to bend forward slightly to reach the foot so take care not to strain your back. An alternative arrangement is to be sitting while carrying out this movement.

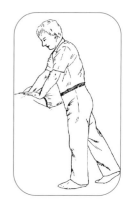

Procedure

Hold the foot by placing the palms of both hands on the dorsal aspect of the foot, and the thumbs on the plantar side (Fig. 6.15). Keep the fingers relaxed and wrapped around the contours of the foot, while holding the thumbs straight and flat to the skin surface. Apply a gentle squeeze between the fingers and thumb of each hand and, starting from the more proximal end (nearer to the ankle) effleurage with both hands in the direction of the toes. Continue the stroke to cover all of the toes and then ease off the pressure and return the hands to the ankle. Repeat the stroke as necessary.

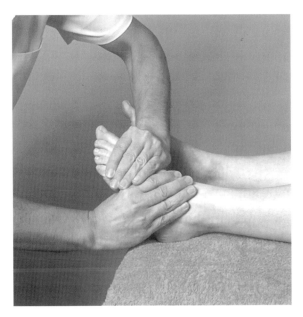

Figure 6.15   Effleurage, with some compression, applied to the foot.

Stroking technique

Fingertip effleurage around the malleoli

Effects and applications

- The tendons and ligaments around the malleoli can benefit from this effleurage stroke. Circulation to the tissues is enhanced and congestion in the area is reduced.

Practitioner's posture

You can either be sitting to carry out this movement or you can stand. If you choose to stand, then the to-and-fro or the upright postures can be adopted. In either case you will need to bend forward slightly; therefore take care not to put too much strain on the back.

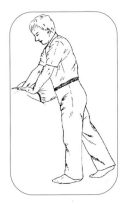

Procedure

Place the hands one on either side of the ankle, with the fingers on the medial and lateral aspects, just above the malleoli (Fig. 6.16). Cross the thumbs over each other or keep them close together. Using the pads of the fingers apply some pressure into the tissues, adjusting it so that it is comfortable to the subject. Stroke around each malleolus, to cover the tendons and ligaments on each side. Maintain the pressure as you go round and repeat the circular movement a few times.

Deep stroking technique

Effleurage *du poing* on the lower leg (anterior)

Effects and applications

- Effleurage *du poing* exerts a heavy effleurage on the lower leg muscles, such as the tibialis anterior, which may be tight—generally owing to exercise or physical work, cycling, or from postural imbalances involving the

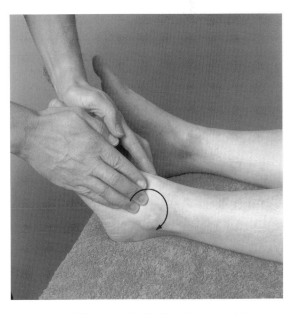

Figure 6.16   Effleurage with the fingertips around the malleoli.

mechanics of the feet. The other muscles that benefit from this movement are the extensor digitorum and the peroneus (longus and brevis). To some extent, the applied pressure transfers also to the deeper tibialis posterior muscle.

• Circulatory problems of the blood vessels, whether systemic or cardiac, can be reflected in the region of the lower leg by the presence of ulcers. Such a situation contraindicates massage.

Practitioner's posture

Stand in the lunging posture. Position yourself in line with the recipient's feet, or just beyond the edge of the treatment table. Adjust your stance if necessary so that you can extend your hands to the proximal region of the lower leg.

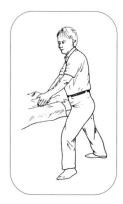

Procedure

Close the more lateral hand into a fist and place it on the distal end of the lower leg, between the tibia and the fibula (Fig. 6.17). Interlock the more medial thumb into the fisted hand. Rest the fingers of the medial hand on the medial region of the lower leg, and effleurage with both hands interlocked in this position. Start at the distal end of the lower leg and travel towards the knee. Lock the wrist and elbow and keep the fisted hand on the anterior region of the lower leg throughout the movement.

Shift your body weight onto the front leg and simultaneously flex your front knee; this manoeuvre enables you to move forward and add pressure behind the movement. Reduce the pressure when your hands reach the region of the knee, then place the hands on the more distal end of the lower leg to resume the technique. Repeat the routine several times.

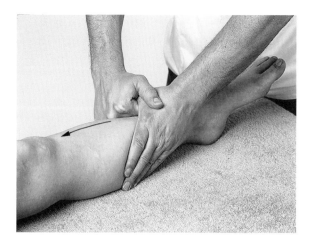

Figure 6.17 Effleurage *du poing* to the anterior aspect of the lower leg.

Deep stroking technique

Deep effleurage on the thigh (anterior)

Effects and applications

• A heavy pressure can be exerted with this effleurage. It may therefore be indicated when the muscles are well developed or very tight. This method of effleurage is also useful in cases of obesity.

Practitioner's posture

Stand in the lunging posture, close to the side of the treatment table. As you carry out the massage, shift your weight onto the front leg to add pressure behind the movement.

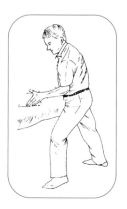

Procedure for effleurage on the anterolateral region

Place the elbow of the lateral arm on your abdomen or pelvis. Rest the lateral hand on the thigh just proximal to the knee (Fig. 6.18). Position the fingers on the lateral region of the thigh, close together and pointing in a cephalad direction. Set the thumb on the anterior side. Position the more medial hand on the medial region of the thigh, to stabilize the leg and as a counterpressure to the movement. Exert even pressure with the fingers, the palm and the thumb as you effleurage in a cephalad direction (towards the upper thigh). Increase the pressure and body weight behind the movement by shifting the body forward onto the front foot and flexing the front knee. Release the pressure when your hand reaches the proximal end of the thigh, then shift the body weight onto the back leg and return the hand to the distal end of the thigh. Repeat the procedure several times.

Procedure for effleurage on the medial region of the thigh

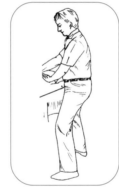

Stand in the t'ai chi posture and in line with the recipient's pelvis. Place the more cephalad hand on the medial region of the thigh, just proximal to the knee. Curve the fingers round

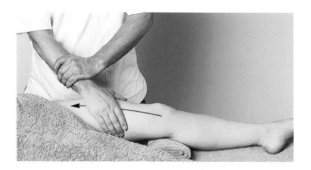

Figure 6.19   Deep effleurage to the medial aspect of the thigh.

the medial side and place the thumb more anteriorly. Hold the wrist with the more caudal hand and use this hold to add pressure to the movement. Effleurage in a cephalad direction with the hands interlocked in this position (Fig. 6.19). Shift your body weight onto the more cephalad leg as you apply the stroke. Trace the effleuraging hand along the medial region of the thigh, and then onto the anterior side before you reach the groin area. Return the hands to the knee area and repeat the movement.

LYMPH MASSAGE TECHNIQUES FOR THE LOWER LIMB

Lymph massage techniques are different from other massage movements in that they are carried out extremely slowly and always in the direction of the lymph nodes; also, very little or no lubrication is used for the movements and only minimal pressure is employed. The two lymph massage techniques described in this text are the intermittent pressure and the lymph effleurage techniques.

The intermittent pump-like action assists in the forward movement of lymph. This is enhanced further by the reflex action of the technique; stretching the tissues in two directions stimulates the receptor organs in the walls of the lymph vessels and causes a reflex contraction of their walls.

Lymph effleurage increases the pressure in the lymph vessels. As a result of the increase in

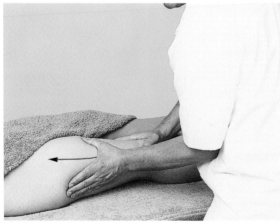

Figure 6.18   Deep effleurage to the lateral and anterior aspects of the thigh.

pressure, the lymph is pushed forward towards the more proximal group of lymph nodes. In addition, the sensory receptors in the vessel walls are stimulated and the vessels reflexively contract. A small amount of lubrication can be used for lymph effleurage to facilitate a smooth movement of the hands over the skin.

Lymph massage movements on the lower limb are carried out using one of the two routines described here. Both routines assist the lymph drainage by enhancing the lymph flow in the thigh before that of the lower leg and foot. Some of the massage movements are demonstrated on the anterior side of the leg, while others are described for the posterior region. The routines, however, are equally applicable to both sides with one or two variations.

Routine A

Perform the intermittent pressure movements on the anterior region of the leg, starting with the area of the inguinal nodes. Continue to the thigh, the knee, the lower leg and, lastly, the foot. Next, apply some lubrication and carry out the effleurage strokes on the same areas, starting again with the thigh, then on to the lower leg, the ankle and foot.

Routine B

Carry out the intermittent pressure movements as well as the effleurage strokes on the thigh, then repeat both techniques on the lower leg, then on the foot and ankle.

Assisting the lymph flow

Place a low cushion or folded towel under the knees when carrying out movements on the anterior region of the thigh with the patient supine. This adjustment raises the thigh and therefore uses gravity to assist drainage into the inguinal nodes. It also encourages relaxation of the thigh and abdominal muscles. When massaging the lower leg and foot, you can reduce the height of the cushion or remove it altogether. When massaging the patient in the prone position, place a cushion or folded towel

under the feet to raise the lower leg and thus use gravity to assist the drainage into the popliteal nodes.

Effects and applications

- The effects and applications are common to all lymph massage techniques. They are used to increase drainage of the lymph through the lymph vessels and nodes. The movements have a direct mechanical influence on the lymph fluid, as well as a reflex effect on the lymph vessels (see Chapter 3). Lymph massage on the lower limb is applied in most cases of oedema, which is most noticeable at the knee and ankle.

Intermittent pressure technique

The thigh (anterior)

Practitioner's posture

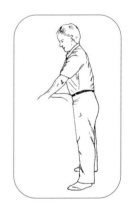

Stand in the upright posture, close to the treatment table and facing towards the patient. Body weight is not required to increase pressure; therefore maintain a relaxed and comfortable stance throughout the movement.

Procedure

Place the hands next to each other and across the upper thigh, close to the inguinal nodes (Fig. 6.20). Angle the fingers so that they point towards the inguinal ligament (between the pubic bone and the anterior superior iliac spine). Without tensing the hands, apply very light pressure with the fingers. Synchronize this action with that of stretching the tissues in two directions: towards the medial region of the thigh and the inguinal nodes. This movement on the anterior thigh translates as a stretch in an anticlockwise direction when massaging the right leg, and a stretch in a clockwise direction when massaging the left leg. Adjust the angle of the fingers to

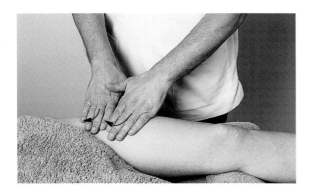

Figure 6.20 The intermittent pressure technique is applied near the inguinal nodes and on other regions of the thigh.

suit your posture, provided that the movement is still carried out towards the inguinal nodes. Prevent the hands from sliding during this manoeuvre, as this hinders the 'pump-like' action of the technique. Release the pressure and the stretch altogether once you have applied the two-way stretch, and allow the tissues to return to their normal relaxed state. Repeat the same procedure several times on the same region, then move the hands to different positions along the inguinal ligament area and the proximal end of the thigh and repeat the technique.

Intermittent pressure technique on the medial and lateral thigh

Adjust your position if necessary and place your hands transversely to the thigh. Continue with the intermittent pressure technique on the medial region of the thigh. To massage the lateral thigh area, move round the treatment table and apply the movement from that side. Adjust the positions of your hands so that you can stretch the tissues in two directions, i.e. away from you and towards the inguinal nodes.

Intermittent pressure technique

The knee

Practitioner's posture

Stand in the upright posture facing towards the recipient, and place one foot slightly behind the other. Sitting on the edge of the treatment table is

an alternative posture for this movement. Carry out the movement with the caudal hand and, therefore, the more medial one.

Procedure

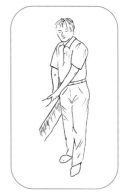

The procedure for this intermittent pressure movement is carried out in one continuous action. However, it is described here in its various stages:

1. Place the thumb on the lateral region of the lower thigh, just proximal to the knee. Keep the fingers straight and relaxed and rest them on the medial side (Fig. 6.21A). Hold the hand more or less upright and the wrist slightly flexed; at this stage the thenar/hypothenar eminences do not touch the tissues. The action of the wrist controls the movement of the hand and therefore plays an important role in this technique.

2. Apply a very gentle and equal pressure with the fingers and the thumb. Note that this pressure is to the superficial tissues only, and that a heavy application will compress the lymph vessels and occlude them.

3. Maintaining this slight pressure, and with the hand in the same position, apply a gentle and simultaneous stretch to the tissues on both sides. The stretch is more or less in a perpendicular direction and is therefore towards the treatment table. It is also a very small stretch, sufficient to take the 'slack' out of the tissues. It is necessary to guard against stretching beyond the 'yield' of the tissues.

4. Next, lower the wrist and swivel it into extension. With this action, you can also move the fingers and thumb in an arc to point them towards the head (Fig. 6.21B). During this manoeuvre, maintain the grip on the tissues to stretch them in the same direction. Avoid any sliding of the fingers and thumb, and do not extend the stretch beyond the 'yield' of the tissues.

5. Release the pressure and the stretch altogether, and flex the wrist so that the hand is in

the upright position once more. Repeat the procedure several times.

Carry out the movement just proximal to the knee, at the very distal end of the thigh, then repeat it over the knee.

Intermittent pressure technique

The foot (anterior)

Practitioner's posture

Sit at the foot end of the treatment table. Rest the calcaneus on a folded towel to raise the

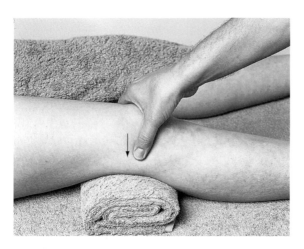

Figure 6.21A The fingers and thumb gently compress the tissues and stretch them towards the treatment table.

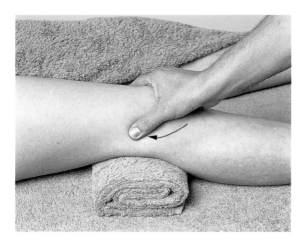

Figure 6.21B The stretch is continued in a cephalad direction before the tissues are released.

foot and to reach comfortably behind the malleoli.

Procedure for the intermittent pressure technique on the anterior side of the malleoli

Position the hands one on each side of the ankle. Place two fingers on the anterior part of the malleolus, making contact with the pads of the fingers and keeping them flat to the skin surface (Fig. 6.22). Press gently with the pads of the fingers to compress the fluid and grip the tissues. Stretch the tissues in an 'arc'; towards the centre of the ankle and towards the knee. Ease off the pressure and allow the tissues to return to their normal state. Repeat the procedure a few times, then reposition the fingers to treat another region. Continue with this method over the anterior surface of the ankle.

Procedure for the intermittent pressure technique on the dorsum of the foot

As this technique is a continuation of the one around the ankle, continue to use the same two fingers. Place them across the dorsum of the foot or at a slight angle to each other. Use a similar method as for the ankle. Exert a small degree of pressure with the pads of the fingers as you

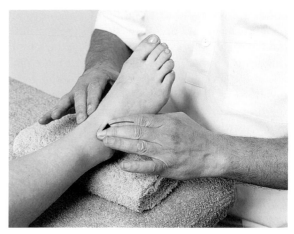

Figure 6.22 The intermittent pressure technique on the anterior side of the ankle and malleoli.

simultaneously stretch the tissues, towards the midline and towards the knee. Having applied the movement a few times on one area, change the position of the fingers to repeat the routine on another area until you have covered the whole region of the dorsum. It may also be practical to extend the movement to the toes, although these will drain once the dorsum and ankle are clear of oedema.

Procedure for the intermittent pressure technique on the posterior side of the malleoli

Carry out the intermittent pressure technique on the posterior part of the malleoli and on each side of the Achilles tendon. Introduce a gentle pressure with the pads of two fingers (Fig. 6.23). Maintain the grip on the tissues as you stretch them in the same 'arc' direction, towards the anterior side of the ankle and towards the knee. Positioning the fingers on each side of the Achilles tendon may prove difficult, especially if the recipient's foot is rotated laterally. You may therefore prefer to treat one side at a time, and to use the non-massaging hand to hold and support the foot. Placing a folded towel under the calcaneus can also make the technique more practical.

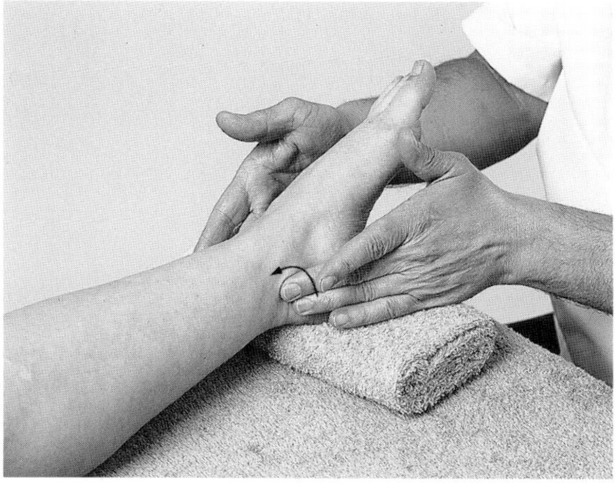

Lymph effleurage techniques

The leg (anterior)

Lymph effleurage on the knee and thigh (anterior)

While you can carry out this movement in the upright posture, you may find it more comfortable to be sitting. It is also easier to maintain contact with the hands and to keep them relaxed when you are in the sitting position. Place the hands on each side of the knee (Fig. 6.24). Make contact with the fingers and palm of each hand, keeping them relaxed and flat to the skin surface. Compress the tissues marginally by exerting a uniform pressure with both hands. Starting below the knee itself, effleurage in a cephalad direction. Trace your hands on each side of the knee, then allow them to meet just above the knee. Continue the stroke along the thigh with the hands next to each other. When you reach a comfortable point on the proximal thigh, remove the hands and return them to the knee area. Repeat the same stroke several times.

Lymph effleurage on the anterior/lateral thigh

Place both hands on the lateral region of the thigh, at the more distal end. Make contact with the fingers, the palm and the hypothenar/thenar

Figure 6.23 The intermittent pressure technique behind each malleolus and on either side of the Achilles tendon.

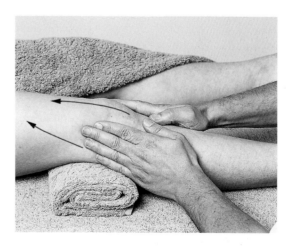

Figure 6.24 Lymph effleurage on the knee and the thigh.

eminences. Angle the fingers to point towards the inguinal area. Use only the weight of the hands for the effleurage, as the movement is more like 'dragging' your hands over the skin. This light pressure is sufficient to drain the fluid through the superficial vessels; a heavier application will compress and occlude them. It may help you to visualize a layer of fluid just below the skin, which is being encouraged to flow through very fine and delicate channels. Effleurage in the direction of the inguinal nodes. Keep the hands close together and move them very slowly; allow about 6 seconds to complete the stroke. End the movement before you reach the inguinal nodes, then remove the hands and return to the more distal position. Repeat the stroke several times, arranging the hands in different positions to massage the whole region of the thigh. Use a small amount of lubrication to help the hands move smoothly over the skin.

Lymph effleurage on the anterior/medial thigh

To massage the anterior/medial region of the thigh, stand in the upright posture and place the hands on the medial region of the thigh. Curve the fingers around the thigh and point them towards the treatment table. Maintain this relationship of the hands to the thigh, and effleurage from the distal end towards the inguinal nodes. An alternative method is to stand at the level of the recipient's pelvis and, placing one hand on the medial side of the thigh, effleurage gently towards the inguinal nodes. Keep the hand relaxed and in full contact with the skin. Use very little pressure, and carry out the stroke very slowly.

Lymph effleurage to the lower leg (anterior)

Sit at the foot end of the treatment table to carry out this effleurage stroke. Place the hands one on either side of the lower leg, making contact with the fingers and palm of each hand (see Fig. 2.15). Start the technique at the distal end of the lower leg, and continue the stroke to either side of the knee. Provided it is comfortable to perform, extend the stroke to include the thigh, as this

helps to drain the fluid towards the inguinal nodes. Next, remove the hands and return them to the ankle area. Repeat the same stroke several times

Lymph effleurage on the ankle and foot

For this movement you can either sit at the foot end of the treatment table or be in a standing position. Either position should enable you to carry out the massage in the same slow manner and without exerting any pressure. Place one hand across the dorsum of the foot, keeping the fingers relaxed and curved round its contour (Fig. 6.25). Support the foot on the plantar surface with the other hand. Effleurage over the dorsum of the foot and the ankle, applying a light pressure, and continue the stroke onto the lower leg. Gently lift the hand and position it on the foot to resume the effleurage. Repeat the procedure a few times.

Intermittent pressure technique

The thigh (posterior)

Practitioner's posture

Stand in the upright posture and at the side of the treatment table. This position is the most suitable when massaging the medial region of the

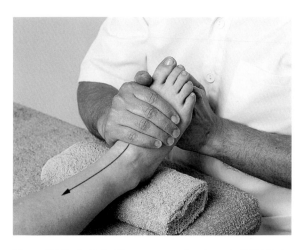

Figure 6.25 Lymph effleurage over the dorsum of the foot.

thigh; however, to massage the lateral side you will need to move round the treatment table and resume the upright posture. Carry out the effleurage from that side of the treatment table, reaching across and placing your hands on the outer thigh region.

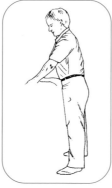

Procedure for the intermittent pressure technique on the medial side of the thigh (prone)

The procedure for this technique is similar to that carried out on the anterior region of the thigh (see Fig. 6.20). Place both hands, next to each other, on the posteromedial part of the thigh and close to the buttocks. Using mainly the fingers, apply a gentle pressure and stretch the tissues in an 'arc' direction, towards the treatment table and the inguinal nodes. This movement can be translated as an anticlockwise direction when massaging the left leg and clockwise on the right. Release the pressure and the stretch altogether, and allow the tissues to return to their normal relaxed state. Repeat the procedure several times, then move the hands further down the thigh and repeat the movement. Continue with this method along the length of the thigh to the knee.

Procedure for the intermittent pressure technique on the lateral side of the thigh (prone)

Move round to the other side of the treatment table and stand in the upright posture. Reach over to the contralateral thigh, and place your hands on the lateral region. Apply the same intermittent pressure to the tissues, and simultaneously stretch them towards the treatment table and towards the pelvis. This is a clockwise movement when massaging the left thigh and anticlockwise on the right. Start at the proximal end and repeat the same procedure along the thigh to the popliteal fossa.

Intermittent pressure technique

The calf

Practitioner's posture

Stand in the upright posture, with one foot behind the other. Position yourself to the side of the treatment table and rotate your body so that you face in a cephalad direction (towards the recipient's head).

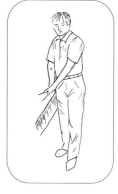

Procedure

With your body rotated towards the head end of the treatment table, place the more medial hand on the patient's calf. Rest the thumb on the lateral side of the calf and the fingers on the medial region (Fig. 6.26A). Use the same intermittent pressure technique as for the knee. Apply a gentle pressure with the thumb and the fingers while the hand is more or less upright. Maintain this gentle grip on the tissues and stretch them towards the plinth and towards the popliteal fossa; the stretch is continuous and forms an 'arc'. To carry out this action, extend the wrist so that you can lower the hand

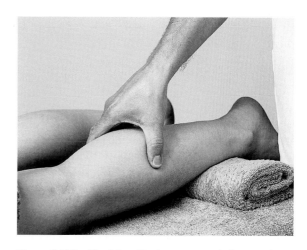

Figure 6.26A The intermittent pressure technique on the calf, using a gentle grip with the fingers and the thumb.

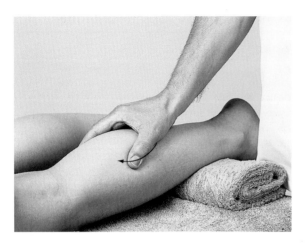

Figure 6.26B The grip is held and the tissues momentarily stretched.

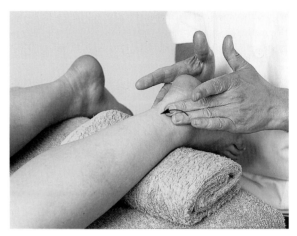

Figure 6.27 Intermittent pressure is applied with the pads of two fingers around the malleolus and Achilles tendon.

and swivel the fingers and thumb together in the direction of the popliteal fossa (Fig. 6.26B). Guard against stretching beyond the 'yield' in the tissues, and against sliding the hands. Next, release the pressure to allow the tissues to return to their normal relaxed state before resuming the procedure once again. Start at the upper end of the calf and, having applied the movement a few times, reposition the hands in a more caudal position (towards the feet). Repeat the movement and continue in the same manner along the length of the calf.

Intermittent pressure technique

The Achilles tendon and malleoli

Procedure

Sit at the foot end of the treatment table. To assist with the lymph drainage, raise the recipient's lower leg by wedging a cushion or folded towel under the foot or ankle. Place the pads of two fingers on each side of the foot, close to the malleoli and the Achilles tendon (Fig. 6.27). Gently press the tissues, with the pads of the fingers close together. Hold this gentle grip and stretch the tissues towards the midline and towards the popliteal fossa. The fascial layers are generally rigid in this region; the range of motion is therefore somewhat limited. Release the grip and

allow the tissues to recoil to the normal resting state, then repeat the procedure over the same area. Continue to the other regions of the malleolus and Achilles tendon.

Lymph effleurage technique

The thigh (posterior)

Practitioner's posture

Sit to the side of the treatment table and position yourself in line with the subject's knees. Rotate your whole body so that you can massage the medial and lateral sides of the thigh without twisting your trunk.

Procedure for lymph effleurage to the posteromedial region

Place your hands on the midline of the thigh, proximal to the popliteal fossa (Fig. 6.28). Adjust the position of the hands so that they are relaxed throughout the movement and you can move them without straining your wrists. It is not necessary for the hands to be parallel to each other when massaging the posteromedial thigh. The more lateral hand, for instance, can be at a slight angle to the medial one; this association can be altered throughout the movement to allow a smooth effleurage stroke. The lymph channels on the posterior region of the thigh follow two directions away from the midline, one medially and one laterally; the lymph effleurage is therefore carried out along the same paths. Massage the posteromedial side, starting on the midline and sliding the hands gently and very slowly diagonally across the thigh. This follows the lymph channel towards the medial side and the inguinal nodes. Continue to the proximal end of the thigh. Next, remove the hands, place them once more on the more distal region, and repeat the stroke. A tiny amount of lubrication may be necessary to facilitate a smooth movement.

Procedure for lymph effleurage to the posterolateral region

As you massage the posterolateral area of the thigh, adjust the position of your hands so that you move them over the outer tissues without straining your wrists (Fig. 6.29). It is not essential for the hands to point towards the pelvis; the lateral hand can lie across the thigh or at a comfortable angle to it. Move the hands together and carry out the same slow effleurage movement, from the midline to the outer border of the thigh towards the greater trochanter. This direction follows the lymph drainage towards the inguinal nodes. Having completed the stroke to the proximal end of the thigh, return the hands to the midline and repeat the procedure.

Lymph effleurage technique

The lower leg (posterior)

Practitioner's posture

Sit at the foot end of the treatment table. Place a low cushion or folded towel under the recipient's foot to promote the lymph drainage towards the popliteal fossa.

Procedure

Place the hands one on either side of the calf and the Achilles tendon (Fig. 6.30). Keep both hands relaxed, with the fingers and palms flat. Effleurage towards the popliteal fossa using slow movements and minimal pressure, dragging the hands over the tissues rather than exerting any weight. Once you complete the stroke to the popliteal fossa, remove the hands and return them to the distal end. Repeat the stroke several times.

PERCUSSIVE TECHNIQUES ON THE LOWER LIMB

Effects and applications

- Percussive strokes can be applied on the larger muscles such as those of the lower limb. It is not necessary, however, to include these

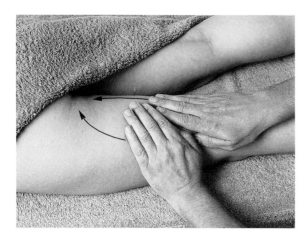

Figure 6.28 Lymph effleurage on the posterior/medial aspect of the thigh.

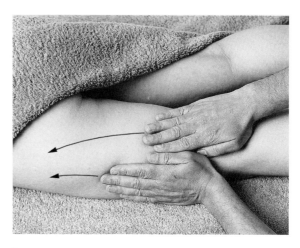

Figure 6.29 Lymph effleurage on the posterior/lateral aspect of the thigh.

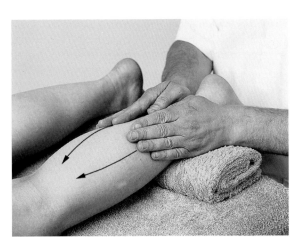

Figure 6.30 Lymph effleurage to the posterior aspect of the lower leg.

techniques in the overall body massage routine, especially if the massage is primarily for relaxation. The effects and applications are common to all methods of percussive strokes.

- Percussive strokes cause hyperaemia in the superficial and muscular tissues.
- They also stimulate the nerve endings, resulting in tiny contractions and an overall increased tone of the skeletal muscles. Consequently, they are frequently used as part of a warm-up or toning routine. They can be applied on most regions of the body, but are used predominantly on the muscles of the lower limb.
- Percussive strokes vary in pressure; they are therefore used according to the state and size of the tissues. The hacking percussive stroke, for example, is applicable on the distal end of the hamstring muscle group, while pounding is of better use in the middle region where the muscle mass is larger.
- Adipose tissue does not require heavy percussive techniques such as pounding with the fist. This type of heavy stroke is in fact contraindicated on adipose tissue, and even more so on cellulite.

Practitioner's posture

Applying percussive strokes is not a tiring exercise, provided you are in the right posture and working with ease. Some of the techniques are best applied on the ipsilateral side of the body, while others are carried out from the contralateral side. The stance is different in each case; stand in the t'ai chi posture to carry out the strokes on the ipsilateral side of the body, and take up the upright posture when massaging from the contralateral side. Hold your arms relaxed and in a comfortable position away from the body. Keep your back straight at all times.

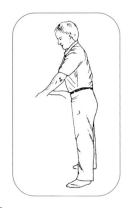

Hacking with the little fingers

Hacking to the lateral and posterior thigh is carried out from the contralateral side. Hold the hands, with the fingers straight and spread apart, above the area to be percussed (Fig. 6.31). The technique of hacking is initiated and controlled by a rapid flicking action of the wrist. Bend the wrist into abduction, thus raising the hand upwards. Next, flex the wrist into adduction and strike the tissues with the little finger, allowing the other fingers to cascade on each other and temporarily close. Abduct the wrist and the fingers again, using a rapid 'flicking' action. Spread the fingers apart once more as you simultaneously strike the tissues with the second hand. Continue with this alternating stroke along the length of the thigh. The medial side of the thigh may be too sensitive for the hacking movement and, consequently, the technique is not usually carried out on this region. If it is applied, it is best carried out from the ipsilateral side.

Hacking with curled fingers

Flex the interphalangeal joints so that the fingers are curled and the fingertips are away from the palm (Fig. 6.32). Hold the fingers close together and, using a similar flicking action to that already described, strike the tissues with the curled little finger of each hand. Use the outer

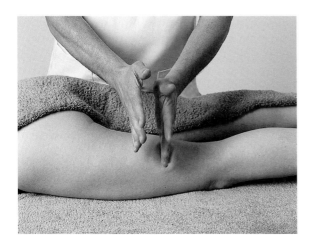

Figure 6.31 Hacking on the posterior thigh muscles.

edge of the fingers only, and not the ulnar border of the metacarpal bones. Continue with the alternating percussive strokes along the length of the thigh. This technique is slightly heavier than hacking with the little fingers, so it is well suited for large muscles like those of the central thigh. You can also carry out the same technique on the calf.

Pounding with a flat fist

Again, stand in the upright posture and on the contralateral side of the treatment table. Flex the interphalangeal joints to make a fist of each hand. Hold the fingertips straight and rest them on the thenar and hypothenar eminences; keep the fingers slightly relaxed and loose. Use the palmar side of the fist to strike the tissues, avoiding the use of the knuckles (Fig. 6.33). Carry out the action with a slight flexion of the wrist. Alternate the stroke with the other hand, and continue with it along the length of the thigh. Pounding with a flat fist offers a heavier or alternative technique to the previous hacking stroke.

Cupping

To apply this percussive stroke, flex the arm at the elbow with very little or no flexion at the wrist. Strike the tissues with the hand in a cupped shape, eliciting a deep sound (Fig. 6.34). Lift the hand without flicking the wrist, and simultaneously strike the same tissue area with the other hand. Continue with this alternating cupping over the whole length of the thigh.

Flicking

Start this technique with the palm open and the fingers together and straight (Fig. 6.35). Strike the tissues with all the fingers. Add a rapid flexion of the metacarpophalangeal joints as you carry out the striking action. This manoeuvre flicks the

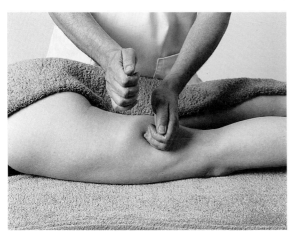

Figure 6.32 A heavier hacking stroke is applied with the fingers slightly curved.

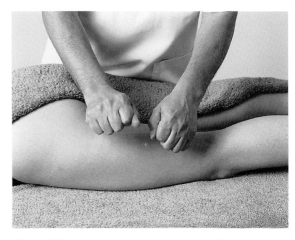

Figure 6.33 Pounding percussive stroke with the palmar side of the fist.

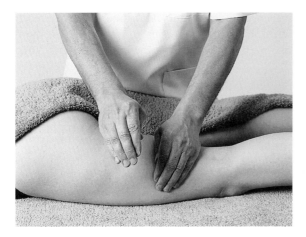

Figure 6.34 Cupping percussive stroke. The elbow is rotated as the cupped hand strikes the tissues.

tissues and shifts the muscles off the underlying layers; consequently, it instigates a reflex contraction of the muscle fibres. Repeat the same flicking movement with the other hand. Continue with this alternating method for a few seconds before moving on to another region.

SUPPLEMENTARY TECHNIQUES FOR THE LOWER LIMB: SUBJECT SIDE-LYING

The patient can lie in the recovery position, with the uppermost leg flexed at the hip and knee.

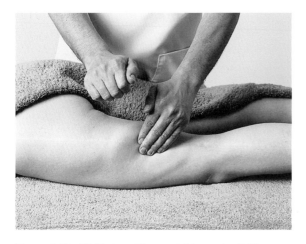

Figure 6.35 Flicking combines a striking and a flicking action on the muscles and tissues.

Support the upper knee on cushions or folded towels, and provide similar padding for the head and trunk. It is vital that the recipient is in a secure position and that this is maintained throughout the treatment. To carry out the massage movements, either stand to the side of the treatment table or sit on a chair. For some movements it may be more practical to be sitting on the edge of the treatment table.

The techniques described in this section are divided into two sets: one set of movements is for the leg resting on the treatment table (the lowermost leg), and the second set is for the uppermost leg. Carry out both sets of movements while the patient is lying on one side, then repeat the techniques when the patient is lying on the opposite side.

Effects and applications

• Massage on the lower limbs can be applied with the patient lying on the side. This practical position is useful in a number of situations: for example, for pregnant women, overweight or elderly subjects, patients following an operation on the abdomen or those with back problems. In most of these conditions the circulation of the lower limb is likely to be impaired. Techniques such as effleurage and petrissage are therefore indicated and are of great benefit. The techniques in this section are synonymous with those carried out when the patient is lying prone or supine. Furthermore, the effects and applications are common to all of the techniques; as these have already been described in the earlier sections they are not repeated here unless additional information is appropriate.

Stroking technique

Effleurage on the lowermost leg

Practitioner's posture

Stand in the lunging posture and to the ipsilateral side of the plinth. Position yourself in line with the recipient's lower leg, and face in a cephalad direction (towards the head). Shift your body weight onto the front leg to exert some pressure behind the movement.

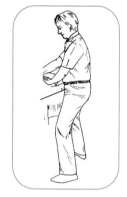

Procedure for effleurage to the posteromedial thigh

Place the more lateral hand on the thigh, with the thumb on the medial region and the fingers approximately on the lateral region. Set the more medial hand on the anterior side of the thigh, and maintain this position to support and stabilize the thigh while carrying out the effleurage with the other hand (Fig. 6.36). Apply some pressure and a gentle compression between the fingers and thumb of the more lateral hand. Effleurage in a cephalad direction, over the posterolateral region of the thigh. Flex your front knee and shift your body weight forward to add pressure behind the movement. When you reach the proximal end of the thigh remove the hand and place it on the lower end, superior to the knee. Repeat the procedure as necessary. The same effleurage method can be applied to the lower leg.

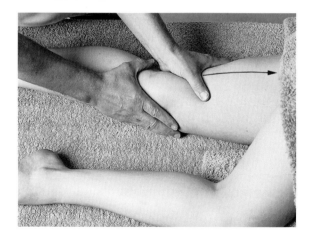

Figure 6.36 Effleurage on the posteromedial thigh is applied with one hand. A similar method is used with the other hand on the anteromedial side.

Procedure for effleurage to the anteromedial side of the thigh

To effleurage the anteromedial region of the thigh, place the hands on either side as for the previous movement. Apply the effleurage stroke with your medial hand, and a counterforce with your lateral hand. Effleurage from the knee to the upper end of the thigh, then remove the hand and return it to the lower end to repeat the effleurage movement. A similar effleurage method can be applied on the lower leg.

Compression technique

Petrissage on the lowermost thigh

Practitioner's posture

Stand in the t'ai chi posture and on the ipsilateral side of the treatment table. An alternative posture suitable when massaging the lowermost leg is to sit on a chair close to the treatment table.

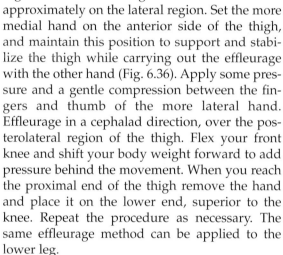

Procedure

Place the fingers of the caudal hand on the anterior region of the left thigh, and the thumb of the cephalad one on the posterior side (Fig. 6.37). Apply pressure with the fingers and the thumb to compress the tissues. It may be necessary to substitute the heel of the hand for the thumb, as this allows for more pressure and lessens the risk of stressing the thumb. Maintain this compression as you lift the tissues and apply a small twist in a clockwise direction (Fig. 6.37). Then release the grip and relax the hands. Allow the hands to slide to the outer borders, the more caudal hand moving to the posterior region of the thigh and the more cephalad hand to the anterior side. Then compress the tissues once more, using the fingers of the cephalad hand to press against the thumb of the caudal one. Maintain the compression as you lift and twist the tissues in an anticlockwise direction.

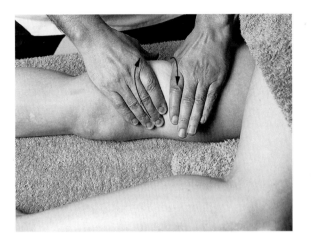

Figure 6.37 Petrissage on the left thigh. The tissues are compressed between the fingers of one hand and the opposite thumb.

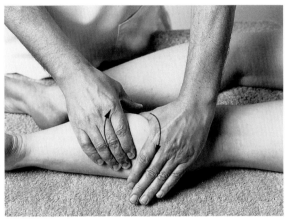

Figure 6.38 The petrissage technique on the calf.

Release the grip and relax the hands once more, then return them to the outer borders and repeat the technique.

Compression technique

Petrissage on the lowermost calf

Practitioner's posture

Stand in the upright posture and on the contralateral side of the treatment table (i.e. on the anterior side of the recipient) to massage the lowermost opposite calf.

Procedure

This technique is similar to that already described for the thigh. For the right calf compress the tissues with the fingers of the more caudal hand against the thumb of the cephalad one (Fig. 6.38). Add a slight twisting action in a clockwise direction, then release the tissues and repeat the compression and the twist with the opposite digits (i.e. with the fingers of the cephalad hand against the thumb of the caudal one). Continue with

this alternating petrissage technique as required.

Lymph massage

Intermittent pressure on the lowermost thigh

Practitioner's posture

Stand in the upright posture and on the ipsilateral side of the treatment table. The patient lies on one side, with the uppermost leg flexed at the knee and the hip, and also shifted forward on the treatment table.

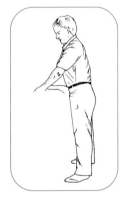

Procedure

Place both hands on the medial region of the thigh, close to the area of the inguinal nodes (Fig. 6.39). Keeping the hands relaxed, apply gentle pressure with the flat fingers, thereby compressing the fluid in the superficial tissues. Maintain this contact with the skin and stretch the tissues towards the anterior thigh and towards the inguinal nodes, describing an arc with your hands. Ease off the pressure, and allow the tissues to return to their normal resting state before

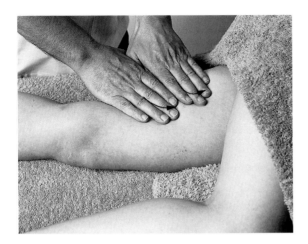

Figure 6.39   The intermittent pressure technique on the lowermost thigh.

resuming the technique. The action of applying the pressure and stretching and releasing the tissues makes up the complete movement; it is, therefore, carried out as one continuous procedure. Apply the technique on the whole region of the thigh. In addition to the intermittent pressure technique, you can apply lymph effleurage on the lowermost thigh (adopt a sitting position for this). Both techniques can also be carried out on the lowermost leg and the ankle.

Stroking technique

Effleurage on the uppermost leg

Practitioner's posture

Stand in the to-and-fro posture and on the anterior side of the recipient. Adjust your position so that you can comfortably extend your arms to the whole length of the thigh, and shift your body weight onto the front foot to add pressure behind the movement. Support the patient's uppermost knee on a cushion or folded towel.

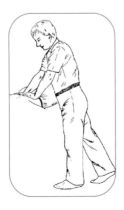

Procedure

Standing in a position facing the patient, place your more cephalad hand on the distal end of the thigh, just above the knee (Fig. 6.40). Rest the other hand on the patient's pelvis or the upper end of the thigh; use this hold to stabilize the leg. An alternative arrangement is to place the more caudal hand on top of the massaging hand to increase the pressure of the stroke.

Curve the fingers of the massaging hand around the anterior region of the thigh, and the thumb round the posterior side. Compress the tissues slightly with the fingers and thumb. Effleurage from the distal end of the thigh towards the proximal region. Lean forwards to apply pressure, raising the heel of the back foot slightly to assist with this manoeuvre. When you reach the greater trochanter, remove the hand and return it to the distal end. Repeat the routine several times.

Deep stroking technique

Effleurage *du poing* on the uppermost thigh

Practitioner's posture

Again, stand in the to-and-fro posture and on the anterior side of the recipient. Shift your body weight onto the front foot to add pressure behind the movement. Support the patient's uppermost

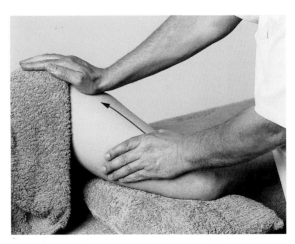

Figure 6.40   Effleurage on the uppermost thigh.

knee on a cushion or folded towel.

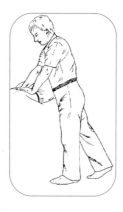

Procedure for the left thigh

Close the fingers and make a fist of the right hand, aligning the fingertips on the thenar and hypothenar eminences. Place the fisted hand on the posterolateral region of the uppermost thigh (Fig. 6.41). Push the thumb of the left hand inside the fisted one to interlock the hands. Rest the palm and fingers of the left hand around the anterolateral region of the thigh. Starting at the distal end of the thigh, effleurage upward with both hands in the interlocked position. Continue the stroke towards the proximal end. Apply pressure with the fisted hand (avoiding digging in the knuckles), and also with the corresponding palm and fingers. Add pressure behind the movement by shifting your body forward onto the front foot and raising the heel of the back foot. When you reach the more proximal end of the thigh, release the pressure and return the hands to the distal end. Repeat the stroke several times. Effleurage *du poing* on this region can

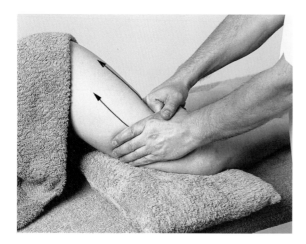

Figure 6.41 Effleurage *du poing* on the uppermost thigh.

also be applied with both hands in a fisted position.

Compression movement

Kneading the uppermost thigh

Practitioner's posture

Stand in the to-and-fro posture and on the anterior side of the recipient. Position the patient's uppermost thigh close to the ipsilateral edge of the treatment table; this arrangement enables you to extend your hands to the thigh without any excessive forward bending.

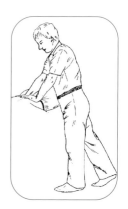

Procedure for the left thigh

Position the hands on the uppermost thigh. Place the thenar/hypothenar eminences of both hands on the iliotibial band. Curve the fingers of the right hand round the posterior region of the thigh, and those of the left hand round the anterior side (Fig. 6.42). Apply pressure with the thenar/hypothenar eminences of both hands, and compress the tissues against the fingers. Maintain this pressure as you roll the tissues forward and over the fingertips. Guard against sliding the hands over the tissues or pulling sharply on the skin. Next, remove the pressure completely and return the thenar/hypothenar eminences of both hands to the more lateral position while maintaining contact with the fingertips. Repeat the procedure over the whole region of the thigh.

Alternative compression movements

1. Instead of using two hands simultaneously as already described, you can apply the same kneading technique with one hand at a time. If you opt for this method, you may find it easier to stand in front of the recipient to knead the poste-

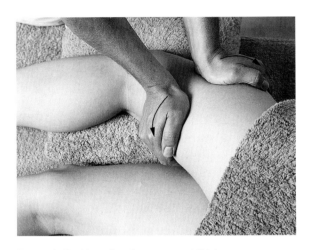

Figure 6.42   Kneading the uppermost thigh.

rior side of the thigh and behind the patient to treat the anterior region.

2. A second alternative method for the compression technique is the petrissage movement, which is similar to that used on the lowermost thigh.

7

Massage for body regions—the abdomen

OBSERVATIONS AND CONSIDERATIONS

In addition to the information obtained while taking the case history, the abdomen is observed and assessed for any conditions that may contraindicate the massage treatment. It is stressed that diagnosis of abdominal problems requires expertise that is beyond the scope of this book. However, the relevant signs and symptoms pertaining to common conditions of the abdomen and its viscera are given, with the aim of providing background knowledge for the therapist. Further information is also given in Chapter 4.

During observation and massage of the abdomen, patients lie with their arms resting on the plinth or on their chest. The arms should not be in a position above their heads, as this stretches the abdominal tissues and makes palpation difficult. Massage is also likely to be uncomfortable for patients if they have a full bladder or a full stomach.

The abdominal viscera

For the purpose of establishing the anatomical location of the structures and viscera the abdomen is divided into a number of regions and planes (Fig. 7.1 and Box 7.1). The contents of the abdominal regions are shown in Box 7.2.

The greater omentum

Deep to the muscular layer of the abdomen is the greater omentum. This can be described as an

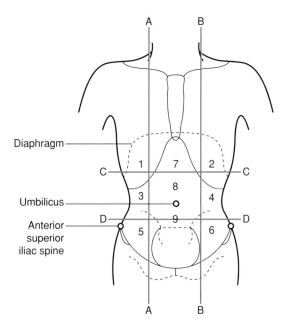

Figure 7.1 Regions and planes of the abdomen.

Box 7.1 Regions and planes of the abdomen

Regions of the abdomen

1. Right hypochondrium
2. Left hypochondrium
3. Right lumbar
4. Left lumbar
5. Right iliac region or fossa
6. Left iliac region or fossa
7. Epigastrium
8. Umbilical region
9. Hypogastrium

Planes of the abdominal wall

A. Right mid-clavicular line—from the middle of the clavicle to the middle of the inguinal ligament
B. Left mid-clavicular line
C. Transpyloric plane—midway between the suprasternal notch and the upper border of the pubic bone. It can also be described as one hands-breath below the xiphisternal joint or at the level of the ninth costal cartilage. In the anatomical position (when standing) the pylorus is from 3 to 10 cm below this line
D. Transtubercular plane. The tubercle (bony prominence) is about 5 cm further back from the anterior superior iliac spine

Box 7.2 The contents of the abdominal regions

Right hypochondriac region
Liver
Gallbladder
Hepatic flexure of colon
Right kidney
Right suprarenal gland

Epigastric
Liver
Stomach and pylorus
Transverse colon
Omentum
Pancreas
Duodenum
Kidneys
Suprarenal glands
Aorta
Lymph nodes

Left hypochondriac region
Liver
Stomach
Splenic flexure of colon
Spleen
Tail of pancreas
Left kidney
Left suprarenal gland

Right lumbar
Liver
Ascending colon
Small intestine
Right kidney

Umbilical
Stomach
Duodenum
Transverse colon
Omentum
Small intestine
Kidneys
Aorta
Lymph nodes

Left lumbar
Descending colon
Small intestine
Left kidney

Right iliac fossa
Caecum
Vermiform appendix
Lymph nodes

Hypogastric
Small intestine
Sigmoid flexure
Distended bladder
Enlarged uterus

Left iliac fossa
Sigmoid flexure
Lymph nodes

extension of the peritoneum, which drapes over the transverse colon and the coils of the small intestines. Due to the large amounts of fatty tissue it contains, the greater omentum is often referred to as the 'fatty apron'. It moves about the peritoneal cavity in response to the peristaltic action of the small intestines and colon. Adhesions can be found within it following surgery, but these are not necessarily palpable. The effect of deep massage to the abdominal wall is likely to extend to the omentum, which benefits from the improved circulation.

The stomach

An empty stomach is almost hidden by the ribs and is therefore not easily palpated. Furthermore, the stomach varies considerably in size, shape and position. It is palpable when full or when the subject is inhaling or standing. A portion of it can be palpated in the epigastric region. When the stomach is full, its circulation and that of the other digestive organs is increased. This is part of the processes of digestion and absorption, which continue for at least an hour or two after ingestion. A heavy and systemic massage is therefore not advisable for 2 h after the intake of food. Local abdominal massage is also inappropriate, as it may be uncomfortable for the recipient.

A disorder of the stomach can refer pain to the central thoracic region of the back, between the spinal vertebrae T4 and T9. Indirect tissue changes can also be observed in the thoracic back, on the left side. The following areas have increased tension:

1. To the lateral side of the vertebral column, in segments T7 and T8.

2. Over the inferior angle of the left scapula.

3. In the infraspinous fossa of the left scapula, inferior to the lateral part of the scapular spine. This area is invariably associated with gastritis and gastric ulcers. It is likely to be very tender to palpation and perhaps even to breathing.

4. The upper fibres of the left trapezius, along its lateral border in the cervical and shoulder areas—tension is not always present here.

5. On the anterior trunk, where some tension can be found along the dermatomes T7 and T8 over the left rectus abdominis.

Another reflex area to the stomach runs from the tip of the tenth costal cartilage on the left side to the sternum and then down the right costal margin. This area is massaged with the fingertips and from left to right. This is most beneficial at securing contractions of the involuntary stomach muscles.

The aorta

The abdominal aorta is palpated in the upper abdomen, slightly left of the midline. A firm pressure is applied with the thumb on one side of the aorta and the fingers on the other side. In the case of a thick abdominal wall (or as an alternative method) both hands are used, pressed firmly on each side of the aorta (Fig. 7.2). The pulsations of the aorta can be observed and identified. A normal aorta would send pulsations in an anterior direction. When the pulsations are prominent and expand laterally, they point to changes that require investigation. The most likely abnormality is an aortic aneurysm (an expansion of the aortic wall and the presence of a mass within the aorta). Until the abnormality is diagnosed by a doctor, deep massage is contraindicated. This precaution is necessary to prevent any possibility of haemorrhaging. Light stroking massage should not cause any damage, and systemic massage can also be applied.

The liver

The liver lies mostly beneath the right rib cage and in the right hypochondrium. Its lower border is often felt below the right costal margin. Palpation of the liver is carried out by placing the left hand in the loin area, parallel to the eleventh and twelfth ribs. The right hand is placed on the right abdomen, lateral to the rectus abdominis muscle and with the fingers below the costal border (Fig. 7.3). The patient takes a deep breath and a firm pressure is applied with the left hand, to push the liver anteriorly. As the diaphragm

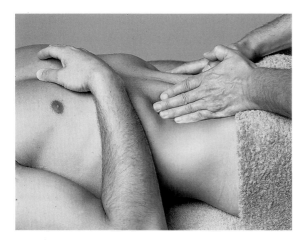

Figure 7.2 Palpating the aorta, using one hand on either side of the upper abdomen.

pushes the liver downwards, the lower edge can be palpated with the right hand. Identification may be easier if the right hand is allowed to ride over the edge of the liver as it descends. It is also helpful to reduce the pressure of the right hand at the peak of inspiration. The manoeuvre is repeated and the edge of the liver can be traced medially and laterally.

In a normal liver, the edge is felt as a firm, sharp and regular ridge with a smooth surface. Tenderness can suggest inflammation, as in hepatitis, or venous congestion, as in right-sided heart failure. Irregularity in the edge or the surface of the liver can indicate some malignant changes. Palpating the lower edge of the liver also facilitates an assessment of its size. Enlargement is indicated by an edge which is palpated well below the costal margin. An enlarged liver is common in some conditions (e.g. emphysema); however, such a change is not always present (e.g. in cirrhosis). At times the liver is elongated or in a downward displacement, but this is not necessarily indicative of pathology. In a young child, for example, the liver is relatively large and its lower border is found at a lower level.

Enlargement of the liver, as well as tenderness and irregularities, are likely to require investigation. One example is jaundice; this can lead to enlargement of the liver as well as the spleen,

and massage to these regions is contraindicated. Chronic hepatitis is a similar condition, and massage to the liver area is best avoided. It is worth mentioning at this point how important it is for the massage therapist to safeguard himself or herself against infectious diseases such as hepatitis (see Chapter 1). Viral hepatitis and jaundice associated with viral infection of the liver may contraindicate massage, or it may be carried out with extreme care.

The massage therapist may encounter an enlarged liver, but must not attempt any diagnosis and is obliged to refer the patient to the doctor. Palpation of the liver may cause a dull discomfort, which is only mild with no muscular rigidity. In most cases this is not a contraindication to massage.

Malfunction of the liver (and the gallbladder) can cause referred pain in the following areas:

1. The right side of the neck, the anterior, lateral and posterior regions extending to the clavicle, and the medial end of the supraspinatus muscle.
2. The lower region of the right scapula.
3. The central epigastric region of the abdomen.

Tissue changes associated with the liver and gallbladder are found as follows:

1. In the right thoracic region of the back.
2. Increased tension over the lateral border of the latissimus muscle, on the right side.
3. Tension over the lateral fibres of the trapezius, extending over the upper end of the deltoid. The tension also travels to the anterior side of both muscles.
4. Tightness in the lateral area of the lower rib cage, on the right side, and extending towards the anterior region of the same subcostal margin.
5. An area between the scapula and the vertebral column at the level of T4–T6.
6. Congestion over the area of C7.
7. In a small area located between the superior angle of the scapula (on the right) and the vertebral column, levels T1–T3. This region tends to be very hypersensitive to palpation, even after several treatment sessions.

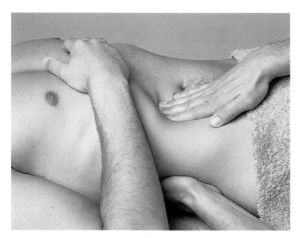

Figure 7.3 Palpation of the liver.

The gallbladder

The gallbladder lies deep to the liver. It is not palpable except for a tiny part of its fundus, which projects below the lower border of the liver. This area corresponds to the tip of the ninth costal margin. At this junction it meets the lateral border of the right rectus abdominis muscle.

- Cholecystitis, or inflammation of the gallbladder, is characterized by tenderness in the right hypochondrium and in the area slightly inferior to the right costal margin. The presence of inflammation is further confirmed by a positive Murphy's sign. One hand is placed just below the right costal margin, and pressure is applied as the subject takes a deep breath. If this action exacerbates the pain and stops the effort of inspiration, it is considered a positive Murphy's sign.
- The smooth muscles of the gallbladder will contract in an attempt to expel a gallstone. When this contraction is intense, it can refer pain to the epigastrium.

Massage to the abdomen is contraindicated if there is severe inflammation of the gallbladder or if the strokes elicit great discomfort. However, massage to the gallbladder must not be ruled out completely. The action of pressing down on the gallbladder area while the patient inhales deeply can help to expel any blockages. This method can only be carried out in the absence of inflammation and tenderness, so it has limited use.

Hepatic portal vein

Portal hypertension can result when the pressure within the hepatic portal vein or its subdivisions is increased. This is generally caused by conditions such as cirrhosis, occlusion of the hepatic or splenic veins, or cardiac disease. Portal hypertension can also be caused by the back pressure of blood which can result in right heart failure. If the portal hypertension is chronic, there is also an enlarged spleen and ascites. As massage improves the circulation through the portal vessels, it also helps to prevent the onset of portal hypertension.

Cautionary note

- Abdominal massage is contraindicated if there is ascites related to portal hypertension. Both ascites and portal hypertension can be related to cirrhosis of the liver or to right heart failure.

The pancreas

The pancreas lies behind the stomach and in front of the lumbar vertebrae L1 and L2. Its head is in the curve of the duodenum, while its tail is in front of the left kidney and touches the spleen. It is not normally palpable unless affected by pathological changes such as chronic pancreatitis or carcinoma. The organ is more accessible when the stomach is empty.

The caecum

The caecum lies in the right iliac fossa and is just below the intertubercular line; it is situated above the lateral half of the inguinal ligament. Anatomically, the caecum is a blind-ended portion of the large intestine positioned below the level of the ileocaecal valve. On its anterior aspect are the greater omentum, coils of ileum, the peritoneum and abdominal wall. It may lie free in the iliac fossa, completely surrounded by peritoneum, or it may be attached to the iliac fossa by peritoneal folds. At the upper end of the caecum is the orifice for the ileocaecal valve.

Below this is a second orifice, for the appendix. The caecum may be sensitive to palpation (dull discomfort and no muscular rigidity), even when functioning normally. It is often congested with intestinal contents (constipation and irregular bowel habit being the main contributory agents), which cause it to dilate and be sensitive to pressure. Massage treatment on the caecal region should only be carried out after that on the descending and transverse colon.

Ileocaecal valve

The ileocaecal valve is situated at the junction of the ileum and the caecum. Localized colicky pain can arise from ileocaecal kinking.

The appendix

The appendix is situated at about the middle of the caecum. It is often slightly behind the caecum, and in front of the psoas and iliacus muscles. Tenderness in the right iliac region, accompanied by involuntary contractions of the abdominal muscles, is indicative of appendicitis. Gentle lifting of the skin folds in this area, using the thumb and first finger, may be unusually painful and could also point to appendicitis.

The colon

The wall of the large colon is felt as a series of folds or sacs (sacculated). When the hand palpates deep into the abdominal structures, it may encounter portions of stool-filled colon. These feel like hardened elongated structures, but are not to be mistaken for tumours. The transverse colon is not fixed to the anterior abdominal wall, and therefore is not always palpable as a transverse structure in the abdomen. It is palpable in the upper umbilical area when the subject lies supine and when its contents are considerable. Carcinoma of the colon is another factor that would make it easily palpable. When the subject is standing, the colon descends noticeably within the abdominal cavity. The ascending and descending colon, as well as parts of the duodenum, are easier to palpate because they are better attached to the abdominal wall. A normal or spastic sigmoid colon can be tender on palpation (dull discomfort and no muscular rigidity).

Indirect tissue changes relating to malfunction of the large intestine can be observed and treated with massage:

1. The lumbar area, around the spinal levels of T12 down to L5.
2. An area of increased tension from the sacrum and running downward and laterally towards the greater trochanter.
3. The iliotibial band is similarly connected and will also be sensitive to palpation.
4. Increased tension and sensitivity in the upper gluteal area.
5. Over the abdomen, with an area of increased tension in the iliac fossa on the left side.

The small intestines

The walls of the small intestines are smooth to the touch. The intestines are fairly mobile, except for their attachment to the posterior abdominal wall. The fixture is by the mesentery portion of the peritoneum. A firm hold on these structures is therefore not easily accomplished.

Dysfunction of the intestines can lead to tissue changes in the following zones:

1. On each side of the spine, at the level of T9 down to L5.
2. Close to the spine, with an area of increased tension at the level of L3–L4.
3. On the abdomen, with an area of increased tension just inferior to the umbilicus.

The kidneys

The kidneys lie on the posterior abdominal wall, surrounded by fat. Each kidney measures about 11 cm in length. In the supine subject, the hilum or hilus of the kidney is found on the transpyloric plane, about 4–5 cm lateral to the midline. The right kidney is lower in the abdomen than the left, because of the amount of space occupied by the liver. It follows that the hilum of the right kidney is also lower on the transpyloric plane than the left one. In the recumbent position the lower poles of the kidneys are found 3–4 cm above the iliac crest, while the upper parts lie deep to the lower ribs. In the upright posture, the kidneys drop further down into the abdominal cavity.

On inspiration, each kidney descends and may be palpated between the hands. One hand is placed on the anterior flank area, below the costal margin and with the fingers pointing towards the midline. The other hand is placed on the posterior loin region, between the rib cage and the iliac crest (Fig. 7.4). Firm pressure is applied with both hands to identify its size, contours and tenderness. It is worth noting that the right kidney can sometimes lie close to the abdominal wall (anteriorly). In this position its lower pole may be prominent (in very thin people) and not easily differentiated from the liver. However, the lower pole of the kidney is more rounded than that of the liver edge and, furthermore, it does not extend medially or laterally. Enlargement of the kidney may indicate hydronephrosis (collection of urine in the kidney pelvis owing to an obstructed outflow). Polycystic disease is another condition with similar results. Tenderness may indicate infection. Any such findings require further investigation by a doctor.

The spleen

The spleen measures about 12 cm (5 inches) and is situated in the left hypochondriac region, under the cover of the ninth, tenth and eleventh ribs. It lies posterior to the stomach, and also inferior to it. The position of the spleen can also be described as being located between the stomach and the diaphragm. An adjacent organ is the pancreas, its tail lying in contact with the hilus of the spleen. As the spleen lies under the cover of the lower ribs, it is not palpable in normal conditions. It is rendered more noticeable by splenomegaly (enlargement), which causes its notched anterior border to protrude downwards and medially. In this position it can be palpated through the anterior abdominal wall.

Palpation is carried out with the right hand, and from the contralateral side of the abdomen. The fingers are placed well below the left costal margin and, on inspiration, they are pressed towards the lower border of the spleen (Fig. 7.5). During this manoeuvre, the left hand supports and pushes forward the lower rib cage. Enlargement of the spleen is confirmed when the tip becomes palpable below the left costal margin on inspiration. Such findings necessitate referral to a doctor.

The spleen is involved with blood production, mostly of lymphocytes and monocytes. It also stores blood and filters out bacteria and worn-out

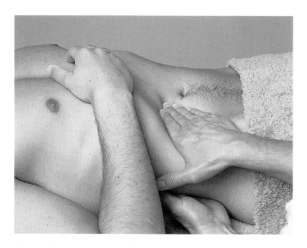

Figure 7.4 Palpation of the kidney.

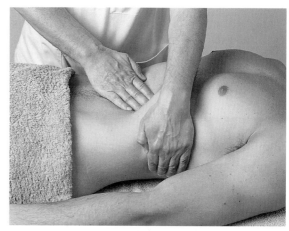

Figure 7.5 Palpation of the spleen.

blood cells. Although the spleen produces white blood cells, it does not filter lymph. Splenomegaly, or enlargement of the spleen, is caused by an increase in the number of red blood cells and/or phagocytes. Chronic infections can lead to hyperplasia (hypertrophy) of its lymphoid tissue or white pulp. These disturbances result from infections such as tuberculosis, typhoid fever and malaria. Another cause is congestion in the portal veins, which can extend to the spleen. The congestion is often associated with conditions such as congestive cardiac failure and hepatic cirrhosis. Splenomegaly is also caused by portal hypertension.

One complication of spleen enlargement is the increased destruction of red blood cells and, therefore, anaemia. This can also be seen in blood disorders such as leukaemia and marrow failure. Massage can be of benefit to the spleen, increasing the circulation to and away from the organ. However, in certain conditions massage is contraindicated or is carried out only with the approval of a medical consultant. For example, it is not advisable to massage a patient with a low platelet count following a bone marrow transplant.

The ovaries

To locate the ovaries a horizontal line is drawn between the left and right anterior superior iliac spines of the pelvis (see Fig. 7.1). A second line (vertical) is drawn from the midpoint of the inguinal ligament, one line on the right and one on the left. Each ovary is roughly located at the point where the horizontal and vertical lines meet.

The abdominal wall

The abdominal wall is made up of the skin, subcutaneous tissue, deep fascia and muscle layers. These superficial structures can undergo changes which may require attention, but which are not necessarily contraindications to massage (Box 7.3).

Other changes in the abdominal wall may be indicative of disorders in the superficial tissues or in the viscera, and these are likely to be diag-

---

Box 7.3 Observable changes in the abdominal wall

- A muscle which is well developed through strenuous physical activity or sports
- Fatty nodules
- Minor adhesions between the fascia or muscular layers
- A muscle spasm which is transient and not associated with such pathology as appendicitis
- A skin blemish, an abrasion or inflamed hair follicle
- The hardened tissue of cellulite
- A haematoma in the lower abdomen from rupture of the rectus abdominis muscle
- Old scar tissue
- Stretch marks

---

nosed and treated by a doctor or a specialist. On the other hand, they may also present for the first time during the abdominal observation carried out by the massage practitioner. Local massage for these conditions is generally contraindicated, and referral to a doctor is imperative. Examples of these changes are:

- Superficial tumours or subcutaneous lipomas. These arise in connective tissue, but especially in subcutaneous fat. They can be observed as a fatty swelling within the abdominal wall.
- A mass within the abdominal cavity. A mass may be felt on palpation of the abdominal wall. If the mass is within the superficial tissues (fascia and muscle), it will remain palpable when the patient tightens the abdominal muscles. The patient can do this by lifting the shoulders off the treatment table or raising the legs slightly. A mass that is within the abdominal cavity, and possibly pathological, will disappear when the abdominal contraction takes place. Pain, as always, is indicative of the seriousness of the problem. While it is advisable not to make a hasty and alarming assessment, such a mass should not be ignored. If there is any doubt about its cause, referral to a doctor is advisable. In the mean time, abdominal massage is contraindicated as manipulation of the tissues may exacerbate the condition even if it does not cause discomfort.
- Inflammation of the abdominal wall. This may be secondary to pathology within the abdomi-

nal cavity. For example, right iliac fossa inflammation can be related to an infection or abscess of the appendix. If the inflammation occurs in the left iliac fossa, it may be associated with diverticular disease of the sigmoid colon or to perforation of a carcinoma of the large bowel.

Reflex zones and trigger points

The abdominal wall can bear a number of reflex zones or trigger points. As noted elsewhere, reflex zones are small areas of hypersensitivity, tightness and so forth, which are caused by stressors. In the abdominal region, most of the reflex zones relate to malfunction of the viscera (see Fig. 1.2) as well as to other regions, organs and systems. Trigger points, on the other hand, are in themselves the source of pain, sensation, dysfunction, etc. in distant tissues or organs. Palpation of the abdominal wall can reveal both reflex zones and trigger points. Reflex zones are treated with massage and the neuromuscular technique, while active and dormant trigger points are addressed with pressure and passive stretching.

Intra-abdominal adhesions

Intra-abdominal adhesions can be present within or around the structures deep to the abdominal wall, such as the omentum. Their history is one of injury, operation, or infection and inflammation. Some may be associated with an ongoing disease or a malfunction such as constipation.

- Although not palpable, these strictures can be stretched when the tissues of the abdominal wall are picked up and pulled gently. Lateral stretching of the abdominal wall and manipulation of the viscera (see Figs 7.9A and B) will likewise exert a degree of transverse stretch. With the usual precautions in mind, these manipulations are only carried out in the absence of any known pathology.

Muscle tension

As the abdomen is one of the most sensitive regions of the body, manipulation of the tissues calls for great caution and gentleness. Very often the patient feels tense and vulnerable when the abdomen is being palpated; consequently, the lightest touch can be met with a spontaneous contraction of the abdominal muscles. This instinctive action provides self-protection and shields the vital abdominal organs. A similar reaction to palpation can also occur when there is underlying pathology, such as inflammation of an organ or of the peritoneum. Local massage is contraindicated in the presence of such inflammation, as it can cause discomfort and exacerbate the underlying pathology. Rigidity of the abdominal muscles must also be considered, and this is often characteristic of general anxiety or premenstrual tension. Massage can be used very effectively to reduce the rigidity of nervous strain. In premenstrual tension, however, abdominal massage may be uncomfortable to the patient, especially if the muscular cramps are severe.

Scar tissue

Recent scars that are still in a 'raw' state are likely to be too tender to palpate. Old scars indicate past surgery or trauma, which can lead to contracted tissues and adhesions. Generally, they are not a contraindication to massage.

Striae

Striae (stretch marks) appear when there is a disruption in the collagen and elastic fibres that act as support to the dermis. The striae are normally silvery or whitish in appearance, and develop because of rapid distension of the tissues. Pregnancy is a typical example, with striae observed on the abdomen and breasts. They also infrequently occur in boys and girls during the growth phase of adolescence. Treatment with steroids, whether topical or systemic, can likewise result in a loss of dermal support and in striae. As these changes in the tissues are usually superficial and uncomplicated, massage is generally safe to apply.

Striae can also show as pinkish purple if the patient is suffering from Cushing's syndrome. This condition results in hypersecretions of corticosteroids (primarily cortisol) by the adrenal cortex. One of the symptoms of the condition is adiposity of the neck, face and trunk. Striae accompany these changes, and can be prominent in the abdominal region. As there is also thinning of the skin and spontaneous bruising, massage has to be carried out with great care, if applied at all. Cushing's syndrome is, however, very rare.

Dilated veins

Dilated veins may be observed in some areas of the trunk. In some instances the veins only appear to be dilated, when in fact they are unusually visible because of a wasting of the subcutaneous fat. This is not of major concern and massage can invariably be applied. When the dilated veins are prominent, they can be a consequence of a serious condition (Box 7.4). Light stroking movements are unlikely to have any detrimental effects; if anything, they can improve the local circulation. However, because of the causative pathology of these conditions, massage is best carried out with the approval of the patient's doctor.

Spider naevi

Spider naevi are similar to dilated veins, but show as a prominent central arteriole with leg-like branches. They are said to occur in skin that is drained by the superior vena cava. Degeneration of the liver causes portal hypertension and, in turn, blockage of the superior vena cava. Spider naevi are therefore associated with

---

cirrhosis of the liver. Some authorities state that distension of the superficial abdominal veins is caused by the tenseness of the ascites. As with dilated veins, light massage is unlikely to be harmful but, owing to the underlying pathology, it is best carried out with the approval of the patient's doctor. Deep massage is contraindicated.

General abdominal swellings

As all medical students are well aware, the 'five fs' associated with a generalized swelling of the abdomen translate as fat, flatulence, fluid, faeces and fetus. While their assessment is perhaps obvious, the use of massage for these conditions should not be freely assumed. For example, a protuberant abdomen may be a sign of obesity, gas or pregnancy and massage is likely to be applicable in these situations, provided that there are no complications. However, a swelling may also be indicative of serious conditions such as ascitic fluid (see ascites), chronic constipation or an ovarian tumour. Patients suffering from severe disorders are probably receiving treatment; furthermore, they are unlikely to seek medical aid from the massage therapist. However, there are always exceptions to the rules and the massage therapist must not be complacent. If there appears to be a prominent or unexplained swelling in the abdominal region, it is advisable to refer the patient to a doctor.

Fat (obesity)

The abdominal swelling observed in obesity is caused by a build-up of fat. A common place for this to occur is in the superficial tissues of the abdominal wall. Adipose tissue can also be deposited in the deeper tissue layers, such as the mesentery and the omentum. Organs are also encased in fat, the kidney being one example. An excessively fat abdomen may obscure an intra-abdominal mass, a tumour or a fetus.

Mild fluid retention

A mild form of fluid retention may be present in the abdominal region in women. During the

---

> **Box 7.4** Disorders causing prominent veins in the abdomen
>
> * Obstruction or compression of the inferior vena cava. This can be caused by a growth inside or outside the vena cava
> * Carcinoma of the oesophagus and the liver
> * Carcinoma of the bladder
> * A mass on the ovaries
> * Portal hypertension
> * Portal vein thrombosis
> * Ascites, perhaps secondary to cirrhosis of the liver

reproductive years this is often associated with menstruation. Although the oedema is not always apparent or easily palpated, it is amendable to massage.

Pronounced fluid build-up

The lining of the abdomen and its contents is called the peritoneum. It is made up of the parietal and the visceral layers, with the peritoneal fluid in between. When fluid accumulates heavily within the abdomen or within the peritoneum, it is referred to as ascites. In the advanced stage, the fluid is observed as a bulge in the abdomen that changes position due to gravity—it is low in the abdominal region when the subject is standing, but moves to the lateral border of the abdomen when lying on one side. Although the fluidity can be observed and palpated, expert advice should be sought for a precise diagnosis.

Ascites is related to conditions such as cirrhosis of the liver, peritonitis, heart failure, obstruction of the vena cava and malignancy. In most of these cases, other symptoms would also be present; for example, cirrhosis of the liver can be accompanied by jaundice. If the ascites is advanced or gross it is very apparent; however, a litre of fluid needs to be present before ascites can be detected clinically. Early ascites may therefore be mistaken for a mild form of obesity. Massage is not likely to have a significant effect on the fluid build-up, which is trapped inside the peritoneal space. Deep massage is certainly inadvisable owing to the underlying pathology causing the ascites.

Transient abdominal swelling

A stress-related condition that causes abdominal swelling and a feeling of distension is sometimes referred to as abdominal proptosis (dropping). Its onset is quite rapid. The patient can easily demonstrate it by pushing down the diaphragm and arching the back while supine. On relaxing, the abdominal swelling reduces but the feeling of distension remains. In its chronic stage it is has the same mechanisms as pseudocyesis (phantom pregnancy). In this condition, the usual signs and symptoms of pregnancy are present without the patient actually being pregnant. The enlargement of the abdomen is present during waking hours. When the patient is asleep, under hypnosis or anaesthesia, the enlargement disappears. Although treatment for abdominal proptosis is usually by psychiatric means, massage is indicated as an adjunct to the therapy. Systemic massage can be used very effectively to encourage relaxation. In most cases, abdominal massage has similar benefits; however, if the condition is chronic, abdominal massage may have an adverse effect. Because of the psychogenic factors involved, it may exacerbate the emotional disturbances. In these circumstances massage is therefore best applied with the approval of the patient's psychiatrist.

Pregnancy

In the early stages of pregnancy the abdomen does not always show any sign of bulging. Abdominal massage is best avoided during this period. This is more of a precaution than a specific contraindication. In the unlikely and unfortunate event of complications, it is best to rule out that these were a consequence of massage.

Constipation

A bloated abdomen is often a sign of constipation. It can be chronic and associated with severe disturbances. An example of such a disorder is megacolon (a colon that is abnormally dilated), which is a rare disorder with chronic constipation and distension. A further example is an accumulation of faeces in the large intestines, which causes the abdominal distension. If severe, massage should not be carried out without the consent of the patient's doctor. Intestinal obstruction (loops of bowel caught in a herniated area) can also be a complication of constipation. In this situation massage is contraindicated, as it can exacerbate the hernia and irritate an already tender colon segment. Diverticular disease or diverticulosis (the formation of distended pockets in the gut wall) is yet another disorder, and is common in the adult population. The only prevailing symptoms of a mild form of diverticulosis are those of obstruction, these being abdominal distension, flatulence and colicky pain.

Flatulence (gas)

A gas-filled intestinal tract is usually associated with the normal process of food digestion. In this situation, flatulence does not normally hinder massage work on the abdomen provided the patient finds the massage comfortable. The patient may, however, tighten up the abdominal muscles in an attempt to control the flatulence; if this happens the massage can become difficult to apply. Distension of the intestines with gas may be a consequence of serious pathology that contraindicates massage. One such condition associated with distended intestines is intestinal obstruction (loops of bowel caught in a herniated area). A further example is the twisting of the sigmoid colon upon itself. Other situations include chronic obstruction of the large colon, and megacolon (a colon that is abnormally dilated).

Pain in the abdominal region

During the case history, the patient may refer to some pain in the abdominal region. It may also be that the patient experiences the pain when the tissues are palpated or during the massage treatment. Having an awareness of the possible causes of abdominal pain (Box 7.5) helps the massage practitioner to assess the complaint and the suitability of massage. However, a diagnosis must of course not be offered; this can only be performed by a doctor.

Some causes of abdominal pain can be self-explanatory and mild; others can indicate more serious disease. The practitioner may conclude that the origin of the pain is easily perceived, such as with flatulence or indigestion, and also assume that assuring the patient of the mildness of the condition is adequate. This may be so, but it is unwise to fall into the trap of minimizing the symptoms, no matter how slight. Caution is of prime importance. At the same time, if the mas-

---

> **Box 7.5** Conditions leading to pain in the abdomen
>
> - Flatulence
> - Indigestion
> - Premenstrual tension
> - Kidney problems
> - Colic
> - Back problems
> - Cancer of the viscera or spine
> - Inflammatory conditions such as gastritis, appendicitis and nephritis
> - Gallstones referring pain to the epigastrium
> - Cholecystitis or inflammation of the gallbladder, giving rise to pain in the right hypochondrium
> - Pancreatitis leading to pain in the epigastrium or the right hypochondrium

---

sage therapist suspects a more serious disorder and concludes that the patient should consult a doctor, this must be suggested to the patient without causing undue alarm.

Assessment of pain

Pain in the abdominal region can arise from a number of organs and can be caused by various conditions. Assessment is therefore not a matter of simple deduction. Most abdominal pain is localized, such as that arising from ulcers and appendicitis. This is in contrast to peritonitis and other conditions, in which the pain is more generalized.

The patient's facial expression gives a good indication of discomfort or pain. Any kind of physical hurt is normally expressed by frowning and tightening of the facial muscles. Pain can be present even if the abdomen is not touched. It can be elicited or made worse when the practitioner's hand is placed on the abdomen, or when pressure is applied.

An assessment of pain is made by placing a hand on the area of hypersensitivity. Pressure is first applied, and then promptly released. This action may elicit a 'rebound response', which can be described as an increase in the tenderness as the pressure is withdrawn (Fig. 7.6). A positive rebound response can indicate the presence of underlying pathology such as peritonitis. Understandably, the novice massage therapist may not feel confident enough to carry out such

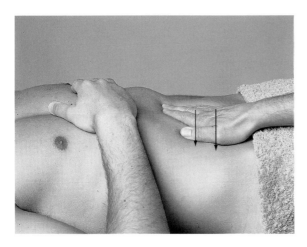

Figure 7.6 The hand is placed gently on the abdomen to conduct a rebound test.

a test. On the other hand, the more experienced practitioner should feel competent to do so.

Colic pain

Abdominal colic describes a 'rumbling' type of pain relating to spasms of the involuntary muscles. Blockage of the bile duct by gallstones is one of its causes, and this is described as biliary colic. It is accompanied by local pain, which increases on inspiration and may also be referred to the right shoulder-tip and scapula. Colic pain may also occur in the kidney, appendix, fallopian tubes, uterus, spleen and liver. The person suffering from colic is generally very restless; this is in contrast to one who lies still as an account of the pain due to peritonitis.

Massage is not always tolerated or indeed advisable in some colicky situations. Although it can be soothing to have the area massaged, sometimes the patient may find this too painful. The massage itself, or the increased pain it may elicit, can set off a reflex response. This is likely to result in further contractions of the involuntary muscles and those of the abdominal wall. Palpation of the abdomen may also elicit pain in conditions involving the passing of stones (calculi), as in renal and biliary colic. Massage may be tolerated in conditions such as menstrual/uterine colic (synonymous with dysmenorrhoea) and infantile colic.

Inflammatory conditions

The following inflammatory conditions must be considered when the abdomen is being assessed for massage treatment. They do not occur often, and the patient is likely to be under the care of a doctor if suffering from one of these conditions. In the unlikely event that a condition has not been diagnosed, the massage therapist may observe unusual pain patterns. In such a case, he or she may need to refer the patient to a doctor. Massage is contraindicated in all these conditions.

1. *Pancreatitis*. Acute pancreatitis (inflammation of the pancreas) is a very serious condition; one of its symptoms is sudden and intense pain in the epigastrium or right hypochondrium. Pain radiating to the back is a further diagnostic feature of inflammation. This pain pattern may also point to the presence of a carcinoma.

2. *Appendicitis*. Tenderness in the right lower quadrant or right iliac region is one of the symptoms of appendicitis. This is invariably accompanied by an involuntary and protective contraction of the abdominal muscles.

3. *Diverticulitis*. The tenderness of acute diverticulitis is similar to that of appendicitis, but it is located in the left lower quadrant or the left lumbar region. The condition is associated with inflammation of a diverticulum or diverticula in the intestinal tract, particularly in the colon. The pain can be made worse by complications of the acute stage; these include inflammation of the peritoneum and formation of an abscess. There is also the possibility that gangrene may develop, which is accompanied by perforation of the intestinal wall.

4. *Peritonitis*. Peritonitis is caused by infectious organisms that gain access to the peritoneum. This can happen in a number of ways, such as rupture or perforation of an infected viscus (intra-abdominal organ) like the appendix or stomach. Peritonitis can therefore accompany appendicitis, ulcers, ulcerative colitis, intestinal obstruction and diverticulitis. Infection can also occur from an adjacent organ that is inflamed. Another pathway is via the blood stream in a patient with septicaemia (the presence of

pathogenic bacteria in the blood). Acute peritonitis can result from injury or infection of a wound in the abdominal wall. The abdominal pain of acute peritonitis can be very intense. Other symptoms include a chill, fever and rapid pulse rate. If the peritonitis is severe enough to involve the abdominal portion of the diaphragm, the pain could be referred to the shoulder-tip. Massage to the shoulder area can have a beneficial reflex effect on the condition, but it is contraindicated on the abdomen.

MASSAGE TECHNIQUES FOR THE ABDOMEN

During massage on the abdomen it is vital that the abdominal muscles, and indeed the patient, are in a relaxed state. To this end, place a bolster under the patient's knees so the legs are relaxed and flexed at the hips. This arrangement encourages relaxation in the abdominal muscles and, moreover, in the patient. Relaxation of the abdominal muscles facilitates easy and effective massage movements.

Practitioner's posture

A number of the massage techniques for the abdomen are described with the practitioner standing on the left or the right side of the recipient. In some cases this format is chosen because it simplifies the instructions; in others, it is used because the technique requires the practitioner to be in a specific position.

Light stroking technique

Effleurage on the abdomen

Effects and applications

- A light stroking effleurage promotes relaxation in the patient. The massage is carried out very lightly and slowly; the slower the rhythm the greater the feeling of tranquillity.
- The massage encourages relaxation of the abdominal muscles, primarily the rectus abdominis, the internal and external obliques and

the transversus abdominis. As the abdomen is very sensitive, the muscles can easily tense from undue or sudden pressure.
- The circulation to the superficial fascia (subcutaneous), the skin and the abdominal muscles is improved. Lymph drainage of the abdominal region is also enhanced. The portal circulation gains from a similar boosting effect, which increases the transportation of absorbed nutrients from the intestines and from the stomach to the liver. The visceral organs, in particular the kidneys, liver and spleen, all benefit from an increased blood supply and drainage.
- Mechanical manipulation of the superficial soft tissues stimulates a reflex mechanism to the digestive organs. Contraction of the involuntary muscles takes place in organs such as the stomach, the intestines and glands. It is worth noting that minimal pressure is required to create a reflex contraction of the involuntary muscles. Too much pressure can have a temporary paralysing effect.
- Most of the beneficial effects from the effleurage can also be attributed to all massage movements carried out on the abdominal area.

Practitioner's posture

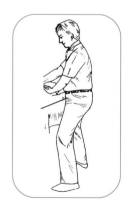

Stand in the t'ai chi posture, and flex your knees slightly to lower your stance. This is a suitable position that enables you to keep your forearms more or less horizontal. Your hands can be relaxed and flat to the skin surface, avoiding extension of the wrist.

Procedure

Place the hands next to each other on the ipsilateral side of the abdomen (Fig. 7.7). Make contact with the palm and fingers, and draw the fingers close together. Keep both hands relaxed while you introduce a slight pressure. Effleurage in a clockwise direction over the whole abdominal region, including the lower rib cage. Continue the effleurage to the ipsilateral side of the abdomen to resume the movement. Repeat the procedure several times.

Maintain a constant and gentle pressure, deep enough to indent the superficial tissues without being heavy. It is worth remembering that pressure applied on the superficial tissue surface is also transferred to the internal abdominal organs. The weight of the stroke therefore needs to be fairly light, to affect the abdominal wall primarily.

Allow about 5 seconds to complete each circular stroke. The rhythm of the massage is necessarily slow to allow for the reflex action to take place. As a result of the effleurage, peristalsis occurs in the involuntary muscles of the digestive tract and organs; the contraction is then followed by a period of relaxation. If this relaxation phase fails to take place, it can lead to a spasm of the involuntary muscles. Maintaining a slow rhythm encourages peristalsis as well as the relaxation phase.

Compression technique

Petrissage on the abdominal muscles

Effects and applications

- Petrissage is used to reduce any rigidity in the abdominal muscles, in particular in the rectus abdominis, the transversus abdominis and the internal and external obliques. Tightness of the abdominal muscles can result from strenuous physical work or exercise. In these situations the petrissage movement can be applied rou-

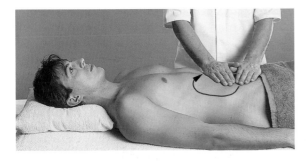

Figure 7.7 Light stroking effleurage on the abdomen.

tinely, and a lessening of the rigidity should be observed. Muscle guarding (tightness) can also occur in response to some underlying pathology. In this case, the petrissage movement is contraindicated until the malady is resolved. If the muscular contraction is caused by tension or anxiety, the muscles (and the subject) need to achieve a level of relaxation before the petrissage is applied. The technique may otherwise cause discomfort or compound the tightness. Effleurage strokes are therefore more appropriate for initiating and deepening the relaxation.

Practitioner's posture

Stand in the t'ai chi posture and to the side of the treatment couch. Hold your forearms horizontal and with minimal extension at the wrists.

Procedure

Place one hand on the ipsilateral side of the abdomen and the other on the contralateral outer border (Fig. 7.8). Compress the central abdominal tissues by applying an equal pressure with both hands and sliding them towards the midline. Use an even weight with the palms and fingers, avoiding excessive force with the thenar/hypo-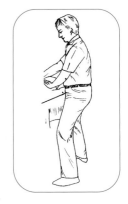thenar eminences. Having applied the compression, ease the hold on the tissues and continue the stroke towards the opposite flanks of the abdomen. Then carry out the same technique as you slide the hands in the reverse direction. Repeat the procedure a few times.

Visceral technique

Manipulation of the viscera

Effects and applications

- This technique helps to mobilize the abdominal viscera, in particular the large and small

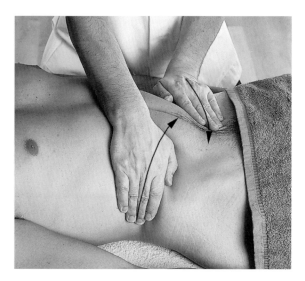

Figure 7.8 Petrissage on the abdominal muscles.

intestines. The effect is mostly mechanical, assisting the forward movement of their contents.
- A reflex response to the manipulation of the superficial tissues results in contraction of the involuntary muscles. The stimulation increases the peristaltic action of the intestines, helps to empty the stomach and facilitates glandular secretions.
- Lymph drainage of the muscular wall and of the visceral organs is also enhanced with this technique.
- The superficial tissues as well as the muscular layers are stretched. Relaxation of the same muscles generally ensues; primarily the internal and external obliques, the rectus abdominis and the transversus abdominis.

Practitioner's posture

Stand in the t'ai chi posture. It may be necessary to flex your knees slightly and lower your stance; this enables you to place your hands on the abdomen without overextension of the wrists.

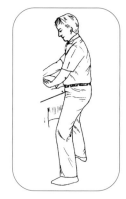

Procedure

Place both hands close together on the abdomen. Extend the fingers to the contralateral side while keeping the thumbs on the ipsilateral area. With your fingers relaxed and fairly straight, compress and 'roll' the tissues towards the midline; avoiding any sliding of the hands (Fig. 7.9A). Apply sufficient pressure to manipulate the viscera as well as the abdominal wall. Having stretched the tissues in this direction, lift your fingers to release the compression and allow them to recoil. Next, roll the tissues from the ipsilateral side towards the midline, using the thumbs (Fig. 7.9B). Make contact with the whole length of each thumb as well as the thenar eminence of both hands. Release the pressure once more, and allow the tissues to recoil as you lift the thumbs. Repeat the whole procedure several times. Add body weight behind the movement by leaning backward as you pull the tissues towards the midline with your fingers, and leaning forward as you roll them with the thumbs.

Visceral technique

Effleurage on the stomach region

Effects and applications

- The effleurage technique on the stomach region assists the movement of the contents of the stomach through the pyloric sphincter and the duodenum. Mechanical emptying of the stomach is also achieved by deep breathing techniques, which can be added to the massage. As the diaphragm descends into the abdominal cavity, it massages the stomach and applies mechanical pressure on its contents.
- Any excessive build-up of hydrochloric acid in the stomach can be removed by the mechanical drainage of massage. This in turn can prevent peptic ulcers from developing. The technique is therefore indicated when there is susceptibility to this condition.
- In addition to the mechanical effect, manipulation of the superficial tissues triggers a reflex mechanism, which causes the stomach muscles

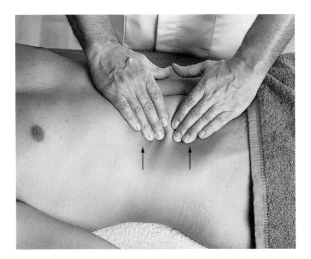

Figure 7.9A The abdominal tissues and viscera are 'rolled' towards the midline with the fingers.

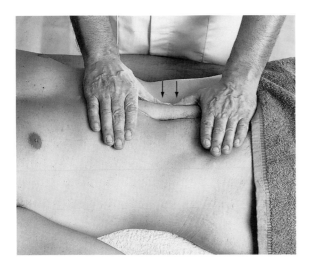

Figure 7.9B The manipulation is repeated in the opposite direction, with the thumbs rolling the tissues forward.

to contract. As a result of the contraction, the contents of the stomach are propelled towards the pyloric sphincter and the duodenum. The surface area where this reflex can be induced spreads from the tip of the tenth costal cartilage on the left side to the sternum, and also down the right costal margin.

Practitioner's posture

Stand in the upright posture and on the right side of the patient. Place a bolster under the patient's knees; this position flexes the hips and relaxes the abdominal muscles. Raise the patient's shoulders slightly with a cushion; you can also lift the head rest of the treatment table if it has such a mechanism. Elevating the trunk in this manner assists with the drainage of the stomach contents. Add some padding under the left side of the thorax to tilt the stomach towards the right side. At this angle, its fluid contents exert a pressure on the pylorus and facilitate easy passage into the duodenum.

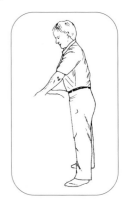

Procedure

Place one hand on the stomach area and position the fingertips just inferior to the left costal margin (Fig. 7.10). Apply a stroking movement with the whole hand, from the left rib cage area towards the midline. The stroking has the effect of pressing and 'squeezing' the stomach against the diaphragm. Add some pressure with the pads of the fingers, particularly near the contralateral costal margin. Increase the pressure as necessary, provided the massage is comfortable to the recipient. Repeat the stroking action a few times, in a very slow motion. Follow this movement with a gentle vibration technique (described below). Another option is to integrate the vibration movement with the stroking. In addition to the mechanical effect, the effleurage stroke is performed for its reflex response; that is, to stimulate contraction of the involuntary stomach muscles. In this case, however, the stroking is much lighter, sufficient only to 'dent' the superficial tissues; furthermore, it is applied at a very slow speed, using an average of 12 movements a minute.

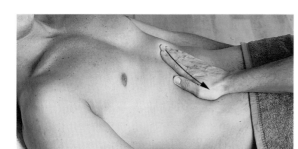

Figure 7.10 Effleurage on the stomach assists the flow of its contents into the duodenum.

Visceral technique

Effleurage for the portal circulation

Effects and applications

- The veins of the portal circulation have no valves, and therefore rely on the intra-abdominal pressure and external forces to assist with the flow of the venous blood. Massage is used to enhance the portal circulation, which drains blood from the gastrointestinal tract, spleen, pancreas, gallbladder and stomach to the liver.
- Lymph drainage in the abdomen is promoted along with the circulation. Drainage takes place towards the central cisterna chyle and the thoracic duct.

Practitioner's posture

Stand in the upright posture and on the left side of the patient. Place a bolster under the patient's knees; this position flexes the hips, which encourages the stomach muscles to relax. Remove any cushions from under the shoulders or the neck. Place some padding under the pelvis so that both the pelvis and thighs are slightly higher than the

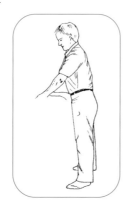

liver; this increases the drainage of the venous blood towards the liver.

Procedure

Place the hands in the region of the left iliac fossa (Fig. 7.11). Carry out the massage strokes with alternating hands. Commence the effleurage with one hand, stroking towards the midline and then continuing towards the right costal margin. As the hand crosses the midline, start the effleurage with the second hand, from the left iliac fossa. This continuous stroking is essential as it creates an uninterrupted flow of blood within the portal veins. As already noted, the portal veins have no valves; the continuous stroking provides a constant pressure and prohibits any back flow of blood. Proceed with the stroking for a short while, perhaps a minute or two. The technique is only feasible when the stomach muscles are completely relaxed and the hands can descend into the tissues. However, the massage itself requires only a gentle pressure.

Visceral technique

Effleurage on the liver area

Effects and applications

- The liver is said to be a semi-solid organ, which is encased by a fibrous capsule. This

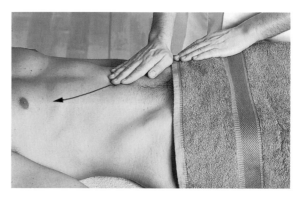

Figure 7.11 Effleurage on the abdomen is applied in the direction of the portal circulation.

being so, the organ is influenced by external pressures—whether from the diaphragm above, an adjoining viscus or, indeed, the compression of palpation. Direct manipulation of the liver itself is not possible as it is largely protected by the rib cage; however, the compression of the massage mechanically assists the portal circulation to the liver through the hepatic portal vein. It also increases the oxygenated blood supply to the liver via the hepatic artery. Circulation is also enhanced through the lobes of the liver and the central and hepatic veins, and to the superior vena cava.

- Secretion of bile is augmented to some extent by the advanced blood flow, and by the mechanical pressure of the technique.
- The likelihood of a reflex action on the liver must not be ruled out. Using the reflex zone theory, manipulation of the superficial tissues over the rib cage may create a reflex mechanism involving the intercostal nerves and the sympathetic system. Any reflex response resulting from the manipulation is, in all probability, confined to the blood vessels supplying the organ.

Cautionary note

- An enlarged liver is often present in jaundice or hepatitis. Massage to this region is therefore contraindicated in both conditions.

Practitioner's posture

Position yourself on the right side of the patient. While sitting down is the most practical arrangement for this technique, it can also be applied from a standing position such as the t'ai chi posture.

Procedure

Place your left hand underneath the patient's right lower ribs, pointing your fingers towards the spine. Set the right hand on the anterior abdominal wall, inferior to the lower costal margin on the right side, and point the fingers of the same hand towards the midline (Fig. 7.12). As the

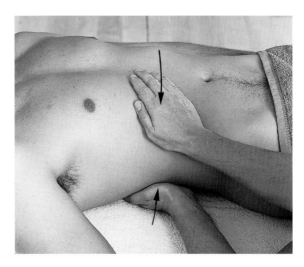

Figure 7.12 Gentle compression and a pumping action are applied on the liver region.

patient takes in a deep breath, apply a squeezing action between the hands; push anteriorly with the left hand and posteriorly with the right. Exert a positive pressure that is not excessive. Next, apply a pumping action on the liver area as the patient exhales. Perform this by compressing and releasing the tissues rapidly between the thumbs, and repeat it several times. Carry out the whole procedure a few more times.

Visceral technique

Compression on the gallbladder area

Effects and applications

- The gallbladder area is located below the costal margin. Its fundus is opposite the ninth costal cartilage. This point is also described as the junction between the lateral border of the rectus abdominis muscle and the costal margin. Pressure on this area can create a reflex mechanism that stimulates the involuntary muscles of the gallbladder. Contraction of the smooth muscle fibres secretes bile into the cystic duct and the common bile duct. This reflex method of bile secretion complements the action of the hormone cholecystokinin, released by the small intestines.

- Bile is also forced through the cystic duct and into the common bile duct by the mechanical compression of the massage.

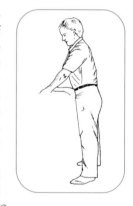

Practitioner's posture

Stand in the upright posture and on the left side of the patient. Maintain a relaxed stance, as no body weight is involved in this technique.

Procedure

Place the left hand just inferior to the right costal margin. Set the fingers close to the ninth and tenth ribs, where the gallbladder is located (Fig. 7.13). Rest the right hand on top of the left and compress the gallbladder area with both hands as the patient inhales. On deep inhalation the diaphragm pushes the liver and gallbladder downward, beyond the edge of the rib cage. Exert the pressure primarily with the right hand, onto the left one. If the abdominal muscles are relaxed, both hands should be able to sink deep into the tissues. Maintain the pressure for a few seconds as the patient exhales. Repeat the procedure a few times.

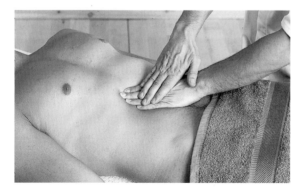

Figure 7.13 Compression is applied on the gallbladder, with the right hand reinforcing the left.

Visceral technique

Effleurage on the colon

Effects and applications

- Massage on the colon has a direct mechanical effect, moving its contents along the digestive tract.
- A reflex mechanism is also involved. Stimulation of the superficial tissues and of the colon itself leads to contractions of the involuntary muscles of the gut wall, and peristalsis is therefore improved.
- It is worth noting that familiarity with the regional anatomy of the abdomen, as indeed of all other regions, is vital for the massage therapist. The significance of locating the organs to be massaged, like the colon, and those to be avoided, such as the ovaries, is beyond doubt.

Practitioner's posture

Stand in the upright posture and on the left side of the patient. Use some padding to raise the patient's head and shoulders slightly; this position assists the drainage of the descending colon. Massage of the colon is carried out along three obvious sections. The first to be treated is the descending colon; this is followed by massage on the transverse colon and, finally, on the ascending colon. An alternative posture for applying this stroke is described later.

Procedure—effleurage on the descending colon

Place the left hand below the left rib cage and the splenic flexure area, with the fingers pointing in a cephalad direction (towards the head). Rest the right hand on top of the left, with the fingers of the right hand pointing towards the contralateral (right) side (Fig. 7.14A). Carry out the effleurage with the hands in this position, keeping the fingers more or less flat throughout the movement. Palpate the colon with the left hand and apply most of the pressure with the right one. The pressure has to be deep enough to exert mechanical drainage of the colon, without pushing it against the posterior abdominal wall. It must also be comfortable for the patient. Massage the descending colon along the lateral border of the abdomen and in the direction of the sigmoid flexure (in the left iliac fossa). Next, continue the stroke medially towards the pubic bone (hypogastric region). As you approach the bladder area, lift the palm and apply the stroking with the fingertips. Release the pressure as you get close to the bladder; avoid any pressure in the region of the left ovary. Repeat the whole procedure several times.

Palpation of the abdomen frequently results in muscle guarding, which limits the massage movements. This can, however, be prevented when the massage takes the form of a regular pattern of stroking. The rhythm of the stroke is therefore slow and even. Furthermore, the rhythm can match that of peristalsis, which occurs about three times a minute. Time is also needed for the relaxation phase to take place in between the peristaltic contractions, and the patient's discomfort is minimized when the stroking is carried out at an unhurried pace.

Additional techniques

1. A vibration technique can be performed in addition to the effleuraging strokes. The method is applicable on all sections of the colon, in particular the iliac region. It helps to stimulate peristalsis, reflexively and mechanically.

2. The effleuraging strokes for the colon can also be carried out with the patient lying on one side (see Fig. 7.24).

3. Another stroke which is of benefit to the colon is the deep circular movement, as described for the small intestines (see Fig. 7.16).

Effleurage on the descending colon—alternative posture

Effleurage on the descending colon can be applied while standing on the right side of the patient. This position enables you to palpate the lateral wall of the descending colon. It also facilitates easy stroking of the sigmoid colon into the hypogastric region. The movement can be applied using only one hand. Reach across the abdomen with the right hand and place it just below the left rib cage (Fig. 7.14B). Add pressure if necessary by placing the left hand on top of the right one. To massage the descending colon, start at the splenic flexure in the left hypochondrium and effleurage to the lumbar region and left iliac region. Continue the stroke medially towards the pubic bone (hypogastric region). Release the

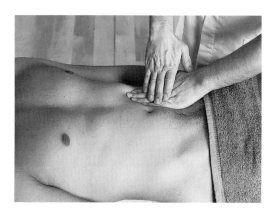

Figure 7.14A Effleurage on the descending colon is applied in a caudal direction.

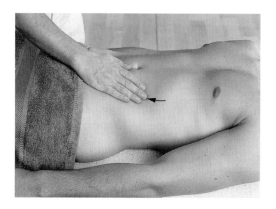

Figure 7.14B Effleurage on the descending colon can also be carried out from the right side of the patient.

pressure before you reach the uterus and bladder. Repeat the movement as necessary.

Massage on the transverse colon

Stand on the left side and place the right hand on the right side of the abdomen, just inferior to the rib cage. Point the fingers towards the same (contralateral) side. Rest the left hand on top and across the right hand so that the fingers are pointing towards the patient's head (Fig. 7.14C). Slide the hands across the abdomen and towards the ipsilateral (left) side, applying most of the pressure with the left hand. As you palpate and drain this region of the colon, it is worth noting that it is a mobile structure and does not transverse the abdomen in a straight line. As you reach the splenic flexure area, change the position of the hands so that the right hand is on top of the left. Follow the descending colon with the right hand into the hypogastric region, as already described. Repeat the whole procedure several times, starting from the transverse colon and finishing on the sigmoid colon.

Massage on the ascending colon

Place the right hand on the ascending colon, in the right lumbar region of the abdomen (Fig. 7.14D). Point the fingers towards the pelvis and set the fingertips in line with the umbilicus. Rest the left hand on top and across the right one, with the fingers pointing towards the contralateral (right) side. Slide the hands together, but apply the pressure mostly with the left hand. Starting at the level of the umbilicus, effleurage the ascending colon in the direction of the hepatic flexure, which is at the inferior angle of the right rib cage. When you reach the hepatic flexure, rotate the position of the hands so that the right one is lined up with the transverse colon, then continue the stroke over the transverse colon as already described. At the splenic flexure area, change the position of the hands once more and continue the massage on the descending colon as already described. Repeat the whole procedure several times.

The ileocaecal valve is just below the level of the umbilicus. Slightly inferior to the ileocaecal valve is the root of the appendix (at McBurney's point) and also the caecum. These structures may be tender when they are first palpated with the massage stroking, and this is probably because of congestion. Palpation may also cause a reflex response, demonstrated as a muscular contraction of the abdominal wall. By way of forestalling these reactions, start the effleurage on the ascending colon at the level of the umbilicus. Follow this method when you carry out the first few strokes, then extend each stroke gradually to

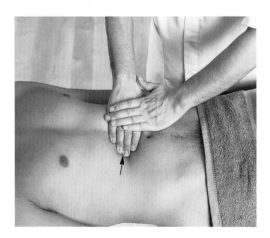

Figure 7.14C The effleurage on the transverse colon is also continued on the descending portion.

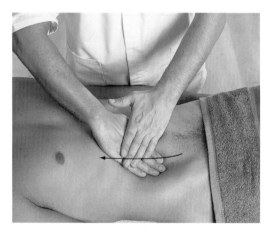

Figure 7.14D Effleurage on the ascending colon starts at the level of the umbilicus and the ileocaecal valve.

include the areas of the ileocaecal valve and the caecum.

Visceral technique

Manipulating the ileocaecal valve area

Effects and applications

- The manipulation is used to stretch the tissues and reduce any restrictions or adhesions in and around the deep fascia, the greater omentum, the peritoneum, the local mesentery and the coils of ileum.
- It also breaks down any congestion in and around the ileocaecal valve and the appendix. To this end, a cushion is placed under the pelvis to elevate it slightly; this allows gravity to assist with the drainage. It follows that massage to this region is only carried out after the ascending and transverse colon have been treated.
- The technique stimulates, by reflex action, the longitudinal muscles of the caecum. As the muscles contract, they push forward its contents and reduce any congestion or overloading. Peristalsis is also promoted in the ileum (the last few centimetres of the intestines). The flow of the intestinal contents has a tendency to slow down in this region; increasing the muscular contractions via the same reflex mechanism counteracts this tendency.

Practitioner's posture

Stand in the upright posture and on the right side of the patient. A similar stance on the left side of the patient is equally suitable for this movement. Remove any oil or cream from the skin surface before you start this manoeuvre. If the skin is very slippery, grip the tissues through a towel placed over the area.

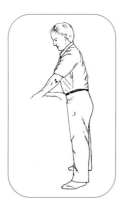

Procedure

Place your hands on the right iliac fossa. Start with the hands flat to the surface, with the fingers and thumbs extended or straight. Compress and grip the tissues between the thumb and the fingers of each hand (Fig. 7.15). Apply pressure with the fingers straight and close together, and counterpressure with the thumb and thenar eminence. As you apply the compression, use the hypothenar eminence as a fulcrum to lift the fingers and thumbs. Maintain the grip and lift the hands further to stretch the superficial and deeper tissues. Hold the stretch for a few seconds, then release the hold gently and allow the tissues to settle in their normal position. Repeat the manoeuvre a few times.

Additional techniques for the ileocaecal valve area

Following the soft tissue manipulation, you can apply some massage strokes to help the mechanical emptying of the caecum. Repeat the effleurage for the ascending colon as already described for the contralateral side. You can also massage the ascending colon while standing on the ipsilateral side. Use the thumbs to apply short strokes, alternating with each other. Continue with this method over the caecum, the ileocaecal valve area and the lower ascending colon.

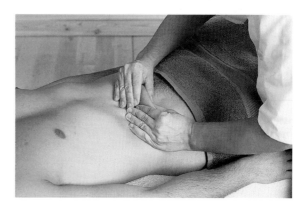

Figure 7.15 Manipulation of the tissues in the region of the ileocaecal valve.

Visceral technique

Spiral stroking on the small intestines

Effects and applications

- This massage exerts a mechanical pressure on the intestinal wall. The small intestines are mobile and are not fixed to the anterior abdominal wall; palpating a specific portion is therefore not easily achieved. Likewise, it is difficult to determine the direction of the flow in the intestinal segments because of their coiled position. Mechanical drainage by massage may take place in the direction of the colon; it is more likely, however, that this will be in an approximate rather than a specific direction. The passage of the contents of the intestines tends to happen without interruption. Blockage is therefore not common unless a mechanical obstruction exists. The flow can be slowed down if the caecum is at fault, or if there is a kink in the intestines. Any hindering of the flow is likely to be in the last few centimetres of the ileum, close to the caecum.
- A reflex contraction of the involuntary muscles is also likely to occur because of the stimulus provided by the manipulation. Palpation of the superficial tissues promotes peristalsis through a similar reflex mechanism.
- Manipulation of the deep tissues and the intestines goes some way towards loosening any adhesions between the intestinal coils. A similar effect is achieved between the intestines and the superficial layers; for example, stretching and loosening old scar tissue.
- The mobilizing technique also stretches the mesentery, which encircles the intestines and attaches them to the posterior abdominal wall.

Practitioner's posture

Because of the location of the intestines, this technique has some minor restrictions but a number of possible methods of application.

1. Stand in the upright posture and on one side of the treatment table. The technique is demonstrated from the left side of the patient (Fig. 7.16).

2. In the case of a well developed or rigid rectus abdominis muscle, apply the movement lateral to its outer borders and therefore not directly on the muscle.

3. You can also attempt to push the muscle mass medially so that you can massage over the central umbilical region.

4. The other abdominal muscles, namely the internal and external obliques as well as the transversus abdominis, may also present a tight barrier of resistance. In this case, increase the pressure without causing a protective spasm.

5. A build-up of adipose tissue offers less resistance because of its relative softness. If the mass of fat is very considerable, you can attempt to push it medially to apply the technique.

6. An alternative arrangement for performing this massage on the intestines is to apply it when the patient is lying on one side (see Fig. 7.25).

7. This deep stroking movement can also be applied over the colon. In a similar manner, it is effective over the stomach and helps to expel its contents.

Procedure

Place one hand on top of the other, and position both on the abdomen. Hold the fingers straight and closed together. Apply the stroking with the pads (distal phalanges) of the lowermost fingers, which are reinforced with those of the uppermost hand. Press your hands into the tissues so that the fingers descend to the deeper layers and compress the small intestines. Simultaneously, perform a spiral sweep with the hands in a clockwise or anticlockwise direction. The aim of this manoeuvre is to apply pressure across the tissues as well as perpendicularly downwards. As you complete the sweep, reduce the pressure and let the hands ascend to the surface. Pause for a second or two before starting another sweeping action; this allows for peristalsis to take place and also for the relaxation phase of the involuntary muscles. Repeat the movement several times over the region of the small intestines.

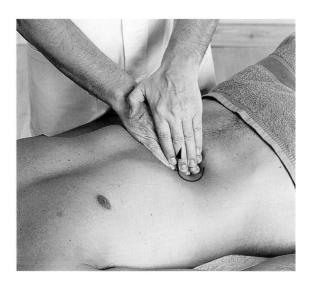

Figure 7.16 Spiral effleurage technique for the small intestine.

Vibration technique

Vibration technique on the abdomen

Effects and applications

- The technique described here is for the colon; it can, however, be applied on most regions of the abdomen. The vibration movement is likely to have a reflex effect, resulting in contraction of the involuntary muscles of the gastrointestinal tract.
- Adhesions between the tissue layers and other structures are reduced with this technique, which also stretches and loosens scar tissue.
- The superficial circulation is improved and, in turn, the superficial fascia is decongested.
- The lymph vessels are gently compressed by the pressure of the movement, and lymph drainage is consequently enhanced.
- Vibration techniques can be used in addition to the other movements already described for the colon and intestines. In some cases they may be preferred to, or be better tolerated than, other techniques.

Practitioner's posture

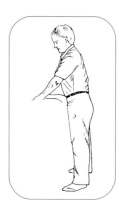

Stand in the upright posture and position yourself on the left side of the patient to massage the ascending colon. Move around to the right side to treat the descending colon. You can be on either side when you massage the other regions of the abdomen.

Procedure

Spread the fingers of one hand and place them over the area to be massaged. Exert a little pressure with the pads of the fingers to grip the tissues. Move the whole hand backwards and forwards or from side to side, so that you vibrate the tissues slowly and without sliding your fingers. Carry out the movement for a few seconds over one area, then position the hand on another segment of the colon and repeat the technique. Continue with the procedure over the ascending colon, then move round the treatment table to massage the transverse and the descending colon.

The technique is described on the calf muscles in Chapter 2 (Fig. 2.25).

Visceral technique

Effleurage and compression on the kidney area

Effects and applications

- The effect of massage to the kidney area is mostly mechanical. It increases the circulation to the organ, and also away from it along the venous return.
- With the improved circulation there is a concurrent increase in the filtration of fluid and the elimination of toxins.
- Locating the kidneys. When palpating the anterior aspect of the abdomen, the hilum of

the kidney lies at the level of the transpyloric plane (just below the rib cage) and at about 4–5 cm lateral to the midline. On the posterior aspect the upper part of the kidney is deep to the lower ribs. The lower pole is about 3–4 cm above the iliac crest.

Practitioner's posture

Stand in the upright posture and reach across the abdomen to massage the kidney area on the contralateral side.

Procedure—compression and effleurage on the kidney area (1)

Insert the caudal hand (the one nearest to the feet) under the contralateral side of the trunk. Position this hand in the loin area below the rib cage, with the fingertips close to the spine. Rest the cephalad hand (the one nearest to the head) on the lower rib cage, slightly higher when on the left side of the trunk than on the right (Fig. 7.17). The kidneys descend into the abdomen during inspiration; accordingly, the movement is best carried out as the patient inhales deeply. Apply some pressure with the caudal hand; this is easily achieved if you lean backwards slightly and let your body weight exert a pull through the arm. Continue to lean backwards as you effleurage with the same caudal hand, over the kidney area and round the lateral border. Engage a gentle counterforce with the cephalad hand to create a wringing action between the two hands. When you reach the anterior abdominal wall, ease the pressure off both hands. Place the caudal hand in the loin area once more to resume the stroke. The kidney is prominent and easily palpable in very slim subjects as there is very little fat surrounding and supporting the organ; conversely, adipose tissue

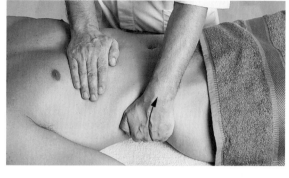

Figure 7.17 Compression and effleurage over the kidney area and the lateral border of the abdomen.

renders the organ less palpable and additional pressure may be required to have an effect.

Procedure—effleurage and compression on the kidney area (2)

An alternative technique is carried out with you sitting to the side of the patient. Adjust your position so that you are in line with the kidney area and facing towards the patient's abdomen. Perform the massage on the ipsilateral kidney. The procedure is demonstrated here on the right side.

Place the left hand on the loin area, just below the lower ribs. Position the fingers close to the spine. Rest the right hand on the anterior region of the abdomen, with the middle finger in line with the umbilicus (Fig. 7.18). The patient inhales deeply as you apply a wringing pressure between the two hands. Maintain the pressure as the patient exhales, and slide both hands towards the lateral border of the abdomen. Ease the pressure once you reach the outer tissues. During inspiration, the diaphragm pushes the kidney distally and makes it more palpable. On exhalation the organ moves in a cephalad direction (towards the head) again, but some compression is still possible. Repeat the movement several times, then position yourself on the left side of the patient to massage the left kidney area. Position your hands more cephalad on the left side, very close to or over the last two ribs.

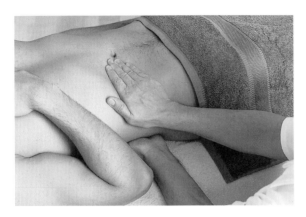

Figure 7.18 Kidney massage is carried out while sitting on the ipsilateral side.

Visceral technique

Compression massage on the spleen

Effects and applications

Compression massage is employed to increase the arterial and venous blood flow in the region of the spleen. The improved circulation serves to stimulate its function, and production of lymphocytes and monocytes can therefore be enhanced with this massage. Filtration of bacteria and of worn-out red blood cells is also stepped up.

The massage produces reflex contraction of the elastic tissue fibres in the spleen capsule. This causes the organ to contract and discharge blood cells into the systemic circulation.

Cautionary note
- The spleen is likely to be enlarged in prehepatic jaundice; massage on the spleen region is therefore contraindicated in this condition.

Practitioner's posture

Stand in the upright posture and on the right side of the patient to massage the spleen on the contralat-

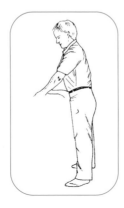

eral side. Alternatively, carry out the movement while standing on the left side. This arrangement enables you to massage the spleen from the ipsilateral side. The technique in this case is similar to the compression movement for the liver.

Procedure

Reach across the abdomen with your left hand and place it on the lateroposterior border of the left rib cage. Place your right hand on the abdomen, below the left costal margin, and point the fingers towards the ribs (Fig. 7.19). As the patient inhales deeply, compress the tissues between the two hands. To accomplish this manoeuvre, pull the rib cage anteriorly with the left hand and push the tissues in a posterior direction and towards the rib cage with the right hand. As the patient exhales, apply one or two intermittent compressions with the right hand to induce a pumping action. Repeat the manoeuvre a few times.

Bodywork technique

Neuromuscular technique on the abdomen

Effects and applications

- The neuromuscular technique (NMT) is used to assess and treat the superficial tissues of the

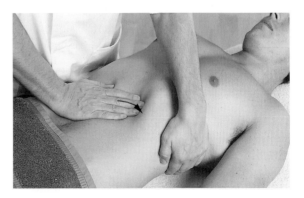

Figure 7.19 Compression on the spleen area is applied as the patient inhales deeply.

abdominal wall. Changes in these tissues are often marked by areas of hypersensitivity, and these reflex zones often relate to a malfunction of an organ. In addition to assessing the tissues for any changes, the NMT helps to reduce the local hypersensitivity and reflexively improve the organ function.

- Hard nodular bands may likewise be palpated in the abdominal musculature. These nodular and hardened areas can have a similar association with organ malfunction. They may also form as a consequence of strains in the local tissues. The NMT is used in both situations, to reverse the contracted state of the tissue and to promote the function of the associated organ.
- The technique is described here as a general assessment and treatment. It does not focus on specific areas relating to particular organs.

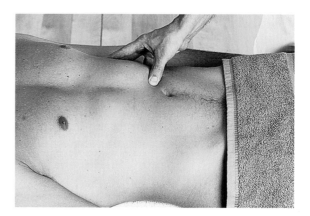

Figure 7.20 The neuromuscular technique on the ipsilateral side of the abdomen.

Practitioner's posture

Stand in the upright posture and position yourself to the side of the patient (demonstrated here on the right side) to massage the ipsilateral side of the abdomen. Move round to the contralateral side of the treatment table to treat the left region.

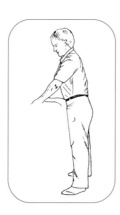

Procedure

Rest the right thumb on the central abdominal area. Spread the fingers of the same hand and place them on the outer border, towards the loin. Hold the thumb straight or slightly flexed at the distal interphalangeal joint (Fig. 7.20). Slide it across the tissues in the direction of the fingers. Cover an area of approximately 5 cm (2 inches) with each stroke. A longer stroke makes it difficult to maintain the thumb in the slightly flexed position, and may even force it into extension.

Using mainly the tip of the thumb, palpate the tissues for any nodular changes or hypersensitive zones. Repeat the thumb strokes over these

areas until the hardness or sensitivity is reduced. Some hypersensitive zones do not diminish easily, or at all. In this situation, continue the treatment for a maximum of 2–3 min; if the tenderness is too severe, omit the area altogether. In the absence of any nodules or sensitive areas, perform the strokes a few times before moving on to another region. Transfer the hand to a position where you can massage another section of the abdomen, and repeat the technique. Continue with this procedure over the ipsilateral side of the abdomen. Move to the left side of the patient and apply the NMT on the left abdominal region, using the left hand.

Lymph massage technique

Effleurage on the abdomen and thorax

Effects and applications

- The lymphatic effleurage facilitates drainage of oedema in the abdominal area. It is of particular benefit when the oedema is associated with cases such as premenstrual tension, after pregnancy, electrolyte imbalances, toxicity and general fluid retention. A back-pressure within the superficial lymph vessels is created by the technique, and this has the effect of moving the lymph forwards. The superficial lymph vessels of the thoracic and abdominal walls drain into the anterior pectoral group of axillary nodes, and the lymphatic effleurage is therefore directed towards this region. The deep vessels of the abdominal and thoracic wall are similarly affected and drained. These vessels empty into the parasternal (internal mammary) lymph nodes.

- The superficial lymph vessels in the lower part of the abdominal wall, from the level of the umbilicus, drain into the inguinal lymph nodes. The lymph effleurage is accordingly directed towards this region.
- When applied on the lower abdomen, the lymph effleurage helps to drain the deep lymphatic vessels. From this region, the deep vessels accompany the circumflex iliac channels and the inferior epigastric vessels to empty into the external iliac lymph nodes.

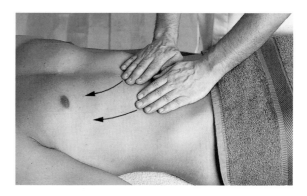

Figure 7.21 Lymph effleurage is applied on the contralateral abdomen and thorax.

Practitioner's posture

Stand in the upright posture, and to the side of the patient. Rotate your body slightly to face the patient. Apply the massage on the contralateral side of the abdomen and chest.

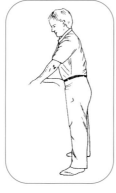

Procedure

Position the hands on the midline of the abdomen and at the level of the umbilicus (Fig. 7.21). Effleurage with the hands relaxed and close together. For men, start at the midline and continue the stroke over the rib cage and the chest towards the axilla. It may be necessary to limit the massage to the lower rib cage area for women. If, on the other hand, it is ethically appropriate, you can continue the effleurage over the lower rib cage and to the outer border of the chest towards the axilla. You can also apply a second stroke over the central area, in between the breasts and towards the clavicle.

Pressure is very light, and amounts to no more than the weight of the hands. It may help you to visualize a thin layer of water in the subcutaneous tissue, which is being moved through the fine and delicate network of lymph vessels. These vessels are easily compressed and occluded if the weight of the stroke is too heavy. Bearing in mind that lymph moves very slowly (as slowly as 10 cm/min), the speed of the movement has to be unhurried. Repeat the movement several times. Move round to the other side of the patient to massage the right side of the trunk. Minimal lubrication is needed for the hands to drag over the skin and push the fluid forwards.

Lymph effleurage on the lower abdomen

Apply the same lymph effleurage on the lower half of the abdomen. Start at the level of the umbilicus and at the midline of the abdomen. Effleurage towards the contralateral inguinal nodes, repeating the stroke several times. You can use both hands, close to each other and with the fingers pointing towards the inguinal ligament. An alternative method is to carry out the stroke using only one hand. In this case, angle the hand so that the ulnar edge is parallel to the inguinal ligament. Maintain this slant as you slide the hand towards the inguinal nodes. Use the other hand to hold down the abdominal tissues superior to the umbilicus.

Lymph massage technique

Intermittent pressure towards the inguinal nodes

Effects and applications

- Like effleurage, the intermittent pressure technique encourages the movement of the lymph towards the inguinal nodes. It is applied to help drain the superficial tissues and, to some degree, the deeper vessels.
- In women, the technique is contraindicated if there is any inflammation or pain in the region of the ovaries.

Practitioner's posture

Stand in the upright posture and to the side of the treatment table. Adjust your position to stand in line with the patient's abdomen, and extend your arms to the contralateral side.

Procedure

Lay both hands on the contralateral side of the lower abdomen. Place the fingers close to the inguinal ligament and pointing in the same direction (Fig. 7.22). Using mostly the pads of the fingers, apply a light pressure to the tissues. Simultaneously, stretch the tissues in an 'arc', i.e. towards the contralateral iliac crest and the inguinal nodes. Then release the tissues and the pressure completely, while maintaining the contact with the hands. Avoid any sliding of the hands throughout the whole process. Repeat the procedure several times, keeping the hands in the same position.

SUPPLEMENTARY TECHNIQUES FOR THE ABDOMEN: SUBJECT SIDE-LYING

Some of the massage movements on the abdomen can be applied with the recipient lying on one

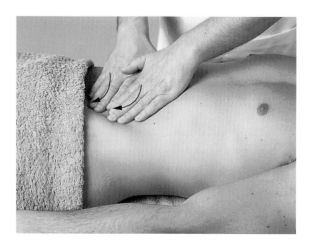

Figure 7.22 The intermittent pressure technique for lymph drainage towards the inguinal nodes.

side. This arrangement is useful for the overweight or the elderly, for example. These side-lying techniques are used as an alternative or in addition to those with the patient supine. When the subject is lying on the right side, for example, the main bulk of the small intestines shifts to the right side of the abdomen. This makes easy palpation of the descending colon and drainage towards the sigmoid region possible.

Support the patient with cushions under the head, as with other massage movements in this position. The patient lies in the recovery position with the uppermost leg flexed at the hip and the knee. Place a cushion under the uppermost knee to support the weight of the leg, and to prevent the patient from rotating and leaning forwards. Use your own body to add further support where necessary.

Effects and applications

- The effects and applications of the following techniques are synonymous with those carried out with the patient in the supine position. As these effects and applications have been described in earlier sections, they are not repeated here unless additional information is relevant.

Stroking technique

Effleurage on the abdomen

Practitioner's posture

Stand in the upright posture and behind the patient, who is lying on one side. Keep your back straight by standing close to the patient. Flex the elbows and place the hands on the abdomen.

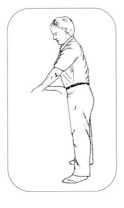

Procedure

Place the hands on the abdomen, with the fingers pointing towards the treatment table (Fig. 7.23). Apply the effleurage stroke primarily with the fingers, but also with the palms if this facilitates an easier movement. Effleurage in a clockwise direction, going over the whole region of the abdomen in one continuous circular movement. Use minimal pressure, and adjust it to suit the patient. Repeat the stroke a few times.

Visceral technique

Effleurage to the descending colon

Practitioner's posture

Massage to the descending colon is carried out with the patient lying on the right side. Stand in the upright posture behind the patient, and use your body to provide additional support if necessary.

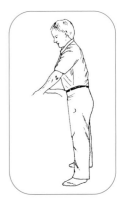

Procedure

Place one or both hands on the left hypochondrium (Fig. 7.24). Palpate the anterior wall of the descending colon with the fingers. In addition to the ridges of the colon wall, you may also palpate hard matter and diverticula, particularly on the lateral wall. These can be gently pressed during the effleurage to encourage drainage, provided there is no inflammation. Starting from the rib cage, effleurage the descending colon along the

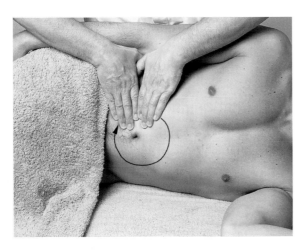

Figure 7.23 Circular effleurage on the abdomen with the patient lying on one side.

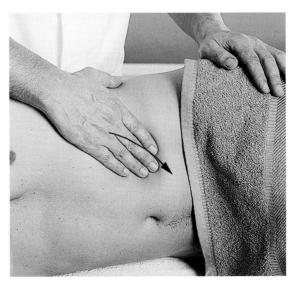

Figure 7.24 Massage to the descending colon.

left lumbar region (of the abdomen); continue along the sigmoid colon in the iliac region. Finish the stroking before you reach the bladder area. Repeat the technique several times.

Alternative method for effleurage to the descending colon

An alternative posture for the effleurage is to position yourself in front of the patient. Apply the same massage stroke, using only one hand. Start from the left rib cage area, and effleurage over the descending colon and the sigmoid colon to the central pubic region.

Additional techniques

1. The transverse colon can be massaged with the patient lying on the left side.
2. In a similar fashion, this position can be used to massage the ascending colon, when the patient is lying on the left side. This position is also suitable for the compression massage to the liver.

Compression technique

Kneading the abdomen

Effects and applications

- This kneading movement can serve as an alternative or an additional technique to the massage on the small intestines carried out with the patient supine. Additionally, it can be performed over other regions of the abdomen, especially if the patient is unable to lie supine.
- The manipulation of the superficial tissues achieved with this technique produces a reflex mechanism. This results in contraction of the involuntary muscles of the visceral organs, in particular of the stomach and the intestines.
- The pressure of this technique on the large intestines leads to mechanical drainage of their contents.
- The kneading movement helps to loosen up adhesions within the deep and superficial structures.

Practitioner's posture

Stand in the upright posture, close to the treatment table and behind the patient.

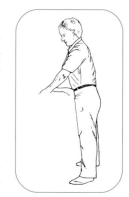

Procedure

Place your hands, one on top of the other, on the abdomen. Carry out the massage movement with the lowermost hand, while applying most of the pressure with the upper one (Fig. 7.25). Press your hands into the tissues, and simultaneously apply a spiral sweep in a clockwise or anticlockwise direction. Exert pressure transversely across the tissues as well as perpendicularly downwards. As you complete the sweep, reduce the pressure and allow the hands to move upwards to the surface. A regular and even rhythm is necessary for this movement, as it prevents muscular contractions of the abdominal wall. Such contractions are otherwise a common reaction to palpation of the tissues. Repeat the manoeuvre over the same area a few times before moving on to another section. Continue with this procedure over the whole area of the abdomen, including the colon, the small intestine and the stomach regions.

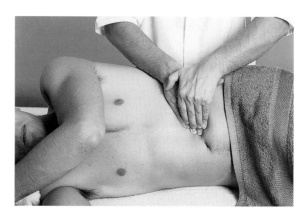

Figure 7.25 Kneading the abdomen involves pressure with the fingers and a circular sweep in a clockwise or anticlockwise direction.

Visceral technique

Effleurage and compression on the kidney area

Practitioner's posture

Stand behind the patient and in the upright posture. Rotate your body so that you are facing in a cephalad direction (towards the head). An alternative position is to sit on the edge of the treatment table, still facing in a cephalad direction.

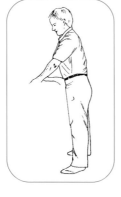

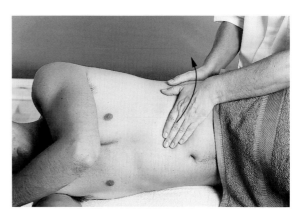

Figure 7.26   Massage on the kidney area.

Procedure

Place the more medial hand on the anterior region of the abdomen, just below the rib cage. Position the more lateral one on the loin area, also below the rib cage (Fig. 7.26). As the patient takes a deep breath in, apply pressure with both hands to compress the tissues over the kidney. Maintain the squeeze and, as the patient exhales, slide the hands up towards the outer border. Repeat the procedure a few times.

Locating the kidneys

1. When palpating the anterior region of the abdomen, the hilus of the kidney lies at the level of the transpyloric plane (just below the rib cage) and about 4–5 cm lateral to the midline.

2. Posteriorly, the upper part of the kidney is deep to the lower ribs while the lower pole is about 3–4 cm above the iliac crest.

8

Massage for body regions—the chest

OBSERVATIONS AND CONSIDERATIONS

The chest area is naturally associated with the heart and the lungs, and some of the signs and symptoms in this region are related to conditions of these two major organs. One or two of the changes that can be observed in the chest occur more frequently than others; for example, those of asthma and emphysema. Other signs indicate the unfortunate presence of more distressing problems, such as the scar tissue of operations and mastectomy. Consequently, observation and any discussion of the chest area require a cautious approach as well as empathy from the massage therapist.

Regional anatomy

One or two of the regional landmarks are listed here to assist with the observation and considerations of the chest area.

1. The apex of the lungs is found 2–4 cm above the medial third of the clavicle.
2. The lower border of the lungs on the anterior chest wall is at the level of the sixth rib, on the mid-clavicular line. From here, it descends round to the lateral side of the trunk and posteriorly towards the tenth thoracic spinous process.
3. The trachea bifurcates at the level of the sternal angle (angle of Louis) anteriorly.
4. Some segments of the lobes of the lungs are palpable through the axillae.

The skin

The skin on the chest area can reveal surgical scar tissue, although in some cases this is very unobtrusive owing to the wonders of keyhole surgery. Engorged veins may be present if a condition such as mediastinal venous obstruction is present.

Observing the breathing

Movement of the rib cage can be observed during normal respiration. Shallow breathing may be associated with stress. As the massage progresses and the patient relaxes, deeper breathing can be observed. The abnormal excursion of the rib cage may be indicative of disorders. Diseases of the lungs, bronchi or pleura may be present if one side of the rib cage appears to move more than the other, and a general restricted movement of the rib cage can be seen in emphysema. It is worth noting that women tend to have greater movement of the chest than men. While women use mainly the intercostal muscles for respiration (thoracic respiration), men make more use of their abdominal muscles (abdominal respiration).

Chest deformities

Barrel chest

In a barrel chest, the ribs can be in a fixed horizontal or inspiratory position. This conformation is generally associated with emphysema, but increasingly it is attributed to overinflation of the lungs. The abnormality can be seen in acute attacks of asthma and in chronic obstructive bronchitis with minimal emphysema.

Pigeon chest

A prominent sternum accompanying an overdevelopment of the pectoralis and sternocleidomastoid muscles gives the 'pigeon chest' of chronic asthma. In comparison, 'pigeon breast', or pectus carinatum, is seen as a bulging forwards of the sternum and rib cage. This condition is common and mostly congenital.

Conditions of the spine

Kyphosis

Kyphosis can result from incorrect postural patterns or from conditions such as ankylosing spondylitis. The flexed position of the spine causes the ribs to angle downwards as in expiration, and movement of the rib cage is limited as a result of the forward bending. Full inspiration is likewise affected, and the viscera are subject to compression. Lymph congestion may also result.

Scoliosis

Scoliosis of the thoracic area is mostly idiopathic (genetic, juvenile or adolescent), and therefore without any apparent cause. About 20% of cases, however, are secondary to various factors. The condition causes displacement of the ribs and, in turn, changes in the chest wall. The ribs appear flattened on the side of the concavity and prominent on the convexity, and the alignment is reversed on the posterior side of the thorax.

Swellings

A variety of conditions, ranging from cancer to tuberculosis, can cause a degree of swelling within the chest wall. If any abnormal distension or changes are observed, the patient is advised to have them investigated by a doctor. Examples of these abnormalities include:

- Tietze's syndrome, which produces a swelling at the costochondral junction (i.e. between the rib and cartilage). It is seen mostly in the second junction, but can also affect others. The subject is usually young, and also suffers from a cough.
- Hodgkin's disease may affect the mediastinal lymph nodes, and it too can produce a local swelling over the chest wall.
- An aortic aneurysm, which can develop in the ascending part of the aorta, may cause a pulsating swelling; this is most commonly located to the right of the sternum and at the level of the upper three intercostal spaces.

Pain in the chest

Chest pain can be located in the central or lateral regions; it can also radiate to the shoulders and the upper limbs. The quality of the pain can vary considerably, from the 'gripping' pain of angina to the sharp, 'stabbing' pain of muscle strain. Equally extensive is the range of pathology that can lead to the chest pain. It includes myocardial infarction, pericarditis, pneumothorax, and mitral or pulmonary stenosis. Consequently, any pain in the chest is treated with extreme caution until its causes are established by the patient's doctor or consultant. The following are some of the more common disorders that give rise to pain and tenderness in the chest.

Pain and tenderness in the superficial tissues

- Tenderness and inflammation of the superficial tissues can be caused by a local lesion or deeper pathology within the chest. Lesions and disorders of the thoracic and abdominal viscera, in particular the heart and lungs, can refer pain or tenderness to the anterior chest wall.
- Trauma to the interspinous ligaments of the spine may refer pain to the corresponding dermatome on the chest.
- Herpes zoster may give rise to pain along one or two dermatomes. It is generally unilateral, and may be present a day or so before the eruptions appear. Post-herpetic neuralgia may persist for long periods after the vesicles and scabs have disappeared, especially in the elderly.
- The inflammation of pleurisy affects mostly the parietal layer. In contrast to the visceral layer, which is insensitive, the parietal layer is supplied with numerous sensitive nerves, which give rise to the pain in the cutaneous tissues. The pain is felt predominantly on inspiration and coughing. It is accompanied by a characteristic creaking sound during inspiration and expiration.
- The breasts can become tender prior to or during a menstrual period. A similar situation can

occur due to medication containing a high dosage of oestrogen.

Pain and tenderness in the rib cage area

- Spondylosis or spondylitis of the thoracic or cervical vertebrae can refer pain to the anterior chest. For instance, tenderness over the sternum and costal cartilages can be related to ankylosing spondylitis.
- Conditions affecting the ribs and sternum, for example fractures, will cause pain that is exacerbated with movement. Injury can also lead to inflammation; sternal or costal osteitis.
- The pain of osteoporosis is also exacerbated with movement or when lying down.
- The upper costal cartilages can become swollen and tender, as in Tietze's syndrome. The main movements that exacerbate the pain of this condition are coughing and deep breathing. Massage is contraindicated unless approved by a doctor.
- Tenderness in the intercostal spaces may be associated with intercostal neuritis. This can result from local pressure on the intercostal nerve, or from intrathoracic pathology such as pneumonia or pleurisy. Massage is contraindicated.
- Congestion of the intercostal lymph nodes can give rise to pain in the intercostal spaces. This build-up of fluid may be secondary to pathology and other disorders like chest infections, to postural imbalances such as kyphosis or obesity, or to menstruation. In a similar manner, congestion can affect the lymph nodes of the breast or the central axillary area. Lymph drainage is indicated, and treatment may be required twice weekly in the initial stages.
- Pain on movement, particularly of the rib cage, can be caused by a strain or injury of the intercostal muscles. In this condition, also known as intercostal myositis, the tissues will become tender to deep pressure. Massage is indicated once the acuteness has subsided. As the healing progresses, effleurage techniques are applied to improve the circulation in the tissues; later on, deeper massage in the intercostal spaces is applied to reduce tightness and adhesions.

Pain in the anterior chest wall

Pain in the anterior chest area is often related to disorders of the circulatory system, in particular of the heart muscles and the coronary arteries. A dissecting aneurysm, for instance, presents as severe anterior chest pain that also radiates to the back, the neck and even the abdomen. Sudden chest pain can also be precipitated by a pulmonary embolism.

Pain and tenderness in the central region

A 'gripping' type of chest pain is generally related to myocardial ischaemia due to angina of effort. Invariably, the underlying cause is either coronary atherosclerosis or a coronary spasm. The pain of angina is central and symmetrical, or may be located slightly to the left of the sternum. It also radiates laterally, towards the axillae and the medial aspect of the arms. Sensations can extend to the epigastrium, the side of the neck, the jaw and the tongue. In angina of effort, the pain is episodic and of short duration, lasting only a few minutes. Typically, it starts during exercise and is relieved by rest; it may also be present after meals and in cold weather. However, if there is severe disease of the coronary arteries, the pain of angina can be elicited with lying down. Furthermore, if the pain is prolonged and occurs at rest it signifies unstable angina. While it may be less common, this condition can be a precursor to myocardial infarction. Midline pain can also originate from a disorder of the oesophagus, usually a spasm. It can be due to achalasia (failure to relax) of the oesophageal muscles or, less commonly, to hiatus hernia.

Pain arising in the abdomen

Conditions affecting the liver and gallbladder, especially gallstones and biliary colic, can refer pain to the right side of the chest and the right shoulder. Other conditions include indigestion, perforated peptic ulcers and acute pancreatitis.

Psychogenic causes of pain in the chest

Anterior chest pain is often present during an acute anxiety attack. These attacks can occur during the day or at night, and the discomfort is generally accompanied by dizziness, palpitations and dyspnoea. These symptoms may be difficult to differentiate from those of more serious pathology such as myocardial infarction, except that in anxiety attacks the patient invariably suffers from stress or emotional trauma. In chronic anxiety states the pain can be anywhere on the left side of the chest and may even radiate to the left arm. The pain of chronic anxiety differs from that of angina, which persists for many hours and generally occurs only after exertion.

MASSAGE TECHNIQUES FOR THE CHEST

The majority of the massage techniques in this section are demonstrated on a male subject. This is to simplify the instructions, and with the expectation that readers will adapt these for female patients. All of the movements are ethically appropriate for either gender. However, if any massage technique is felt to be otherwise, it can simply be omitted from the routine. For all of the massage movements on the chest, the patient lies supine with a cushion placed under the head. A bolster or folded towel can also be placed under the knees.

Stroking technique

Effleurage on the chest

Effects and applications

- The effleurage is carried out to improve circulation, and also for relaxation.
- Palpation or massage of the anterior chest wall is likely to stimulate the thoracic viscera via a reflex mechanism.

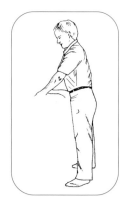

Practitioner's posture

Stand in the upright posture and lean against the treatment table. Alternatively, take up the t'ai chi position. If you opt for this stance, shift the body weight onto the cephalad leg as you effleurage in the same direction, then onto the other foot as you move in a caudal direction (towards the feet).

Procedure

Place both hands on the central region of the chest and at the level of the lower ribs. Hold your hands close together and flat to the surface (Fig. 8.1). Apply an even and light pressure with both hands as you effleurage the contralateral side of the chest. Glide your hands in a cephalad direction and over the contralateral shoulder. Continue the stroke down the lateral border, in the direction of the iliac crest. When you reach the lower rib cage, trace the hands to the front of the chest again. Starting from this position, carry out the same effleurage stroke on the ipsilateral side of the thorax, ending the movement with the hands back in the central region. Repeat the routine several times.

Stroking technique

Deep effleurage on the pectoralis muscles

Effects and applications

- Deep effleurage is used to ease tightness in the pectoralis muscles. These are major respiratory muscles and, consequently, are often tight and overused in the asthmatic subject.
- The pectoralis muscles can also be in a contracted state because of postural imbalances, primarily that of kyphosis. With the thorax fixed in the forward flexion position, there is compression of the rib cage and the tissues in the anterior wall of the chest. The massage is therefore applied to improve the function of the pectoralis muscles and, in turn, to facilitate deep and easy respiration.

Practitioner's posture

Stand in the to-and-fro posture and to the side of the patient. Use your body weight to add pressure behind the movement as you effleurage towards the contralateral shoulder. Lean forward and raise the heel of the back foot to add pressure through your arm. The technique is demonstrated with the cephalad hand; however, it can also be carried out with the caudal hand.

Procedure

Place the cephalad hand (the one nearest to the head) on the contralateral pectoralis muscle, lateral to the sternum and at the level of the fifth rib. Rest the caudal hand on the central region of the chest (Fig. 8.2). Apply some pressure with the cephalad hand; use the whole hand, but mostly the thenar and hypothenar eminences. Effleurage from the sternum towards the contralateral shoulder, along the fibres of the pectoralis major. Cup the hand to effleurage around the shoulder, tracing the hand over the deltoid and supraspinatus muscles. Next, reduce the pressure and return the hand to the sternal area. Repeat the routine a few times. For some of the repetitions, change your starting position to the level of the third rib to cover the whole muscle width.

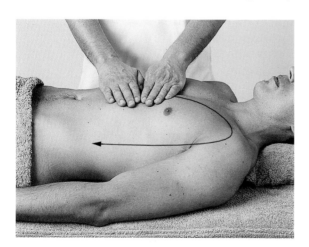

Figure 8.1 Effleurage on the chest.

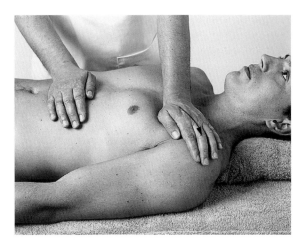

Figure 8.2 Deep effleurage along the fibres of the pectoralis muscle.

Compression technique

Kneading the pectoralis muscles

Effects and applications

• This technique is used in addition to the deep effleurage to further the circulation and relaxation of the pectoralis muscles. As the action of the movement stretches the muscles across their fibres, it helps to reduce any tightness and shortening.

Practitioner's posture

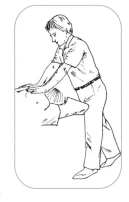

Stand in the to-and-fro posture at the head end of the treatment table. The technique is equally practical when standing in the leaning posture. Position yourself at a slight distance away from the treatment table; this enables you to lean forward and apply body weight through your arms. Another option for this technique is to stand to the side of the treatment table and carry out the massage to the contralateral side of the chest.

Procedure

Lean forward and position your hands one on either side of the chest, on the pectoralis muscles. Lay the fingers on the lateral region of the chest, in the axillary space. Place the thenar/hypothenar eminences on the upper side of the pectoralis muscles, inferior to the clavicles (Fig. 8.3). Compress each muscle by applying pressure through the arms onto the thenar/hypothenar eminences. Introduce a degree of counterpressure with the fingers. Maintain this hold, and stretch each muscle towards the axilla. As this is mostly a compression and stretch movement, take care not to slide the thenar/hypothenar eminences. Next, release the pressure and reposition the thenar/hypothenar eminences to resume the technique.

Deep stroking technique

Fingertip effleurage on the intercostal muscles

Effects and applications

• Tightness in the intercostal muscles restricts the excursion of the rib cage and, in turn, the expansion of the lungs. The deep effleurage is applied to ease and stretch these muscles, sub-

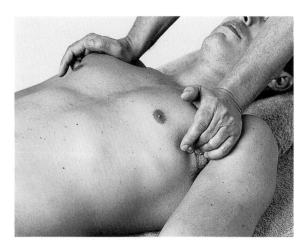

Figure 8.3 Compression and transverse stretching of the pectoralis muscle.

sequently improving internal and external respiration.

- Similarly affected is the transversus thoracis muscle, which is situated on the lateral side of the sternum and diverges to the second and fifth ribs.
- Massage techniques on the anterior lower rib cage are likely to have a reflex action on the involuntary muscles of the spleen, and a further reflex effect on the liver.

Practitioner's posture

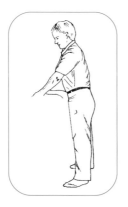

Stand in the upright posture and reach over to the contralateral side of the rib cage. If you apply the technique in the direction of the lateral border, add body weight behind the movement by leaning forwards. You may, however, prefer to use the method of gliding the fingers towards the midline. In this case, lean backward slightly to assist with the movement. The ribs can be more prominent in some people than others, and the angles of the ribs also vary from person to person. Massage of the rib cage can therefore be somewhat intricate, and a choice of techniques is useful.

Procedure—deep effleurage to the intercostal muscles

The technique is applied with the first finger, which is reinforced by the middle digit. Place the fingers in one of the intercostal spaces. Flex the distal interphalangeal joint slightly to add pressure with the pad of the first finger as you effleurage (Fig. 8.4). Slide the reinforced finger from the lateral border towards the midline. Alternatively, start at the midline and push the finger around the rib cage. In this case, effleurage from the sternal end (just lateral to the costal cartilages) and continue round to the lateral border to include the serratus anterior muscle. Having

treated the muscles in one of the intercostal spaces a few times, move your fingers to another space and repeat the routine. Start the massage at the upper rib cage and work your way down to the lower ribs, or vice versa. Adjust the pressure of the fingers according to the tenderness in the tissues and the tightness in the muscles; some feedback from the recipient is therefore very useful.

Deep effleurage on the intercostal muscles— alternative methods

The deep effleurage stroke can be applied from the contralateral side of the treatment table, but using two or three fingers instead of one. Position the fingers in two or three adjacent intercostal spaces, and use the pads of each finger for the effleurage. Carry out the stroking either from the midline towards the lateral border or in a reverse direction. Once you have carried out the movement a few times, move your hand and position the fingers in another group of intercostal spaces and repeat the routine.

A further method for this deep effleurage is to stand at the head end of the treatment table. Place the hands one on either side of the chest, and apply the massage with the fingertips of all the fingers closed together. Perform the technique on both sides of the rib cage simultaneously, one hand on either side. Effleurage from

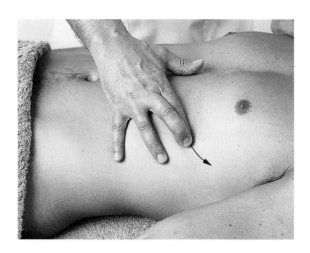

Figure 8.4 Deep effleurage on the intercostal muscles.

the midline towards the lateral border, with all the fingertips in one of the intercostal spaces. Repeat the stroke a few times, then move the fingertips to the next intercostal space and repeat the routine.

Vibration technique

Vibration technique on the intercostal spaces

Effects and applications

- The vibration technique assists the blood and lymph circulation of the superficial tissues. The benefit extends to the intercostal muscles, improving their function. This in turn has a positive effect on respiration.
- A reflex mechanism is also in operation, and produces a stimulating effect on the intrathoracic organs.
- Manipulation of the superficial tissues, particularly those close to the sternum, has a further reflex effect; it enhances the lymphatic drainage of the same viscera.

Practitioner's posture

Stand in the upright posture and to the side of the treatment table. Lean against the treatment table and hold your back straight while reaching over to the contralateral side of the chest.

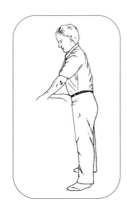

Procedure

Spread the fingers of the caudal hand and position the fingertips in the intercostal spaces on the contralateral side of the rib cage. Rest the cephalad hand on the ipsilateral shoulder, or on another convenient area. To apply the vibration with the caudal hand, employ an on-and-off pressure of very small amplitude. Perform this fairly rapidly for a few

seconds, and without gliding the fingers, then move the hand to another area and repeat the technique. Continue in this manner over the whole region of the rib cage. It may be necessary (or an option) to use the cephalad hand alongside the right. A further alternative method is to place one hand close to and behind the other, then apply the technique with both hands simultaneously. The vibration technique is demonstrated on the calf muscles in Chapter 2 (see Fig. 2.25).

LYMPH MASSAGE TECHNIQUES

Lymph massage techniques are carried out on the chest area to affect the primary group of lymph nodes and vessels (Box 8.1). Methods for applying the techniques are similar to those described for other regions, e.g. the lower limb. The intermittent pressure technique is generally used for areas such as the intercostal spaces and the clavicle, but can similarly be applied elsewhere. Lymph effleurage is also performed on some regions of the chest.

Lymph massage technique

Intermittent pressure on the infraclavicular area

Practitioner's posture

Stand in the upright posture and in line with the clavicle. Move close to the treatment table to reach the ipsilateral side of the chest without extending your arms or straining your back. Hold the cephalad hand and forearm in a comfortable and relaxed position.

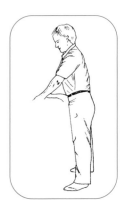

Procedure

Place the cephalad hand on the inferior region of the clavicle and position the fingers medial to the

---

Box 8.1 The main lymph nodes and vessels of the chest and axilla

The rib cage area
- The intercostal vessels and nodes drain into the collecting ducts
- The more central collecting ducts drain into the parasternal nodes and the thoracic duct
- The costal portion of the pleura and the diaphragm drain into the parasternal nodes (internal mammary nodes)
- The parasternal nodes drain into the subclavian trunk
- The thoracic duct and the right lymphatic duct drain into the venous system
- The superficial vessels on the anterolateral wall of the trunk, as far down as the umbilicus, drain to the anterior (pectoral) group of axillary nodes
- The deep vessels of the thoracic wall, as far posterior as the angles of the ribs, drain into the parasternal nodes
- Deep vessels from the anterior abdominal wall, above the umbilicus, drain into the parasternal nodes

The breast
- Lower lateral and lower central portions drain into the subscapular nodes of the axilla
- Upper lateral portion drains into the pectoral nodes
- Upper central portion drains into the lateral and apical nodes
- Medial portion drains into the parasternal nodes

The axilla
The axillary lymph nodes are made up of five groups which are scattered throughout the tissues of the axilla extending also to the breast:

- Anterior or pectoral group, at the lower border of the pectoralis minor. These drain into the apical group
- Posterior or subscapular group, at the lower end of the axilla. They drain into the lateral nodes, some via the central nodes
- Central group deep within the axilla and at its base. These drain into the lateral nodes
- Lateral group at the upper lateral border of the axilla, on the medial side of the upper arm. These drain into the apical lymph nodes
- Apical group, between the clavicle and pectoralis minor muscle; also deep to the clavipectoral fascia and to the infraclavicular fossa. The main vessels of the apical group form and drain into the subclavian trunk

The clavicular area
- The subclavian trunk is situated between the clavicle and the first rib. It forms the exit channel for the lymph into the venous system; sharing this function with the thoracic and right lymphatic ducts. The trunk drains into the venous system at the junction of the subclavian and internal jugular veins. Because of this drainage arrangement, the lymph massage for the subclavian duct is carried out before that of the chest and the abdomen
- The infraclavicular nodes are situated on the clavipectoral fascia and in the infraclavicular fossa; they drain lymph to the apical nodes

---

pectoralis minor (Fig. 8.5). In this region are situated the infraclavicular nodes, which drain into the apical nodes. As a group, the apical nodes are found between the clavicle and the pectoralis minor muscle; their vessels form the subclavian trunk. Hold the fingers flat to the surface and apply a very gentle pressure. Combine this action with a very small stretch of the tissues, towards the contralateral side and towards the clavicle. Next, release the pressure and the stretch so that the tissues return to their resting state, and resume the procedure. Repeat the intermittent pressure technique a few times, then move the hand closer to the midline and carry out the movement once more; this helps to drain the subclavian trunk.

Lymph massage technique

Intermittent pressure close to the sternum

Practitioner's posture

Stand in the upright posture and to the side of the treatment table. Carry out this movement on the ipsilateral side of the sternum, then move round the treatment table and repeat it on the other side.

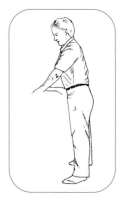

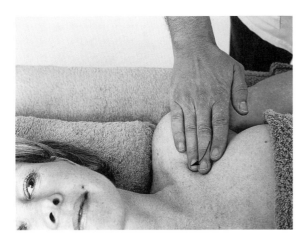

Figure 8.5 The intermittent pressure lymph technique on the infraclavicular area.

Procedure

Place the hands close together on the ipsilateral side of the sternum (Fig. 8.6). The parasternal nodes are situated in this region, and deep to these nodes are the thoracic duct and the bronchomediastinal trunk. Line up the fingers close together and, using only the pads of the fingers, apply a gentle pressure to the tissues. Next, ease off the pressure and repeat the procedure. This on-and-off movement is extremely light and gentle; the action itself is comparable to the 'patting' of a cat's paw. Carry out this technique a few

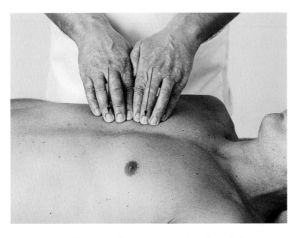

Figure 8.6 The intermittent pressure lymph technique on the region of the parasternal nodes.

times along the length of the sternum. Shift your hands up or down as necessary to treat the whole area.

Intermittent pressure on the intercostal spaces

Spread the fingers of both hands and place them in the intercostal spaces on the contralateral side of the rib cage. Arrange the hands one behind the other, or next to each other. Using only the pads of the fingers, apply a quick on-and-off pressure to the tissues. Carry out this movement for a few seconds, and then move the hands to another position and repeat the technique. Continue with the procedure over the whole area of the rib cage on the contralateral side. This movement stimulates the drainage of the intercostal lymph nodes and vessels as well as the deeper ones that drain the pleura. An alternative technique to the on-and-off pressure is the vibration movement. Use a similar arrangement for the hands, or carry out the movement with only one hand. The action of the vibration is applied in one of two directions; up and down (into the tissues and release) or in a forward–backward direction.

Lymph effleurage on the anterolateral wall

Place both hands, relaxed and close together, on the central area of the lower rib cage. Carry out the effleurage with both hands simultaneously and flat to the surface. Apply minimal pressure by 'dragging' the hands over the skin surface rather than sliding them. Effleurage towards the contralateral axilla, and repeat the stroke a few times. An optional method is to carry out the movement using only one hand. For this technique, hold and stabilize the superficial tissues of the lower abdomen with one hand while applying the effleurage with the other.

With men you can massage over the whole region of the chest, although the nipple should be avoided. The technique, however, has to be adjusted for women. From the central area, direct the effleurage stroke below the breast and onto the contralateral border of the trunk, then continue to the axilla. Apply a second stroke, starting again from the central area; guide the hands in between the breasts, onto the superior region and then towards the axilla.

SUPPLEMENTARY TECHNIQUES FOR THE CHEST

A number of supplementary techniques can be applied to the chest and the rib cage. One or two of the movements are best applied with the subject lying on one side and, consequently, they serve as good alternatives when the patient is unable to lie supine. Others are additional to those massages already described with the patient in the supine position. All of the techniques can be integrated into the massage routine to the chest.

Deep stroking technique

Effleurage to the intercostal muscles

Effects and applications

- Deep stroking to the intercostal muscles has already been described with the recipient lying supine. This method, in the side-lying position, can therefore be carried out in addition or as an alternative procedure. Tightness in the intercostal muscles restricts the excursion of the rib cage and, in turn, the expansion of the lungs. The deep effleurage is applied to ease and stretch these muscles, subsequently improving internal and external respiration.

Practitioner's posture

Stand in the to-and-fro posture and at the head end of the treatment table. Set your stance further by standing slightly to the side and behind the patient. When the patient lies on one side, the arm is abducted above the head. This helps to expand the rib cage and gain access to the intercostal muscles. If this position is uncomfortable, the patient can rest the arm across the chest.

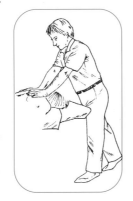

Procedure

Place the hands next to each other on the lateral border of the rib cage. Hold the tips of the fingers together, and place them in the intercostal space (Fig. 8.7). Effleurage with the fingertips and trace the hands in opposite directions, one hand towards the sternum and the other towards the spine. Next, lift the fingers off and position them on the lateral border of the rib cage once again. Repeat the movement in the same intercostal space and then in the adjacent ones, which are easily accessible. Aim to keep the fingertips in the intercostal spaces, and to follow the curves and angles of the ribs. Most of the pressure is applied with the fingertips, but a degree of body weight can be introduced by shifting forwards onto the front foot or by leaning forwards slightly.

Effleurage to the intercostal muscles: standing to the side

An alternative method for this technique is to stand to the side of the treatment table in front of the recipient. You may also find it more comfortable to sit on the edge of the treatment table. Place the fingertips of both hands close together in one of the intercostal spaces on the lateral border of the rib cage. Apply some pressure with the

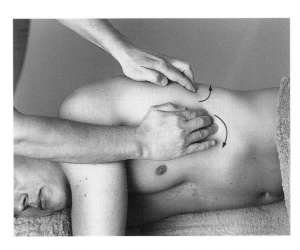

Figure 8.7   Effleurage with the fingertips in the intercostal spaces.

pads of the fingers as you slide the hands in opposite directions, one towards the sternum and the other towards the back. Repeat the stroke several times, and then apply it in the other intercostal spaces. Aim to follow the angles of the ribs, although this may be difficult in some areas.

Effleurage to the intercostal muscles: subject sitting

The deep effleurage to the intercostal muscles can also be applied with the patient sitting on the treatment table. This arrangement is useful if the patient is elderly or has a condition such as emphysema. The upper ribs are the most easily accessible, but the technique can be used on the whole rib cage. The patient sits on the treatment table while you stand behind. Place a folded towel or thin cushion on your chest so the patient can lean back and rest against you. If the treatment table is too high or impractical, the patient can sit on a chair.

Position the hands one on either side of the rib cage, and place one or two fingers in the lower intercostal spaces. Use the pads of the fingertips to effleurage the intercostal muscles, working from the central area (or costal cartilages) towards the lateral border. Repeat each stroke several times before moving up to the next intercostal space. Quite often it is difficult to follow

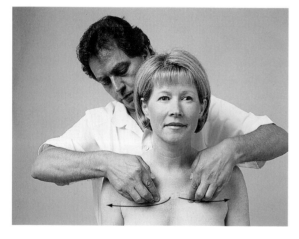

Figure 8.8 Massage to the intercostal spaces with the patient in a sitting position.

the line of the ribs because of their angles and junctions with the costal cartilages. If the fingers slip out of the intercostal spaces, simply realign them and repeat the stroke. The patient is encouraged to take some deep breaths in between the strokes; this encourages movement and expansion of the rib cage. Massage below the level of the breast tissue in women, then, omitting the breast area, work also on the upper ribs. Effleurage from the sternum towards the shoulders (Fig. 8.8).

Bodywork technique

Stretching the respiratory muscles

Effects and applications

- The passive stretch of this bodywork technique increases the effects of the deep effleurage to the intercostal muscles. It also stretches some of the other muscles of respiration: the latissimus dorsi, trapezius, quadratus lumborum and pectoralis minor.

Practitioner's posture

For this movement, the patient lies on one side with the arm abducted over the head. Stand at the head end of the treatment table, in the to-and-fro posture.

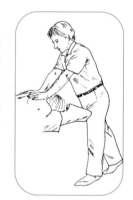

Procedure

Hold the patient's upper arm with both hands; alternatively, use one hand on the forearm and one on the upper arm (Fig. 8.9). Keep the arm locked straight at the elbow, and angle it a touch forward in line with the patient's face; this avoids an excessive pull on the triceps.

Observe the patient's breathing and, as the patient inhales deeply, apply a gentle pull on the arm by leaning backward. This basic traction technique expands the rib cage and

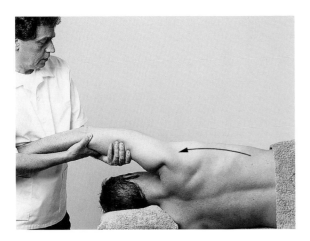

Figure 8.9 Bodywork technique applied to the muscles of respiration, creating a passive stretch.

stretches the muscles of expiration, mainly the latissimus dorsi, serratus posterior inferior and abdominal muscles. These muscles are relaxed during inspiration, and can therefore be passively stretched.

Repeat the same traction technique as the patient exhales deeply. This applies a stretch essentially to the muscles of inspiration, namely the pectoralis minor, serratus anterior, trapezius and the external fibres of the intercostal muscles. The origins of these muscles are somewhat 'fixed', as the rib cage moves downward during expiration. This permits the muscles to be stretched in the direction of their insertions when the arm is under traction.

Bodywork technique

Expanding the rib cage

Effects and applications

• This bodywork technique can be carried out as an alternative or an additional method to the passive stretch of the previous movement. It expands the rib cage and exerts a further traction on the respiratory muscles.

Practitioner's posture

Stand in the upright posture and at the head end of the treatment table. The patient lies supine,

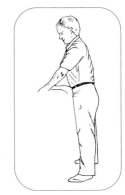

extends the arms above the head and gently holds onto your lower back. Bend your knees as you lean backward and pull on the patient's arms.

Procedure

Grip the recipient's arms proximal to the elbows (Fig. 8.10). With the arms still in extension, ask the patient to inhale deeply. As the patient inhales, lean backward slightly and simultaneously flex the knees. This manoeuvre lowers your body and helps you to expand the patient's rib cage as they inhale. The muscles of expiration, especially the rectus abdominis, are also stretched with this action. Maintain this hold and the traction on the rib cage as the patient exhales; during this phase the muscles of inspiration are stretched. At the end of expiration, straighten your knees and ease off the traction while maintaining the grip on the upper arms. Resume the procedure as the recipient inhales deeply once again.

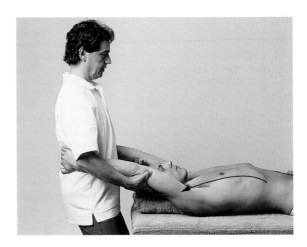

Figure 8.10 Expanding the rib cage with the patient supine.

9

Massage for body regions—the upper limb

OBSERVATIONS AND CONSIDERATIONS

As a general rule, assessment of the arm does not reveal any serious contraindications to massage. There are no underlying organs in this region of the body and, unlike the lower limb, the arm is not subject to circulatory problems such as varicosity. It is none the less important to pay some attention to the arm before the massage, and to be aware of possible conditions.

Cyanosis and clubbing of the fingers

Cyanosis is a blue coloration of the skin or mucosa caused by severe oxygen deficiency. The condition results from a disturbance in the distribution or oxygen content of haemoglobin, and is primarily associated with malfunctions of the respiratory/circulatory systems. Peripheral cyanosis, for instance, occurs when there is a reduced cardiac output or when there is vasoconstriction in the peripheral vessels (e.g. from cold temperatures). The blue coloration of the tissues can be observed in the extremities, the fingers, toes, lips and ears. Clubbing of the fingers is a further sign of disturbances in the lungs, and also in the heart and alimentary system. The soft terminal portion of the finger becomes bulbous, and there is excessive curvature of the nails. These changes in the soft tissues are said to occur because of a disturbed peripheral blood flow. While conditions of the heart and lungs require appropriate treatment, massage can be applied to assist the peripheral and, in many cases, also the systemic circulation.

Raynaud's disease

This condition, which is more common in women than in men, is caused by an impairment of the blood supply to the extremities and, therefore, the fingers, toes and ears. The most common cause is spasm of the blood vessels in response to cold temperatures, which is relieved by heat. Other causes include vascular conditions such as arteriosclerosis, a cervical rib (extra rib) which occludes the blood supply, and collagen diseases such as rheumatoid arthritis. Stress is also said to cause the symptoms, which are seen in the fingers or toes. The affected part becomes pale, cold and numb, and this is soon followed by redness, heat and tingling. In most cases, the attacks are transient and do not affect the tissues; in severe cases, gangrene can set in. Massage is gently applied to the hand to improve the circulation. Systemic massage prevents attacks that can be brought about by stress.

Dupuytren's contracture

In this condition, there is a severe and permanent contracture of the palmar fascia. As a result, the ring or little finger (or both) are forced into flexion and bend towards the palm. The onset can be spontaneous, and affects mostly men of middle age; both sexes are affected equally after the age of 60 years. A history of physical trauma to the hand can be important; other possible factors include alcohol abuse and liver problems. The fascia contracts over a period of months, and the finger has to be surgically released. In the early stages, massage can be applied to stretch the palmar fascia and slow down the process.

Oedema

Oedema in the arm, extending also to the face and neck, is often caused by obstruction of the superior vena cava or its main branches. The primary conditions that contribute to this obstruc-

tion are thoracic aneurysms, thrombosis and tumours. Oedema can also result from other disorders such as nephritis, local trauma, heart failure and obesity, or from hormonal effects during the menstrual cycle. Lymphoedema, particularly in the upper region of the arm, may result from mastectomy or from the removal of lymph nodes in the chest or axilla. Lymph massage techniques can be applied to reduce fluid retention. In some cases, such as lymphoedema and heart problems, the treatment is limited and is only applied with the consent of the patient's doctor.

Pain in the arm

Pain in the arm can have a number of causes. The quality and type of pain may be comparable in all cases, but the onset and frequency may be associated with a number of conditions. Movements of the head and the arm are common and are typical examples of exacerbating factors. Most of the conditions leading to pain in the arm require referral, and are perhaps beyond the scope of massage. However, an awareness of the more common causes is none the less of value to the massage therapist.

Pain originating in the cervical spine

An exceedingly common cause of pain in the arm is disorders of the cervical spine, such as misalignments, arthritis and intervertebral disc herniation. Spondylosis (vertebral ankylosis) may be a further complication. Invariably, these problems cause compression or irritation of the nerve roots supplying the muscles, blood vessels and connective tissue of the upper limb. For example, a dull pain can arise from an impairment of the brachial plexus, which involves the ulnar, median and radial nerves and their branches. Stiffness in the neck is often present, as is pain in the muscles deep to the scapula and in the pectoralis major muscles; these are supplied by the spinal roots from C5/6 and C6/7. From the cervical area, the pain generally radiates to the back of the shoulder, the forearm, wrist and hand. Paraesthesiae are also common, mostly in the fingers.

Pain originating in the wrist

Some of the pain and sensations in the arm, particularly those which occur at night, may be caused by compression of the median nerve at the wrist. Paraesthesiae in the hand, but not beyond the wrist, may be a result of carpal tunnel syndrome.

Pain arising in the joints

The pain of arthritis is felt mostly on passive or active movement of the suspected joint. Arthritis affects any joint in the arm, but is perhaps more common in the shoulders and the hands. If the condition is of the rheumatoid type, the pain is more widespread and is accompanied by bouts of inflammation. In the shoulder joint, the degeneration can also extend to some of the tendons associated with it – primarily the supraspinatus and the long head of the biceps. Calcification may also affect these tendons, thereby exacerbating the pain. Most movements of the shoulder joint, but in particular abduction, will cause the discomfort. The elbow is also susceptible to arthritic changes and inflammation, and undergoes changes that render it painful, inflamed and limited in movement. Prominent rheumatoid nodules on the posterior aspect of the elbow and the tendons of the forearm are common in rheumatoid arthritis. The hands are similarly affected and become ankylosed, with the fingers flexed and fixed in ulnar deviation. Massage is indicated to ease the muscles and help mobilize the joints; however, it is only carried out during the non-inflammatory periods and then with great care.

Heberden's nodes

These are bony protuberances that can be seen in the interphalangeal joints of the fingers. They are usually painless, but occasionally ache. The nodes are characteristic of osteoarthritis. Some deformity of the fingers is also common in this condition.

Gout

Gout is not uncommon in the elbow, wrist and fingers. It presents with tophi (hard deposits of sodium urate in the skin and cartilage), which appear similar to the nodules of arthritis (rheumatoid and osteoarthritis) except that tophi are reddened, inflamed and painful. Acute arthritis and inflammation can also accompany a gout attack. Apart from the use of medication, the treatment for gout is somewhat unclear. While cold packs would be an obvious choice to counteract the inflammation, heat and radiant energy are needed to disperse the build-up of urates. Massage can be employed for a similar effect, although it is not easily tolerated.

Ganglion

This is a cyst that forms within the capsule of a joint or a tendon sheath. It is commonly observed on the dorsum of the wrist. The cyst is benign and contains clear fluid, which sometimes disperses into the joint. Although ganglia can be excised, they frequently recur. Massage is not indicated for this condition.

Pain arising from injuries of the soft tissues

Soft tissue injury is another cause of pain, which is generally sharp, localized, and is exacerbated by contraction of the muscles or by passive or active stretching. The injury itself may be sufficiently severe to require specialist treatment. Massage is used to relax associated muscles that may be in spasm as part of the protective mechanism.

Pain arising from the heart

Pain down the medial aspect of the arm indicates a heart problem, generally angina. Tightness, gripping or pressure are words used by the patient to describe this pain, which occurs usually in the left arm and lasts for a few minutes during an attack. Massage is contraindicated locally and during an attack. Coronary thrombosis is another heart condition with a similar effect.

Pain arising in the abdominal viscera

In the absence of local trauma, pain in the tip of the shoulder could be referred from abdominal pathology such as peritonitis.

MASSAGE TECHNIQUES FOR THE UPPER LIMB

For the following massage routines on the arm, the patient lies supine with the head supported on a cushion or folded towel. It may be more comfortable for the patient if there is also some support under the knees and the lumbar area. Cover the patient with a towel, and bare only the arms. For some of the movements you can sit on the edge of the treatment table as indicated below, while for others you need to adopt a comfortable standing posture. In some cases you can sit on a chair or stool of a suitable height. Carry out all the massage movements on one arm before moving round the treatment table to the other.

Stroking technique

Effleurage on the whole arm

Effects and applications

- The effleurage is generally carried out at the start of the massage routine for the arm. It is used to induce relaxation and to warm up the tissues. At the end of the massage routine, the stroke is repeated several times very lightly as a soothing finishing movement.
- When applied with a degree of pressure, the technique is used to enhance the circulation. Lymph drainage is likewise increased.

Practitioner's posture

Stand in the lunging posture and to the side of the treatment table. Flex both knees a little to lower your stance and reach the patient's arm without too much bending forwards. Stay in this posture, and shift your body weight onto the front foot as you effleurage towards the shoulder. Change to a more upright stance as you apply the effleurage towards the wrist.

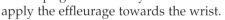

Procedure

Commence the effleurage with the patient's arm resting on the treatment table and with the hand pronated (palm facing downward). Hold the wrist with the more medial hand and effleurage with the lateral one, using the palm and fingers (Fig. 9.1A). Carry out the stroke from the distal end of the forearm along the extensor muscles and over the lateral border of the upper arm, and continue to the shoulder. Apply pressure behind the movement by shifting your body weight onto the front foot as you effleurage in a cephalad direction. Next, cup the hand to effleurage around the shoulder.

The effleurage is continued along the arm and towards the hand. Raise the patient's arm a little distance off the treatment table using the more medial hand, which is holding the patient's wrist (Fig. 9.1B). Next, apply a gentle compression with the lateral hand at the proximal end of the patient's upper arm. Maintaining this squeezing action, effleurage down the arm and towards the wrist. This stroking encourages the arterial circulation. Use your body weight to assist the movement by shifting it onto the back foot and leaning backward slightly. Continue the stroke over the wrist and the hand, then rest the arm back on the treatment table and repeat the whole procedure.

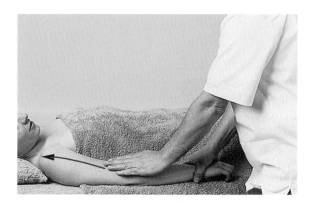

Figure 9.1A Effleurage along the arm and towards the shoulder to assist the venous return.

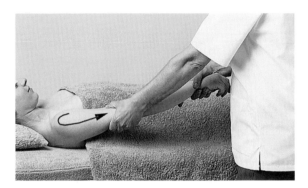

Figure 9.1B Effleurage towards the hand to promote the arterial blood flow.

forearm by supinating the hand and resting it on the palm and fingers of your lateral hand. Place your more medial hand on the patient's palm, interlinking your thumb with the patient's (Fig. 9.2). Apply pressure with the whole hand, but mostly with your thenar and hypothenar eminences. Using the interlinked thumbs as an axis, effleurage in a semicircular direction from the patient's thenar eminence area to the fingers. Next, lift your hand slightly and reposition it to resume the movement. Repeat the procedure several times.

Stroking technique

Effleurage on the forearm

Effects and applications

- This effleurage on the forearm helps the venous return as well as the lymphatic drainage.
- It benefits all the forearm muscles, and is therefore very effective for the sports person. A typical example of its use is for an athlete involved in racket sports, where both the flexor and extensor groups of muscles are likely to be overused.

Stroking technique

Deep effleurage on the palm

Effects and applications

- As with other massage movements on the hand, this effleurage is very relaxing as well as being effective in improving the circulation. Its deep stroking movement helps to ease the muscles on the palmar aspect, especially those of the hypothenar and thenar eminences.

Practitioner's posture

Stand in the upright posture and to the side of the treatment table, facing the patient. Body weight is applied through your arms in a vertical direction; therefore, keep your back comfortably straight during this movement.

Procedure

Hold the patient's wrist with your lateral hand. Raise the forearm by flexing their elbow and resting it on the treatment table. Support the weight of the patient's

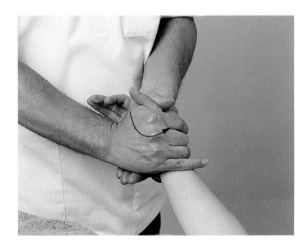

Figure 9.2 Deep effleurage on the palmar side of the hand is applied with the thenar and hypothenar eminences.

Practitioner's posture

Stand in the to-and-fro posture and to the side of the treatment table. Shift your body weight to the front foot as you carry out the massage to the forearm; this adds pressure behind the movement. Should you find it necessary to increase the pressure further, raise the heel of the back foot as you shift your body weight forward.

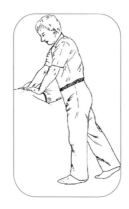

Procedure

Using the more medial hand, flex the patient's elbow and support it on the treatment table (Fig. 9.3). Hold the raised forearm at the wrist, or as if shaking hands with the patient. Effleurage the forearm with the more lateral hand; add gentle compression to encourage the venous return. Start at the wrist and slide the hand towards the elbow. Lean forward or flex the front knee to add some body weight behind the effleurage. When you get to the elbow, relax the grip and slide the hand to the wrist without lowering the patient's forearm. Repeat the movement a few times. The effleurage to the forearm can also be carried out with the more medial hand, either as an optional or an additional stroke.

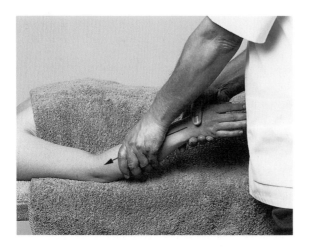

Figure 9.3 Effleurage with the forearm raised.

Compression technique

Kneading the forearm

Effects and applications

- The muscles of the forearm, in particular the extensor group, are often in a contracted state. This is generally related to overuse and strenuous physical activity such as sports. Kneading movements are applied to increase the circulation to the muscles, thereby reducing any congestion of metabolites. A transverse stretch to the fibres is also applied with this technique. This helps to ease any tightness in the muscles that may impair their full function.

Practitioner's posture

Although this technique can be applied from a standing position, it may be more practical to sit on the edge of the treatment table. Flex the patient's elbow and place a cushion or folded towel under the upper arm; this raises the whole arm and enables you to massage the forearm without bending forward too much.

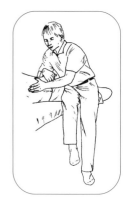

Procedure

Steady the patient's forearm by gripping the wrist with your lateral hand. Curve your medial hand around the forearm so that the thenar and hypothenar eminences are on the inner side and the fingers on the outer aspect (Fig. 9.4). Knead the muscles by applying pressure with the thenar/hypothenar eminences. Simultaneously, roll the tissues forward towards your fingers, which remain stationary. Maintain the pressure throughout the kneading action to avoid sliding over the tissues. You can also use the hand holding the wrist to apply a counter-rotation of the forearm. As you roll the tissues in one direction gently rotate the forearm in the opposite direction, thus adding a twisting action to the kneading. Ease the pressure once the compression and the stretch are completed, then lift the heel of the hand (thenar/hypothenar eminences) and return it to the inner region of the forearm, leaving your fingers in the same position. Repeat the technique a few times. Next, swap the positions of your hands so that the more medial hand grips the patient's wrist. Apply the kneading with the more lateral hand, starting with the thenar and hypothenar eminences on the outer region of the forearm and the fingers on the inner side. Roll the tissues towards your fingers, i.e. towards the inner region of the patient's forearm.

Bodywork technique

Neuromuscular technique on the forearm

Effects and applications

- The bodywork technique on the forearm muscles exerts a deep pressure in between the muscle layers and also on the fascia. The muscles most affected are the brachioradialis and the extensor group, which includes the extensor carpi radialis, longus and brevis; the extensor digitorum communis; the extensor digiti minimi; and the extensor carpi ulnaris.

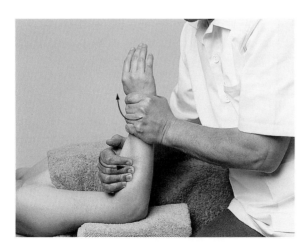

Figure 9.4 Kneading the forearm.

- A similar action is also carried out on the flexor group of muscles, on the anterior region of the forearm.
- Strenuous physical activity and sports, especially racket games, can lead to any one or more of the following states within the muscles and fascia: tightness and rigidity, nodular areas, microadhesions, scar tissue and fibrotic tissue. Unless treated, these changes can make the muscles susceptible to injury, the most common being tennis elbow. The neuromuscular technique (NMT) is used (along with other techniques) to address these changes, thereby helping to improve the function of the muscles and prevent injury.

Practitioner's posture

Stand in the to-and-fro or the upright posture, and to the side of the treatment table. Carry out the movement by extending your arm and add some body weight by leaning forward slightly.

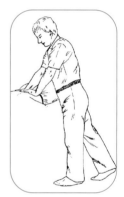

Procedure

Hold the patient's hand with your medial one, as if shaking hands. Raise the patient's forearm by flexing the elbow and resting it on the treatment table. Place the thumb of your lateral hand on the posterior region of the patient's forearm, close to the wrist. Curve the fingers of the same hand around the forearm towards the anterior side; flex the distal interphalangeal joint of your thumb, and press the tip into the tissues (Fig. 9.5). Maintain the pressure and, applying a very short stroke, slide the thumb along the forearm towards the elbow. Next, ease off the pressure and slide the thumb gently back to the starting point. Repeat the same movement several times over one area, until the resistance and tightness in the tissues are reduced, and then move your hand further along the forearm and repeat the procedure. Continue over the whole area of the posterior region of the forearm. Next, carry out the NMT on the anterior aspect. Use the same thumb, or change the hand positions and engage the more medial hand.

Friction technique

Thumb friction on the elbow

Effects and applications

- Friction movements reduce adhesions between tissue layers such as fascia and muscle or fascia and bone, and between muscle bundles.
- They also stimulate the circulation to the tendon and ligaments around the elbow joint.

Practitioner's posture

- To apply this technique, stand in the upright posture to the side of the treatment table; alternatively, sit on a chair or stool. Support the patient's elbow and upper arm on a cushion or folded towel.

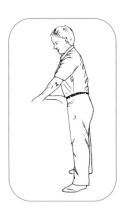

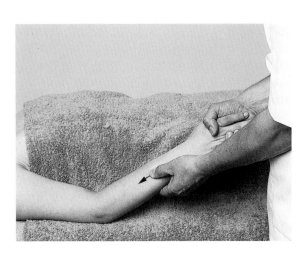

Figure 9.5 The neuromuscular technique on the extensor and flexor groups of the forearm.

Procedure

Raise the patient's forearm, and support it with your more caudal hand at the wrist. Place the thumb of your more cephalad hand on the lateral epicondyle of the patient's humerus (Fig. 9.6). This area is the common origin for the extensor muscle group. Round your fingers under the patient's elbow (the medial side) and apply a counterforce with them against the thumb. Flex your thumb at the interphalangeal joint, and apply pressure with the very tip. Maintain the pressure to grip the tendon as you move it backwards and forwards across the elbow, without sliding over the tissue surface. Apply very short strokes, across the width of the tendon, and continue with the treatment for a minute or two. As the technique can cause some discomfort, it should only be carried out to the patient's tolerance level. Having worked over the lateral epicondyle, move the hand to trace the tendon into the forearm, at the tendon–muscular junction, and repeat the same procedure.

Alternative method for the friction technique

The friction technique can be applied using the first and middle fingers instead of the thumb. This serves as an alternative or additional method, and saves the thumb from excessive fatigue. You may find it more practical to be in a sitting position when applying friction with the fingers.

Stroking technique

Effleurage on the upper arm

Effects and applications

- The effleurage enhances the venous return and the lymph drainage of the upper arm. Further assistance is supplied by a gravitational pull, as the arm is in a raised position during this movement.
- The technique reduces carbon dioxide, lactic acid and fluid, the by-products of muscle activity. It is therefore of great benefit where the muscles are exercised regularly or are overworked; for example, the triceps, deltoid, biceps brachii and brachialis.

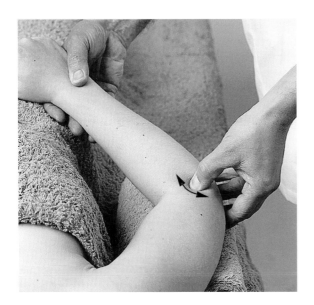

Figure 9.6 Friction movement over the elbow.

Practitioner's posture

Stand in the to-and-fro or the upright posture, close to the patient's shoulder. Adjust your position so that you can reach the upper arm comfortably without bending forwards too much. Lean forward to add some weight behind the movement.

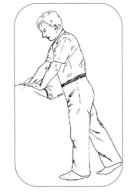

Procedure—effleurage on the posterolateral region of the upper arm

Raise the patient's arm, and hold and support it at the elbow with your medial hand. Rest your lateral hand on the posterolateral region of the upper arm, just superior to the elbow (Fig. 9.7A). Effleurage upwards while applying a gentle compression of the tissues with your palm and fingers. Continue the stroke to include the lateral region of the shoulder. When you reach the shoulder, reduce the pressure and effleurage

lightly towards the elbow. Repeat the procedure a few times.

Procedure—effleurage on the anteromedial side of the upper arm

Hold the patient's arm at the wrist with your lateral hand and raise it to a comfortable position. Support the arm on your upper chest or shoulder, provided that this is comfortable and ethically correct; otherwise, hold the arm slightly away from your body. Place your more medial hand on the anteromedial side of the patient's upper arm (Fig. 9.7B). Apply a slight compression with the palm and fingers, and effleurage from the elbow towards the axilla. Lean forwards to add some weight behind the movement. When you reach the deltoid and axillary region, reduce the pressure and slide the hand gently to the elbow. Repeat the routine several times.

Compression technique

Kneading the upper arm

Effects and applications

- Kneading applies a transverse stretch to the muscle fibres, which has the effect of easing any tightness. It is therefore indicated when the muscles are well developed or very rigid.

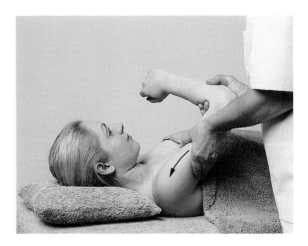

Figure 9.7A Effleurage on the posterolateral aspect of the upper arm and shoulder.

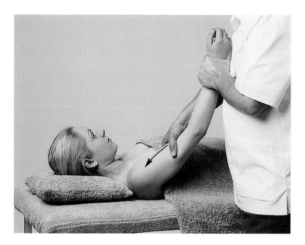

Figure 9.7B Effleurage on the anteromedial side of the upper arm.

The compression increases the circulation through the muscles; in so doing, it reduces congestion and any build-up of metabolites.

Practitioner's posture

Stand in the upright posture, beside the treatment table and in line with the patient's upper arm.

Procedure—kneading the biceps area

Hold the patient's forearm with your lateral hand. Flex the patient's elbow and raise the arm so that you can reach the biceps area with your medial hand while keeping the forearm more or less horizontal. Place the thenar/hypothenar eminences of your medial hand on the medial region of the patient's upper arm, and curve your fingers round the lateral side. Compress the tissues, applying pressure mostly with the thenar/hypothenar eminences (Fig. 9.8). Maintain the pressure and roll the tissues forward and towards your fingers; avoid any sliding of the fingers as you roll the muscles over the fingertips. Next, release the pressure

and resume the kneading position with the thenar/hypothenar eminences on the medial region of the biceps. Repeat the technique a few times.

An optional manoeuvre is to rotate the forearm medially and simultaneously with the kneading action; this exerts a slight torsion to the tissues and extends the stretch.

Compression technique

Kneading the posterior region of the upper arm

Practitioner's posture

Sit on the edge of the treatment table and rotate your trunk so that you can comfortably reach the lateral region of the patient's upper arm. Rest the patient's upper arm and elbow on a folded towel or cushion, and support this on your thigh. Flex the patient's elbow so that the hand rests on the chest or abdomen.

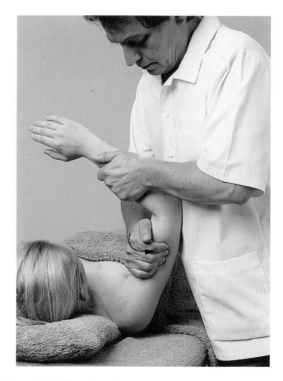

Figure 9.8 Kneading the anterior upper arm muscles.

Procedure for the right arm

Place the fingers of your left hand on the posterior region of the patient's upper arm, and the thumb of your right hand on the medial side (Fig. 9.9). Compress the tissues with the thumb and fingers as you apply a gentle lift and an anticlockwise twist. Release the grip altogether and move the hands in opposite directions so that the fingers of the right hand are pressing the posterior region of the upper arm, and the thumb of your left hand is on the anterior aspect. Apply the same technique of compressing and lifting, this time with a clockwise twisting action. Repeat this alternating petrissage a few times over the deltoid and triceps muscles.

Kneading the upper arm

A kneading movement can be carried out as an alternative method to the petrissage or in addition to it. Remain sitting on the edge of the treatment table. Support the patient's elbow and upper arm on a folded towel or cushion resting on your thigh. Flex the patient's elbow and steady the forearm by holding it at the wrist with your lateral hand (Fig. 9.10). Knead the deltoid muscle with the more medial hand. Position the thenar/hypothenar eminences on the ante-

rior aspect of the deltoid muscle, and the fingers on the posterior side. Compress the tissues between the heel of the hand and the fingers. Simultaneously, use the heel of the hand to roll the tissues forward and towards your fingers. Keep the fingers stationary as you roll the tissues over the fingertips. Release the grip on the tissues and repeat the technique. Extend the procedure over the triceps muscle.

LYMPH MASSAGE TECHNIQUES

Effects and applications

* The applications of lymph massage are constant for all techniques and for all regions of the arm, as for the rest of the body. A direct and mechanical effect is achieved with the lymph effleurage, which helps to drain the lymph fluid; in some cases this is assisted by the pull of gravity.
* The intermittent pressure movement has a similar mechanical effect, but it also involves a reflex mechanism. The pump-like action of the technique causes a reflex contraction of the muscular walls within the lymph vessels.
* Before applying the lymph massage to the arm, it is essential to drain the vessels and nodes

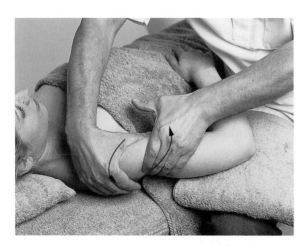

Figure 9.9 Petrissage on the posterior muscles of the upper arm.

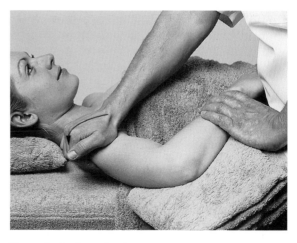

Figure 9.10 Kneading the upper arm.

that are closer to the exit point—that is, the right and left lymphatic ducts and the supra-clavicular and infraclavicular nodes. Lymph massage techniques for these structures are described with the neck and the chest routines, respectively.

Lymph massage technique

Intermittent pressure in the region of the axilla

Practitioner's posture

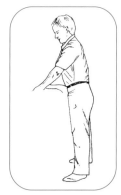

Stand in the upright posture, close to the patient's shoulder. You can also apply this movement whilst sitting on a chair. Extend your hands to the patient's upper arm while keeping your shoulders and arms very relaxed.

Procedure

Flex the patient's elbow and rest the upper arm on the treatment table, with the patient's hand resting on the abdomen. Rest your hands on the patient's upper arm and position your fingers on the lateral region, close to the axilla (Fig. 9.11). Keep the fingers close together, flat to the skin surface and relaxed. To apply the intermittent pressure technique, press gently with both hands together. Simultaneously, stretch the tissues in an arc towards the midline and towards the clavicle. This helps to drain the fluid into the axillary and infraclavicular nodes. Maintain contact with the skin during this manoeuvre, and prevent the hands from sliding by leaving the skin unlubricated. Once you have completed the movement, release the pressure and allow the tissues to return to their normal resting state before repeating the same technique. Treat one area a few times, then move closer to the axilla to resume the procedure, and again over the anterior deltoid area.

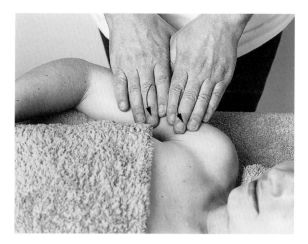

Figure 9.11 The intermittent pressure technique in the region of the axilla.

Lymph massage technique

Intermittent pressure on the upper arm and forearm

Practitioner's posture

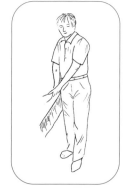

Stand in the upright posture and to the side of the treatment table. Adjust your position so that you are facing more or less towards the patient's head.

Procedure—intermittent pressure on the upper arm

Hold the patient's right arm at the wrist with your left hand. Raise the patient's arm to a vertical position and, if it is comfortable, rest it against your upper chest or shoulder. Place the fingers of your right hand on the medial side of the patient's upper arm, and your thumb on the lateral region (Fig. 9.12). Keep your fingers and thumb straight and very relaxed. Start with your hand at the distal end of the upper arm, and with your wrist in a flexed position. Apply gentle compression with your fingers and thumb; this is very brief and lasts for the same duration

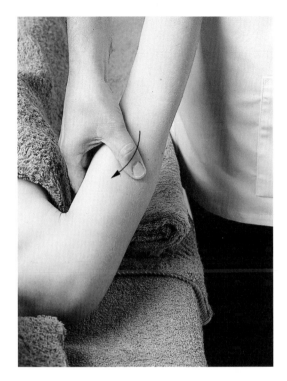

Figure 9.12 The intermittent pressure technique on the upper arm.

as the stretch that is to follow. Lower your wrist and maintain a gentle grip on the tissues as you stretch them in an arc towards the posterior and proximal regions of the arm. The combination of the pressure and the stretch encourages lymph drainage towards the axillary nodes. As in the previous movement, maintain contact with the skin during this manoeuvre and prevent the hands from sliding by leaving the skin unlubricated. When you have completed the stretch, release the pressure and allow the tissues to return to their resting state. Repeat this intermittent pressure movement on each area a few times before moving to a more proximal region along the upper arm, and continue until you reach the axilla.

Intermittent pressure technique—on the forearm

The same intermittent pressure technique is applied on the forearm. Continue to stand in the upright posture, but position yourself closer to

the patient's pelvis. Hold the patient's right wrist with your right hand and apply the technique with the left hand. Rest the patient's upper arm and elbow on the treatment table, then flex the elbow and raise the forearm slightly (Fig. 9.13). Hold the patient's arm in this position as you carry out the same intermittent pressure movements from the wrist to the elbow.

Lymph massage technique

Effleurage on the upper arm and forearm

Practitioner's posture

Stand in the upright posture and to the side of the treatment table. Rotate your body to face the patient; guard against too much twisting of your trunk. Keep your shoulders and arms relaxed.

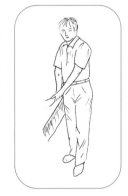

Procedure—effleurage on the upper arm

Use your right hand to hold and support the patient's right forearm (Fig. 9.14). Maintain this grip and flex the patient's elbow to raise the

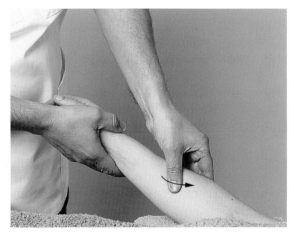

Figure 9.13 The intermittent pressure technique on the forearm.

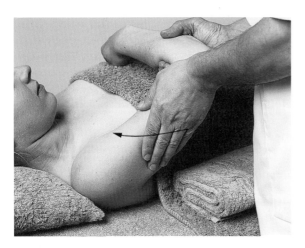

Figure 9.14 Lymphatic effleurage on the upper arm and towards the axillary nodes.

upper arm, keeping the forearm in a horizontal position. Effleurage with your left hand, using a very light stroking action. Slide the hand from the elbow towards the shoulder. As you approach the shoulder, direct your fingers towards the axilla to follow the direction of the lymph flow into the axillary nodes. Next, remove the hand and place it in the region of the elbow to resume the effleurage. Repeat the procedure a few times. A small amount of lubrication can be applied to facilitate the hand sliding over the skin.

Procedure—lymph effleurage on the forearm

Rest the patient's right upper arm and elbow on the treatment table, and flex the elbow to raise the forearm, holding the wrist with your right hand. Apply the very light stroking movements with your left hand, from the wrist to the elbow. Repeat a few times.

Lymph massage technique

Intermittent pressure on the hand

Practitioner's posture

Sit on the edge of the treatment table. Place a folded towel or cushion on your lap or on the treatment table, and rest the patient's hand on this. While sitting is very comfortable and practical, the movement is equally feasible from a standing posture.

Procedure

Place your thumbs on the dorsum of the patient's hand and your fingers on the palmar side (Fig. 9.15). Using minimal pressure, stretch the tissues with each thumb in an arc, towards the midline of the hand and towards the shoulder. The curved direction of the stretch is synonymous with that of the intermittent pressure technique.

This movement is somewhat different in that you can allow the thumb to slide slightly while you are applying the stretch; in this manner you are combining an effleurage stroke with the intermittent pressure technique. Alternate the thumbs, and complete one stroke and stretch before starting again with the other thumb. Continue over the dorsum of the hand, then extend the strokes over the wrist.

SUPPLEMENTARY TECHNIQUES FOR THE UPPER LIMB

In cases where recipients are unable to lie down, for instance if they are elderly or physically dis-

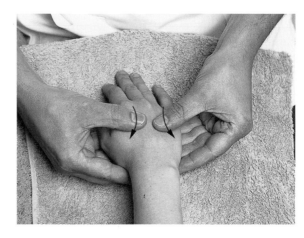

Figure 9.15 Intermittent pressure and effleurage is applied with each thumb on the dorsum of the hand.

abled, effleurage and other massages on the arm can be carried out while they are sitting on the treatment table or on a chair. The latter is a more practical arrangement, as it enables the patient to rest the arm on the treatment table. Support the patient's elbow on a folded towel and, if necessary, place a cushion under the patient's upper arm. The techniques described here are for the upper arm and forearm. Massage techniques for the hand described earlier in this chapter can be adapted and carried out when the patient is in this sitting position. The benefits gained from these techniques to the arm are the same as with those movements carried out when the patient is lying down; their effects and applications are therefore not listed in this section unless particularly relevant.

Stroking technique

Effleurage on the arm

Practitioner's posture

Sit close to the treatment table and face the patient, who adopts a similar sitting position and rests the elbow on top of the treatment table. Should this arrangement prove uncomfortable or impractical, disregard the treatment table and support the patient's arm on your own forearm and hand.

Procedure

Hold and support the patient's forearm with one hand, and place it in a position that is comfortable for the patient and facilitates the massage. Place your other hand on the upper arm, with the palm and fingers pointing towards the shoulder. Apply a steady pressure as you slide your hand upward, towards and over the patient's shoulder. Next, curve the hand to compress the upper arm gently and effleurage in the direction of the elbow (Fig. 9.16). This stroke is

relaxing and enhances the arterial blood flow. As you near the distal end of the upper arm, relax the hand and rotate it round to point towards the shoulder once more. Resume the effleurage with the palm and fingers flat to the surface, and pointing in the direction of the shoulder.

Effleurage on the forearm

Effleurage on the forearm of a seated patient is applied in a similar manner to that used when the patient is lying supine. Carry out the effleurage while still in a sitting position; alternatively, stand close to the treatment table and face towards the patient. Hold and support the patient's forearm with your more medial hand, gripping either the wrist or the patient's hand. Place the palm and fingers of your lateral hand around the posterolateral side of the forearm with your thumb on the medial region. Apply a gentle compression and effleurage from the wrist to the elbow. Ease the grip as you near the elbow and return the hand to the wrist, then repeat the same stroke.

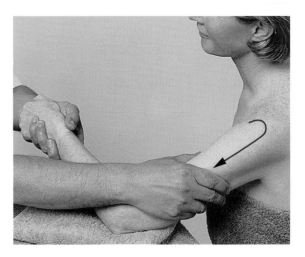

Figure 9.16 Effleurage on the upper arm.

Compression technique

Petrissage on the upper arm

Practitioner's posture

Stand in the upright posture while the patient remains seated. Position yourself close to the patient so that you can comfortably place the hands on the patient's upper arm without bending forward. Support the patient's elbow on a cushion; this also raises the upper arm and facilitates an easier movement.

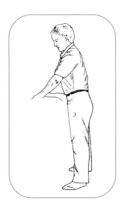

Procedure for the left arm

Place the fingers of the left hand on the posterior aspect of the upper arm. Rest the thumb of the right hand on the anterior side (Fig. 9.17). Apply an equal pressure with the fingers and the

thumb, and synchronize this movement with a gentle lift and a twisting action of the tissues. Next, release the tissues completely and move the hands so that the thumb of the left hand applies pressure on the anterior side of the upper arm and the fingers of the right hand press on the posterior aspect. Repeat the compression with the fingers and thumb, as well as the gentle lift and twisting action. Carry out the procedure a few times and move the hands more cephalad to include the deltoid muscle.

Bodywork technique

Mobilization of the shoulder girdle

Effects and applications

- Movement of the shoulder girdle (the scapula, clavicle and humerus) can be restricted if its associated muscles are tight and contracted. This bodywork technique is applied to loosen and stretch these muscles, which include the trapezius, rhomboids, levator scapula, supraspinatus and latissimus dorsi.
- The technique is supplementary and is therefore not necessarily included in the massage routine for the arm. It is, however, very relaxing, and promotes a feeling of 'release' as the shoulder girdle is mobilized and freed up.

Practitioner's posture

Stand in the lunging posture, and to the side of the massage plinth. The patient lies supine and close to the edge of the massage table. Shift your body forward and your weight onto the front foot, then reverse the position. Keep your back straight throughout the movement.

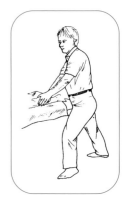

Procedure for the right arm

Lift the patient's arm and grip their hand between your right upper arm and the lateral

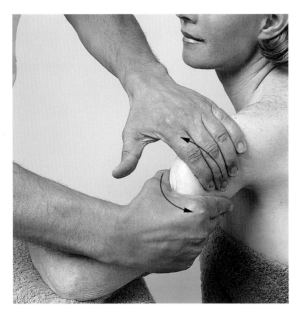

Figure 9.17 Petrissage on the upper arm.

region of your trunk. Grip the patient's elbow with your right hand; use this hold to lock the elbow in extension and to support the weight of the arm. Next, grip the patient's ipsilateral shoulder with your left hand (Fig. 9.18). Keep your left arm in this locked straight position throughout the movement. Carry out the following actions to describe a continuous rotation manoeuvre of the shoulder girdle:

1. Push the patient's shoulder girdle away from you, upward and towards their ear as in the 'shrugging' position. Carry out this action by shifting your body forward and your weight onto the front leg.

2. Press the shoulder girdle down with your left hand, towards the treatment table; this moves the shoulder posteriorly.

3. Pull the whole arm towards you, to 'depress' the shoulder, by leaning backward and shifting your weight onto the back foot.

4. With the patient's arm locked straight, lift it up so that you also lift their shoulder and move

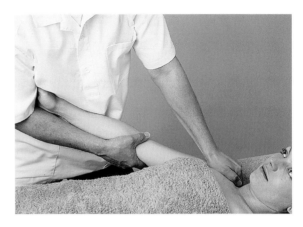

Figure 9.18 Mobilization of the shoulder girdle.

it anteriorly. This completes one circular mobilization.

5. Resume the circular mobilization by pushing the shoulder girdle upward.

10

Massage for body regions—the face, head and neck

OBSERVATIONS AND CONSIDERATIONS

The face is a picture of health or disease, and observation can reveal a great deal about the person. The expression itself may give information about the patient's state of mind and physical health. A healthy person is alert and bright-eyed. In disease, the expression can be apathetic and drowsy. A considerable number of pathological conditions present with abnormalities in the face and the head. These range from hyperthyroidism, Down's syndrome, Grave's disease and thyrotoxicosis to Cushing's syndrome and simple obesity. While a thorough examination is beyond the scope of this book, it is worth bearing in mind a few of the more common signs.

Skin colour and vascular signs

Pallor

A pale skin is not necessarily synonymous with anaemia. Depigmentation may be one explanation; another is vasoconstriction of the blood vessels or a fall in haemoglobin. However, anaemia can present with different degrees of pallor. In pernicious anaemia, for instance, the paleness is very distinct and is seen in the whole face, lips, conjunctivae, eyelids and even the hair.

Jaundice

The skin and eyes have a yellow tinge.

Butterfly rash

The change of colour in this instance is in fact a vascular dysfunction and is associated with an acute onset of systemic lupus erythematosus (SLE). The rash is observed across the nose and the cheeks.

Hypothyroidism

A patient with hypothyroidism has an expressionless and podgy face, pallor, thickened skin, dull eyes, thin hair, a hoarse voice and slow speech.

Swellings

- The commonest swellings in the neck are those of the lymphatic nodes, which indicate inflammatory processes and pathological changes in the associated tissues.
- Thyroid gland swellings are the second commonest masses, and differ in that they nearly always move up and down with deglutition (swallowing). Located at the front of the neck, deep and medial to the sternocleidomastoid muscles, swellings can be acute or chronic and arise from such causes as goitre, myxoedema, autoimmune thyroiditis (Hashimoto's disease) and carcinoma. Thyrotoxicosis is a toxic condition which is caused by hyperactivity of the thyroid gland, and is synonymous with exophthalmic goitre. In goitre, the enlarged thyroid gland has a bi-lobed appearance. Caution is needed in all of these conditions and massage to the enlarged glands is strictly contraindicated.
- A lymph node enlargement seen as a bilateral swelling in the upper cervical nodes can be a sign of Hodgkin's disease.
- A lump in the supraclavicular fossa may indicate a swollen gland from pathology of the stomach, e.g. carcinoma. This can occur because the lymphatic drainage of the stomach is to the supraclavicular glands.
- The deep cervical nodes are largely obscured by the sternocleidomastoid muscle, but the tonsillar nodes and the supraclavicular nodes can be palpated at the two extremes of the deep cervical chain. The posterior cervical nodes and the superficial cervical nodes (which extend along the external jugular vein) are easier to palpate.

Oedema

- Facial oedema accompanied by pallor is likely to be caused by kidney problems such as the nephrotic syndrome. Swelling appears around the eyes and spreads to the face and, in some cases, to other regions of the body.
- Another cause of oedema around the eyes is hypothyroidism, or myxoedema.
- A round or 'moon' face with red cheeks is the result of the increased adrenal hormone production in Cushing's syndrome.

Muscle atrophy or paralysis

Atrophy or paralysis of the facial muscles involves the cranial nerves. In a similar manner, atrophy of the upper fibres of the trapezius or sternocleidomastoid muscles indicates problems with the eleventh cranial (spinal accessory) nerve. Lesions in the brain can also affect the facial muscles. A blunt expression, decreased facial movements and a mask-like face describe the features associated with Parkinson's disease.

Tenderness and pain

Pain arising in the respiratory organs

Malfunctions of the respiratory system, particularly of the lungs and diaphragm, can refer pain to the left side of the neck. Tenderness can also extend to the shoulder, particularly to its medial aspect. Conditions such as bronchitis and asthma may lead to increased sensitivity or tenderness in these tissues (certain pathology, such as bronchial or oesophageal carcinoma, can also refer pain to the back).

Nerve pain

Pain that travels along a specific route invariably originates from a nerve. One example is the pain associated with the trigeminal cranial nerve, which is experienced along its sensory fibres as follows:

- from the side of the nose to the temple (ophthalmic)
- from the mouth to the cheek and temple (maxillary)
- from the chin to the jaw and ear (mandibular).

Sinus pain

The paranasal sinuses are air-filled cavities within the bones of the skull; they drain into the nasal cavities. Congestion of the sinuses causes a heavy, blocked-up feeling, and pain in the forehead and face. Tenderness is elicited on palpation of the frontal sinuses in the locality of the medial eyebrows, and the maxillary sinuses in the cheek bones.

Headaches

The signs and symptoms of headaches are discussed with the application of massage (see Chapter 4). As the neck is discussed here, it is of value to highlight the fact that the anatomy and mechanism of the cervical area is very complex and treatment therefore needs to be carried out with utmost care. The brachial plexus, vagus nerve, sympathetic trunk and the vertebral artery (running through the foramen transversarium of most of the cervical vertebrae) all contribute to its complexity.

Dizziness

Degeneration of the cervical vertebrae is common, particularly in elderly patients. This causes the vertebral artery, which runs along the cervical spine, to be compressed. Patients may experience dizziness, a light head, fainting, headache, tinnitus and disturbances of speech or vision.

Pain and stiffness in the neck

This has many causes.

- Torticollis, or wryneck, is generally a congenital condition, resulting from problems at birth.

There is a permanent contraction of the sternocleidomastoid muscle on one side, and this shortening and thickening causes the muscle to be prominent as a tight band and the head to be pulled towards the same side. As a result of the same contraction, the face and chin are tilted towards the non-affected side. Movement of the head and neck are restricted, not only because of the malfunction of the musculature but also because of the related curvature of the spine.
- Inflammation or enlargement of lymph nodes, in acute cases of inflammation from infection, may also be accompanied by muscle stiffness.
- The pain of trauma to the muscles, ligaments or joints is necessarily accompanied by a limitation of movement of the neck.
- Chilling of the tissues from exposure to wind or a draught, for example when driving or sleeping close to an open window, often results in rigidity of the neck.
- One of the acute systemic infections that can cause stiffness of the neck, particularly in children, is meningitis. The neck may be in a fixed position of extension. Poliomyelitis is less common but equally debilitating, and neck stiffness may be an early sign. Stiffness and spasmodic neck retraction can also occur in tetanus infection.

Cervical arthritis

Arthritic conditions that may affect the cervical spine include rheumatoid arthritis and chronic juvenile arthritis (Still's disease). Other forms of arthritis include:

- *Spondylitis.* Acute episodic pain is found in cases of cervical spondylitis (osteoarthritis with inflammation) of the cervical spine; this is most common in those over 60 years. It is caused by degeneration of the facet joints with osteophyte formation and inflammation. In this condition there can be almost constant pain, which is exacerbated with movements. The pain is often referred from the neck into the occiput and towards the shoulders.
- *Spondylosis.* Stiffness in the cervical spine may be caused by the arthritic changes of spondylosis.

This refers to degeneration of the vertebral bodies and discs with outgrowths of osteophytes around the edges. Disc protrusion may be a complication. The proliferation of osteophytes may be extensive enough to affect the longitudinal ligament, leading to ankylosing (spondylosis deformans). The stiffness itself is periodic and has its onset around middle age.

MASSAGE TECHNIQUES FOR THE FACE, HEAD AND NECK

The techniques in this section are mostly applied to balance the muscles and release tightness. While a relaxing effect is gained from these techniques, other massage movements can be added (especially to the face) to induce deep relaxation. The patient lies supine with a cushion support under the knees and one under the head, and all other regions of the body are covered with a towel or blanket to maintain body temperature.

Massage movements on the left side of the neck (anterior, lateral and posterior regions) can have a referred beneficial effect on the lung and diaphragm. The reflex area extends to the clavicle and the medial end of the supraspinatus. It also covers the greater part of the left side of the neck, extending beyond the midline to the right. Massage on the corresponding right side of the neck can be of benefit to the liver and gallbladder.

Stroking technique

Effleurage on the neck and shoulders

Effects and applications

- This effleurage technique is of great value as a relaxing stroke, and is particularly indicated when the patient can only lie in the supine position.
- The movement is very effective in stretching the posterolateral muscles of the neck, especially the trapezius and levator scapulae. The splenius capitis and cervicis are similarly affected, albeit to a lesser degree. As the technique involves a degree of side-bending of the neck, it cannot be applied if there are con-

traindications such as spondylosis or osteoporosis.

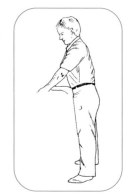

Practitioner's posture

Stand at the head end of the treatment table, in the upright posture and with your feet slightly apart. This wide stance enables you to shift your body to the left and right.

Procedure for the right side

Hold and support the patient's head by placing your left hand under the occiput. Place your right hand on the lateral side of the patient's neck, close to the mastoid process. Apply a slight pressure with the palm, fingers and thenar/hypothenar eminences of your right hand (Fig. 10.1). Effleurage along the muscle fibres on the posterolateral side of the neck. Continue the stroke over the superior region of the shoulder, following the trapezius fibres, and finish at the upper end of the arm. As you apply the effleurage with the right hand, introduce a degree of side-bending of the neck with the left hand by maintaining your grip on the occiput and gently taking the head towards the left side. The combined action of the side-bending in one direction and the effleurage in the opposite direction applies a moderate stretch to the muscles fibres. Repeat the procedure a few times, and then apply it to the left side of the neck.

Bodywork technique

Transverse stretch to the neck and upper shoulder muscles

Effects and applications

- This technique applies a stretch across the fibres of the trapezius, the levator scapulae and, to some degree, the splenius capitis and

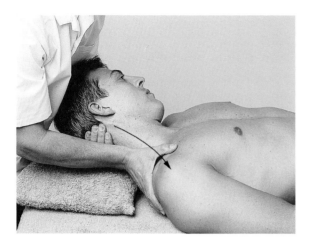

Figure 10.1 Effleurage and stretch to the posterolateral muscles of the neck.

cervicis. With the fingers extended to the upper back, the stretch can also include the rhomboids minor. Freeing these muscles improves the mobility of the neck and the shoulder girdle.
- As the technique also releases tension in the muscles, it is very relaxing and is applicable in most situations.

Practitioner's posture

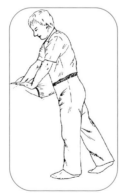

Stand in the to-and-fro position and to the side of the treatment table. Rotate your body to face towards the patient; this allows you to reach the contralateral shoulder comfortably with your more medial hand. Lock your arm straight and lean back to exert pressure from in front of the movement. Rest your more lateral hand on the ipsilateral arm.

Procedure

Place your more medial hand on the upper side of the shoulder and the base of the neck. Curve your fingers round the shoulder, in the region of

the upper fibres of the trapezius and the levator scapulae (Fig. 10.2). Provided it is comfortable, extend your fingers so they also reach the rhomboids minor. Grip the tissues by applying pressure, mostly with the fingers. Maintain this grip and keep your arm straight as you stretch the muscles in an anterior direction. Increase the stretch gradually as you lean backward and shift your body weight onto the back foot. Hold this stretch for a few seconds before transferring your body weight to the front foot and releasing the grip. Repeat a few times.

Deep stroking technique

Effleurage on the masseter muscles

Effects and applications

- The masseter muscle (from the Greek word *masétér*, meaning chewer) is situated over the temporomandibular joint. In mind–body terms, this muscle is associated with unexpressed tension, frustration and anger. As these are the regrettable yet common stresses of everyday living, the muscle is frequently in a state of contraction. The deep effleurage stroke helps to reduce some of this tightness.
- Releasing the tension in the masseter muscle will also improve the mobility of the

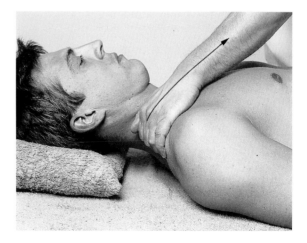

Figure 10.2 Transverse stretch to the neck and upper shoulder muscles.

temporomandibular joint, and reducing restrictions in this will in turn assist the mechanisms of the other cranial bones.

Practitioner's posture

Sit on a chair or stool at the head end of the treatment table, and place your forearms on either side of the patient's head. Support the patient's head on a folded towel or thin cushion. Massage both sides of the face simultaneously.

Procedure

Locate the temporomandibular joint. Instruct the patient to open and close the mouth while you feel the prominent condyle of the mandible move under your fingers. Flex the distal interphalangeal joints of the index and middle fingers and place the fingers in the temporal fossa, superior to the zygomatic arch and the temporomandibular joint. Apply pressure with the pads of the fingers, keeping the distal interphalangeal joints flexed (Fig. 10.3). Effleurage downward over the joint and towards the inferior border of the mandible, tracing the muscle fibres. Ease off the pressure and return the fingers to the temporal bone, and repeat the stroke.

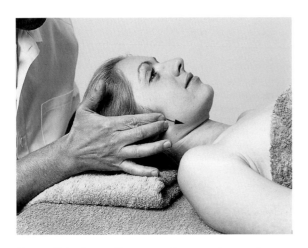

Figure 10.3 Deep effleurage on the masseter muscle.

Friction technique

Massaging the scalp

Effects and applications

- The scalp lies over the cranium. It is a multi-layered tissue, made up of the skin, a dense subcutaneous connective tissue, an aponeurosis (epicranial or galea), loose connective (sub-aponeurotic) tissue, and the periosteum covering the cranial bones. The occipitofrontalis muscle forms part of the temporal and occipital borders, and nerves and blood vessels are also plentiful within the scalp. Congestion can occur within these layers, and adhesions are also common. This friction technique is used to increase extracranial circulation, thereby reducing congestion.
- Improving the extracranial circulation is also likely to benefit the intracranial blood flow.
- Additionally, the technique helps to free up any restrictions. Tightness in the scalp can be associated with disorders such as general tension, impaired systemic circulation, toxicity and viral infections. The friction movement improves the mobility of the scalp over the cranial bones, and is therefore indicated to prevent or improve these conditions.
- The friction massage to the scalp can also act as a preventative method for headaches. However, as it can bring about a sudden increase in circulation, it needs to be carried out with care or omitted altogether if the subject is susceptible to migraines. It is certainly contraindicated during a migraine attack.

Practitioner's posture

Stand in the upright posture and at the head end of the treatment table. Support the patient's head on a low cushion or folded towel.

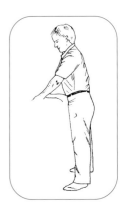

Procedure

Position the hands one on either side of the patient's head. Spread your fingers and place them on the temporal and parietal bones. Flex the distal interphalangeal joints and apply pressure with the pads of all the fingers; using the thumb may exert too much pressure and is therefore best avoided (Fig. 10.4). Increase the pressure with the fingertips sufficiently to grip the scalp and move it over the cranial bones. Apply small circular movements, clockwise or anticlockwise, and with both hands simultaneously. Guard against sliding of the fingers over the scalp as this causes you to lose the grip. Continue with the stroke for a few seconds, then place the hands on another region of the cranium and repeat the routine.

Friction movement to the back of the head

To massage the back of the head, rotate it to one side and support it with one hand. Rest the same hand on the treatment table, and brace the forearm against the forehead to stabilize the head. Spread the fingers of the free hand and massage the back of the head, applying the same movements and pressure with the pads of the fingers. Next, gently rotate the head to the other side, swap the position of the hands, and repeat the movement.

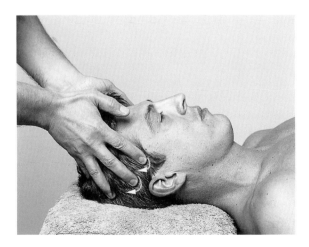

Figure 10.4   Friction massage on the scalp.

Bodywork technique

Cranial vault: supporting hold

Effects and applications

- This is an extremely relaxing technique for the patient, and it has a number of indirect yet beneficial responses throughout the body.
- Supporting the head in this manner communicates a feeling of caring and, in particular, emotional empathy to the patient.
- The stillness and relaxation brought about by this technique has the effect of balancing the body, mainly the autonomic nervous system towards a parasympathetic state.
- The technique has a normalizing effect on the cerebrospinal fluid and a tendency to lower the intracranial pressure. It can also be of benefit to the interrelated mechanisms of the cranial bones.
- It is likely that the technique causes an 'unwinding' or release of tight fascial planes in the cervical area. Very occasionally such tightness may be associated with a history of trauma, and the unwinding may cause unease and restlessness in the recipient. While this is a normal reaction and should eventually subside, the patient may find it unpleasant; in such a case, discontinue the application and allow the patient to rest for a short while.

Practitioner's posture

Sit at the head end of the treatment table. Rest your forearms (including the elbows) on top of the table, with your hands beneath and on each side of the recipient's head. As your hands are under the patient's head, it is not necessary to support it on a cushion or folded towel.

Procedure

Position the hands, which are supinated and resting on the treatment table, under the patient's head. Place the fingers under the occipital border and the upper end of the neck (Fig. 10.5). Avoid exerting pressure on the tissues with the fingertips.

Place the thumbs either above the patient's ears or close to your palm and fingers. Keeping the hands relaxed, use the palms and thenar/hypothenar eminences to support the occiput and take the full weight of the head.

Hold this position of stillness and support, accommodating any adjustments the patient may want to make to be more comfortable. Observe the patient's breathing, which may become deeper on relaxation. Allow your own body to relax and be free of tension. Continue with this technique for a few minutes, or until it feels appropriate to release the hold gently and remove the hands.

LYMPH MASSAGE TECHNIQUES FOR THE NECK

Lymph massage technique

Effleurage on the supraclavicular region

Effects and applications

- Lymph massage to the supraclavicular areas promotes drainage of the thoracic duct on the left side and the right lymphatic duct on the right. Both ducts provide the exit for all systemic lymph into the venous system.
- The lymph massage also encourages drainage of the deep cervical nodes into the jugular lymphatic trunk. This vessel in turn opens into either the junction between the subclavian and internal jugular veins on the right side, or into the end of the thoracic duct on the left side (Box 10.1).
- Because of its significant effect, the lymph massage on this region is carried out before and between other lymph massage movements. This procedure is followed whether the movements are employed on the chest, abdomen or face and neck, and for any condition requiring lymph drainage.
- Minimal lubrication is required for this technique.

Practitioner's posture

Stand in the upright posture, to the side of the treatment table and in line with the patient's shoulder. Adjust your position so that you face across the treatment table, i.e. towards the contralateral side. Place a low support under the patient's head, both for comfort and to assist with the lymph drainage in the cervical area.

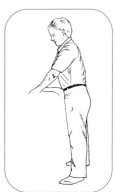

Procedure for the left side

Rest your left hand on the upper side of the patient's shoulder, more or less parallel to the clavicle. Place your fingers in the supraclavicular fossa, which is superior to the clavicle and also lateral and posterior to the sternocleidomastoid. It also forms the lower border of the posterior triangle of the neck (Fig. 10.6). Carry out this movement with the distal phalanges of the index and middle fingers (or with the middle and ring fingers). Apply a light stroking movement with the pads of both digits.

Start at the anterior margin of the trapezius and massage towards the clavicle. The stroke is therefore carried out across the scalenus medius

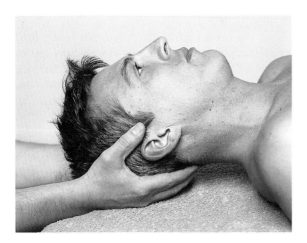

Figure 10.5 Cranial vault-supporting hold.

Box 10.1   Cervical lymphatic nodes and vessels

- The deep cervical nodes run along the internal jugular vein. The majority of the nodes lie under the cover of the sternocleidomastoid muscle. Other deep cervical nodes extend laterally beyond the border of the sternocleidomastoid, some forming a posterior cervical chain
- Some of the lower deep cervical nodes extend downward behind the clavicle
- The deep cervical nodes drain into the jugular lymph trunk
- The jugular trunk opens into:
    a. the junction between the subclavian and internal jugular veins on the right side
    b. into the end of the thoracic duct on the left side
- The thoracic duct on the left side is located slightly lateral and deep to the sternocleidomastoid muscle. It is also lateral to the internal jugular vein and superior to the clavicle. Located on the corresponding right

side is the right lymphatic duct. The ducts receive lymph from the jugular and subclavian lymphatic trunks. The right lymphatic duct also receives the bronchomediastinal trunk.
- The superficial cervical nodes are situated along the external jugular vein which runs over the sternocleidomastoid at its upper end and slightly posterior to it lower down. The superficial cervical nodes drain into the deep cervical nodes
- The face and head drain into a number of primary nodes, e.g. the submental, submandibular and the parotid, as well as the cervical nodes
- Pathological disorders can cause the cervical nodes to adhere to the internal jugular vein, and may be observed as enlarged nodes along the posterior border of the sternocleidomastoid muscle. The retroauricular and the occipital nodes can also be enlarged and prominent in German measles

---

and scalenus anterior towards the sternocleido-mastoid insertion into the clavicle. Stroking along this region encourages drainage of the thoracic duct on the left, and the lymphatic duct on the right. Keep your fingers more or less straight, and your hand in the same horizontal position. As you apply the stroke in the direction of the clavicle, supinate the hand slightly to perform a 'scooping' action with the fingers. Once you have completed the stroke, remove your fingers and place them on the anterior margin of the trapezius to repeat the stroke.

Lymph massage technique

Draining the cervical nodes

Effects and applications

- Lymph massage on the anterolateral border of the neck drains the superficial cervical nodes, which lie superior to the sternocleidomastoid muscle, as well as the deeper ones, which are almost obscured by it.
- The improved lymph flow therefore benefits the nodes situated around the head and face, including the submental, submaxillary, tonsillar, occipital, retroauricular (mastoid) and

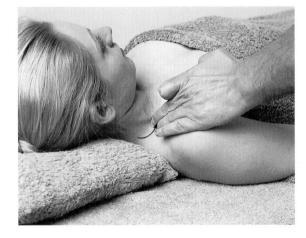

Figure 10.6   Lymph massage to the thoracic duct is carried out from the anterior border of the trapezius towards the clavicle.

preauricular nodes, most of which drain into the superficial and deep cervical nodes.
- The technique can be used in a number of situations, such as the treatment of congested sinuses, after a cold (not during an attack), or following inflammation of the glands. In cases of serious pathology, the technique may be contraindicated.
- Use very little or no lubrication for this movement.

Practitioner's posture

Sit at the head end of the treatment table and place your hands on either side of the patient's neck. Place a cushion or folded towel under the patient's head; this elevates the head and assists the flow of the lymph.

Procedure — effleurage on the cervical nodes

Position your hands one on either side of the patient's neck. Support one side of the head and neck with the non-massaging hand. Place the massaging hand on the upper region of the neck, and place the fingers in a slight transverse position (Fig. 10.7). Make contact with the palm and fingers, and keep these relaxed throughout the movement. Extend the neck slightly and rotate the head away from the side being massaged; this provides you with easy access to the lateral tissues of the neck. Carry out the light effleurage strokes in the following directions:

1. Stroke down the neck towards the clavicle, along the scalenus medius and the scalenus anterior. The external jugular vein and the superficial cervical nodes are in this region. As you near the clavicle, remove the hand and position it once more on the upper region of the neck to resume the stroke.
2. Repeat the same stroking action along the sternocleidomastoid. The upper and lower deep cervical nodes are located in this area; massaging towards the clavicle enhances the lymph flow in the same direction.
3. Apply a similar stroking movement starting further up the neck, on the mastoid process. The movement encourages drainage of the mastoid nodes (retroauricular), which are located in this area. Place the hand on the occipital border and repeat the stroke; this also assists the drainage of the occipital nodes, which are situated on the cranial attachment of the trapezius. Both these groups empty into the deep cervical nodes.

Once you have completed the series of strokes on one side of the neck, reverse the position of

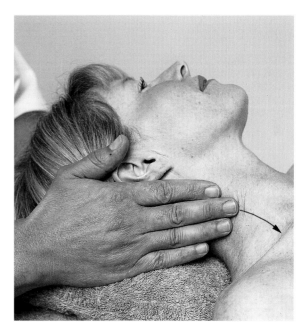

Figure 10.7 The hand position for the lymph effleurage remains unchanged for the intermittent pressure technique.

the hands and continue with the massage on the opposite side. In addition to the effleurage strokes, apply the intermittent pressure technique described next.

Draining the cervical nodes — intermittent pressure technique

With the position of the patient's head unchanged, continue to support it with one hand. Place the other hand on the opposite side of the neck, as for the previous effleuraging stroke. Start with the hand close to the clavicle, and gradually move it upward towards the mastoid process. Using mostly the pads of the fingers, apply a gentle pressure to the tissues. Simultaneously, stretch the tissues towards the midline and towards the clavicle, describing an arc with your fingers. This manoeuvre has the effect of stretching the lymph vessels, which creates a reflex contraction of their muscular walls, causing the lymph to move forward. Furthermore, the applied pressure encourages movement of fluid through the lymph nodes.

Release the pressure to return the tissues to their resting state, and repeat the movement several times on the same tissue area. Next, place the hand slightly further up the neck and apply the intermittent pressure technique once again. Continue with this procedure on the same regions of the neck as those for the lymph effleurage strokes. Having completed the technique on one side of the neck, repeat the procedure on the opposite side. No lubrication is needed for this movement.

SUPPLEMENTARY TECHNIQUES FOR THE NECK

Stroking technique

Effleurage on the lateral side of the neck

Effects and applications

- An effleurage stroke to the anterolateral aspect of the neck can be applied with the patient lying on one side. The technique can be used as an effective substitute or alternative method to that used on a supine patient. It is therefore of particular use when recipients can only lie on their side.
- If the effleurage is carried out very lightly, it assists the lymph flow through the cervical nodes and vessels. A stronger pressure is of benefit to the muscles, primarily to the sternocleidomastoid, scalenus medius and scalenus anterior.

Practitioner's position

Sit at the head end of the treatment table. As the patient lies on one side, support the head on a cushion or pillow. The head should be horizontal and there should not be any flexion or extension of the neck.

Procedure for the left side

Place the left hand on the side of the neck. Adjust the angle of the hand so that it is slightly transverse to the neck, more or less in line with the fibres of the scalene muscles (Fig. 10.8). Effleurage with the pads of the fingers, from the mastoid process towards the clavicle.

Apply very little or no pressure to influence the lymph drainage; use very slow movements and keep your hand relaxed. Effleurage along the scalenus medius and the scalenus anterior to help drain the superficial cervical lymph nodes. Apply the massage along the sternocleidomastoid to drain the deep cervical nodes. As you repeat the massage, include also the mastoid process and the occiput to drain the mastoid and occipital nodes.

To benefit the muscles, apply the effleurage stroke using a slightly deeper pressure. Follow the fibres of the scalene muscles with the stroke, then repeat it along the sternocleidomastoid. These muscles are often tight, but can be encouraged to relax with this effleurage movement. Avoid too much pressure on the external jugular vein.

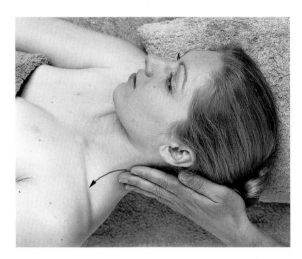

Figure 10.8   This effleurage stroke is used for easing muscles or for lymph drainage.

References

Acolet D, Modi N, Giannakoulopoulos X et al 1993 Changes in plasma and catecholamine concentrations in response to massage in preterm infants. Archives of Disease of the Child 68:29–31.

Adamson-Macedo EN, Alves-Attree JL 1994 TAC-TIC therapy: the importance of systematic stroking. British Journal of Midwifery 2:264–269.

Bach CS, Lewis GP 1973 Lymph flow and lymph protein concentration in skin and muscle of the rabbit hind limb. Journal of Physiotherapy (London) 235:477.

Barr JS, Taslitz N 1970 The influence of back massage on autonomic functions. Journal of Physical Therapy 50(12).

Bartels EM, Danneskiiold-Samsíe B 1986 Histological abnormalities in muscle from patients with certain types of fibrositis. Lancet 8484:755–756.

Bélanger AY, Morin SP, Pin P et al 1989 Manual muscle tapping decreases soleus H-reflex amplitude in control subjects. Physiotherapy Canada 41:192–196.

Bell AJ 1964 Massage and the physiotherapist. Physiotherapy 50:1679–1691.

Benson H 1976 The relaxation response. New York, Avon.

Brobeck JR (ed.) 1979 Best and Taylor's Physiological Basis of Medical Practice 10th edn, Section 4. Williams and Wilkins, p92.

Brunton T, Tunnicliff T 1894–1895 On the effects of the kneading of the muscles upon the circulation, local and general. Journal of Physiology 17:364.

Bühring M 1984 Physikalische Medizin bei chronischen Schmerzzuständen. In Schmerzkonferenz (D. E. Gross, G. Schmitt and S. Thomalsk eds) Fischer, pp. 13–32.

Caenar JS, Pflug JJ, Reig NO, Taylor LM 1970 Lymphatic pressures and the flow of lymph. British Journal of Plastic Surgery 23:305.

Cailliet R 1980 The Shoulder in Hemiplegia. FA Davis.

Cailliet R 1995 Low Back Pain Syndrome. FA Davis.

Chaitow L 1987 Soft Tissue Manipulation. Thorsons.

Chaitow L 1996a Modern Neuromuscular Techniques. New York, Churchill Livingstone.

Chaitow L 1996b Muscle Energy Techniques. New York, Churchill Livingstone.

Chamberlain GJ 1982 Cyriax's friction massage—a review. Journal of Orthopaedic and Sports Physical Therapy 4(1):16–22.

Chamberlain GJ et al 1993 Pain and its relief in childbirth—the results of a national survey conducted by the National Birth Trust. Churchill Livingstone.

Cuthbertson DP 1933 The effect of massage on metabolism: a survey. Glasgow Medical Journal 120:200–213.

Cyriax J 1945 Deep Massage and Manipulation. Hamish Hamilton.

Danneskiiold-Samsíe B, Christiansen E, Lund B, Anderson RB 1982 Regional muscle tension and pain (fibrositis). Scandinavian Journal of Rehabilitation Medicine 15:17–20.

Day JA, Mason RR, Chesrown SE 1987 Effect of massage on serum level of beta-endorphin and beta-lipotropin in healthy adults. Journal of Physical Therapy 67:926–930.

De Bruijn R 1984 Deep transverse friction; its analgesic effect. International Journal of Sports Medicine (suppl.) 5:35–36.

De Watteville A 1885 The cure of writer's cramp. British Medical Journal 1:323–324.

Dicke E 1953 Meine Bindegewebsmassage. Marquardt.

Dicke E 1956 Meine Bindegewebsmassage. Stuttgart, Hippokrates-Verlag.

Dieter JNI 1999 The effects of tactile/kinaesthetic stimulation on the physiology and behaviour of preterm infants. Dissertation Abstracts International, B 60/05 (November), 2335.

Dubrovsky V 1982 Changes in muscles and venous blood flow after massage. Teoriya i Praktika Fizicheskoi Kultury 4:56–57.

Ebner M 1962 Connective Tissue Massage: Theory and Therapeutic Application. E. & S. Livingstone.

Ebner M 1968 Connective tissue massage: therapeutic application. New Zealand Journal of Physiotherapy 3(14):18–22.

Ebner M 1978 Connective tissue massage. Physiotherapy 64:209–210.

Edgecombe W, Bain W 1899 The effects of baths, massage and exercise on the blood-pressure. Lancet 1:1552–1557.

Engelmann GJ 1994 Massage and expression or external manipulations in the obstetric practice of primitive people. Massage Therapy Journal Summer. (Reproduced from an article first published in 1882, in American Journal of Obstetrics and Diseases in Women and Children 15:601–625).

Ernst E, Matrai A, Magyarosy IE et al 1987 Massages cause changes in blood fluidity. Physiotherapy Journal 73(1).

Ferrell-Torry AT, Glick OJ 1993 The use of therapeutic massage as a nursing intervention to modify anxiety and the perception of cancer pain. Cancer Nursing 16(2):93–101.

Field T 1990 Newborn behaviour, vagal tone and catecholamine activity in cocaine-exposed infants. Symposium presented at the International Society of Infant Studies, Montreal, Canada, April 1990.

Field T 1998 Massage therapy effects. American Psychologist 53:1270–1281.

Field TM 2000 Touch Therapy. Edinburgh, Churchill Livingstone.

Field TM 2002 Massage therapy for immune disorders. In: Rich JG (ed). Massage Therapy: The Evidence For Practice. Edinburgh, Mosby, pp. 47–55.

Field T, Schanburg SM, Scafidi F et al 1986 Tactile/kinaesthetic stimulation effects on preterm neonates. Pediatrics 77:654–658.

Field T, Morrow C, Valdeon C et al 1992 Massage reduces anxiety in child and adolescent psychiatric patients. Journal of American Academy Child Adolescent Psychiatry 31:1, 125–131.

Field T, Ironson G, Scafidi F et al 1996a Massage therapy reduces anxiety and enhances EEG pattern of alertness and math computations. International Journal of Neuroscience 86:197–205.

Field T, Grizzle N, Scafidi F et al 1996b Massage and relaxation therapies' effects on depressed and adolescent mothers. Adolescence 31:903–911.

Frazer FW 1978 Persistent post-sympathetic pain treated by connective tissue massage. Physiotherapy 64(7): 211–212.

French's Index of Differential Diagnosis, 12th edn, 1985 Edited by F. Dudley Hart. Bristol, John Wright.

Ganong WF 1987 Review of Medical Physiology, 13th edn. Appleton and Llange.

Gatterman MI 1990 Chiropractic Management of Spine Related Disorders. Maryland: Williams & Wilkins.

Goats G 1994 Massage—the scientific basis of an ancient art: Part 1. The techniques. British Journal of Sports Medicine, 28(Sept):149–152.

Goldberg J, Sullivan SJ, Seaborne DE 1992 The effect of two intensities of massage on H-Reflex amplitude. Journal of Physical Therapy 72(6).

Gorsuch R, Key M 1974 Abnormalities of pregnancy as a function of anxiety and life stress. Psychosomatic Medicine 36:353.

Greenman PE 1989 Principles of Manual Medicine. Williams and Wilkins.

Grupp DR 1984 Lymphatics in Edema. New York, Raven.

Guyton AC 1961 Textbook of Medical Physiology, 2nd edn. WB Saunders.

Hall G, Winkvist L 1996 Hall V-Tox, a treatment for the removal of metal and environmental toxins. Positive Health Magazine, April 26–28.

Harrison L, Olivet L, Cunningham K et al 1996 Effects of gentle human touch on preterm infants: pilot study results. Neonatal Network 15:35–42.

Hartmann F 1929 Funktionelle Stoerungen der zentralen Kreislauf-organe bei geloester Erkrankung der Koeperdecke. Wien Klin Wosenschrift 41:272.

Head H 1889 Die Sensibilitaetsstoerungen der Haut bei Viszeral Erkrankungen. Berlin.

House SR 1879 Archives of Medicine, as cited by Engelmann GJ 1994 Massage and expression or external manipulations in the obstetric practice of primitive people. Massage Therapy Journal 1994:34–110.

Hovind H, Nielsen SL 1974 Effect of massage on blood flow in skeletal muscle. Scandinavian Journal of Rehabilitation Medicine 6:74–77.

Intyre AK 1975 Perception of Vibration. Australian Ass Neurologists 3:71–176. Melbourne.

Ironson G, Field T, Scafidi F et al 1996 Massage therapy is associated with enhancement of the immune system's cytotoxic capacity. Journal of Consulting and Clinical Psychology 84:205–218.

International Journal of Neuroscience 84(1–4): 205–217.

Jacobs J 1996 The encyclopedia of alternative medicine: a complete family guide to complementary therapies. Boston: Journey Editions.

Jacob M 1960 Masage for the Relief of Pain: Anatomical and Physiological Considerations. Physical Therapy Review 40:93–98.

Jacobson E 1939 Variation of Blood Pressure with Skeletal Muscle Tension and Relaxation. Annals of Internal Medicine 12:1194–1212.

Jenkins R, Rogers A 1997 Managing stress at work: an alternative approach. Nursing Standard 11(29):41–44.

Kaada B, Torsteinbo O 1989 Increase of plasma beta-endorphins in connective tissue massage. Gen Pharmacology 20(4): 487–489.

Klauser AG, Flaschentrager J, Gehrke A, Mull-Lissner SA 1992 Abdominal wall massage: effect on colonic function in healthy volunteers and in patients with chronic constipation. Z Gastroenterol 30: 247–251.

Kuhn CM, Schanberg SM, Field T et al 1991 Tactile-kinesthetic stimulation effects on sympathetic and adrenocortical function in preterm infants. Journal of Pediatrics 119:434–440.

Kurosawa M, Lundenberg T, Agren G, Lund I, Uvas-Meberg K 1995 Massage-Like Stroking of the Abdomen Lowers Blood Pressure in Anaesthetized Rats: Influence of Oxytocin. Journal of the Autonomic Nervous System 56:26–30.

Labrecque M, Eason E, Marcoux S et al 1999 Randomized controlled trial of prevention of perineal trauma by perineal massage during pregnancy. American Journal of Obstetrics and Gynecology 180(3 Pt 1): 593–600.

Le Bars D et al 1979 Diffuse noxious inhibitory controls (DNIC): effects on dorsal horn convergent neurons in rats. Pain 6:283–304.

Leone JA, Kukulka CG 1988 Effects of tendon pressure on alpha motoneuron excitability in patients with stroke. Journal of Physical Therapy 68(4).

Lewit K 1991 Manipulative Therapy in Rehabilitation of the Locomotor System. Oxford, Butterworth–Heinemann.

Licht E, Licht S 1964 A Translation of Joseph-Clement Tissot's Gymnastique Medicinale et Chirurgicale. Elizabeth Licht.

Lloyd DPC 1955 Principles of nervous activity, Section 1. In JF Fulton (ed.) Textbook of Physiology. Philadelphia, Saunders.

Lutgendorf S, Antoni MH, Shneiderman N, Fletcher MA 1996 Psychosocial counseling to improve quality of life in HIV infection. Patient Education and Counseling 24:217–235.

MacKenzie J 1923 Angina Pectoris. London, Henry Frowde and Hodder and Stoughton.

Matrai A, Ernst E, Dormandy JA 1984 Die Rolle der Hämorheologi in der Medizin. In Klinische Rheologie und beta–1-Blockade (E Heilman, H Kieswetter and E Ernst eds). Zuckschwèrdt.

Melzek R, Wall P 1988 The Challenge of Pain 2nd edn, Penguin.

Menard MB 2002 Methodological issues in the design and conduct of massage therapy research. In: Rich JG (ed). Massage Therapy: The Evidence For Practice. Edinburgh, Mosby, pp. 27–41.

Mennell James MA 1920 Massage: its Principles and Practice. Churchill.

Milan MJ 1986 Multiple opioid systems and pain. Pain 27:303–347.

Mislin H 1976 Active contractility of the lymphangion and coordination of the lymphangion chains. Experienta 37:820.

Montagu A 1986 Touching, The Human Significance of the Skin 3rd edn. Harper and Row.

Morelli M, Seaborne DE, Sullivan SJ 1990 Changes in H-Reflex amplitude during massage of triceps surae in healthy subjects. JOSPT 12(2):55–59, August.

Mortimer PS, Simmonds R, Rezvani M et al 1990 The measurement of skin lymph flow by isotope clearance-reliability, reproducibility, injection dynamics and the effect of massage. Journal of Inv Derm 95(6): 677–681, August.

Moyer-Mileur L, Leutkemeler M, Boomer L, Chan GM 1995 Effects of physical activity on bone mineralization in premature infants. Journal of Pediatrics 127:620–625.

Müller EA, Esch JS 1966 Die Wirkiung der Massage auf die Leistungsfähigkei von Muskeln. Int Z Angew Physio 22:240.

Murphy LR 1996 Stress management in work settings: a critical review of the health effects. American Journal of Health Promotion 11(2):112–135.

Olszewski WL, Engeset A 1979/80 Intrinsic contractibility of prenodal lymph vessels and lymph flow in the human leg. American Journal of Physiology 239:H775.

Ostgaard HC, Andersson GBJ et al 1989 Prevalence of back pain in pregnancy. Spine Journal January 17(1):53–55.

Overholser LC, Moody RA 1988 Lymphatic massage and recent scientific discoveries. Massage Therapy Journal, pp.55–80, Summer.

Parsons RJ, McMaster PD 1938 The effect of the pulse upon the formation of the flow of lymph. Journal of Experimental Medicine 68:353.

Peterson FB 1970 Xenon disappearance rate from human calf muscles during venous stasis. Danish Medical Bulletin 17:230.

Read D 1972 Childbirth without fear: the principles and practices of natural childbirth. New York Press, New York.

Reddy NP 1987 Lymph circulation: physiology, pharmacology, and biomechanics. Critical Review of Biomedical Engineering 14:45.

Reed BV, Held JM 1988 Effects of sequential connective tissue massage on autonomic nervous system of middle-aged and elderly adults. Journal of Physical Therapy 66/8:1231–1234.

Richards A 1998 Hands on Help. Nursing Times 94(32):69–75.

Russell IJ, Orr MD, Vipraio GA et al 1993 Cerebrospinal fluid Substance P is elevated in fibromyalgia syndrome. Arthritis and Rheumatism 36:223.

Scafidi F, Field TM, Schanger SM et al 1986 Effects of tactile/kinaesthetic stimulation on the clinical course and sleep/wake behaviour of preterm neonates. Infant Behaviour and Development 9:91–105.

Scafidi F, Field TM, Schanger SM et al 1990 Massage stimulates growth in preterm infants: a replication. Infant Behaviour and Development 13:167–188.

Schliack H 1978 Theoretical basis of the working mechanism of connective tissue massage. In: A Manual of Reflexive Therapy of the Connective Tissues (E Dicke et al eds). Sidney S. Simon Publishers, pp.14–33.

Selye H 1984 The Stress of Life. McGraw Hill.

Shipman MK, Boniface DR, Tefft ME, McCloghry F 1997 Antenatal perineal massage and subsequent perineal outcomes: a randomised controlled trial. British Journal of Obstetrics and Gynaecology 104(7):787–791.

Sirotkina AV 1995 (As cited by Zhena Kurashova Wine). Material for the study of massage influences on paresis and paralysis of different etiology. Massage 55:100–102.

Smith RO 1949 Lymphatic contractility, a possible intrinsic mechanism of lymphatic vessels for transport of lymph. Journal of Experimental Medicine 90:497.

Solomon EP, Schmidt RR, Adragna PJ 1990 Human Anatomy and Physiology 2nd edn. Saunders College Publishing (Harcourt Brace, Florida USA).

Stewart MA, Wendkos Olds S 1973 Raising a Hyperactive Child. Harper and Row.

Stoddard A 1969 Manual of Osteopathic Practice. London, Hutchinson Medical Publications.

Stone C 1992 Viscera Revisited. Tigger Publishing.

Sullivan SJ, Williams RT, Seaborne DE, Morelli M 1991 Effects of massage on alpha motoneurone excitability. Journal of Physical Therapy 71(8).

Sunshine W, Field T, Schanberg S et al 1996 Massage therapy and transcutaneous electrical stimulation effects on fibromyalgia. Journal of Clinical Rheumatology 2:18–22.

Taber's Cyclopedic Medical Dictionary 13th edn. (C. L. Thomas, ed.). FA Davis.

Tappan F 1988 Healing Massage Techniques. USA, Appleton & Lange.

Taylor GH 1860 A sketch of the movement cure. Reprinted in Massage Therapy Journal 1993.

Tisserand R 1992 Success with stress. International Journal of Aromatherapy, Summer.

Tovar MK, Cassmere VL 1989 Touch—the beneficial effects for the surgical patient. AORN Journal 49:1356–1361.

Tracy C 1992/93 Massage then and now. Massage Journal 7(3):10–12.

Travell JG, Simons DG 1983 Myofascial Pain and Dysfunction (1), Williams and Wilkins.

Uvnas-Moberg K, Widstrom AM, Marchini G et al 1987 Release of GI hormones in mother and infant by sensory stimulation. Acta Paediatrica Scandinavia 76:851–860.

Vander JA, Sherman JH, Luciano DS 1970 Human Physiology 5th edn. McGraw-Hill.

Vander AJ, Sherman JH, Luciano DS 1990 Human Physiology. New York, McGraw-Hill Publishing Company.

Van Why R 1991 Cornelius E. De Puy MD. Massage Therapy Journal 31.

Van Why R 1994 Charles Fayette Taylor. Massage Therapy Journal, 32.

Wale JO 1983 Tidy's Massage and Remedial Exercises. Bristol, John Wright.

Walsh D 1991 Nociceptive pathways, relevance to the physiotherapist. Physiotherapy Journal 77(5).

Wang G, Zhong S 1985 Experimental study of lymphatic contractility and its clinical importance. Annals of Plastic Surgery 15:278.

Watson J 1981 Pain mechanisms—a review. Characteristics of the peripheral receptors. Australian Journal of Physiotherapy 27(5):135–143.

Watson J 1982 Pain mechanisms—a review. Endogenous pain control mechanisms. Australian Journal of Physiotherapy 28(2):38–45.

Webner KM 1991 Massage for drug-exposed infants. Massage Therapy Journal 62–65, Summer.

Wittlinger G, Wittlinger H 1990 Dr. Vodder's Manual Lymph Drainage. Karl F. Haug.

Xujian S 1990 Effect of massage and temperature on the permeability of initial lymphatics. Lymphology 23:48–50.

Yates J 1989 Physiological Effects of Therapeutic Massage. Therapists Association of British Columbia.

Yoffey JM, Courtice FC 1970 Micromanipulations of Pressure in Terminal Lymphatics, Lymph and Lymphomyeloid Complex. New York Academic Press.

Zorrilla E, McKay J, Luborsky L, Shmidt K 1996 Relation of stressors and depressive symptoms to clinical progression of viral illness. American Journal of Psychiatry 153:626–635.

Zweifach BW, Prather JW 1975 Micromanipulation of pressure in terminal lymphatics in the mesentery. American Journal of Physiology 228:1326.

Bibliography

Agur A 1991 Grant's Atlas of Anatomy. Baltimore, Williams and Wilkins.

Alter M 1988 The Science of Stretching. Illinois, Human Kinetics Books.

Bates B 1983 A Guide to Physical Examination (Harper International Edition). Philadelphia, JB Lippincott.

Benson H 1976 The Relaxation Response. New York, Avon.

Berkow R (ed.) 1982 The Merck Manual of Diagnosis and Therapy, 14th edn. New Jersey, Merck Sharp & Dohme Research Laboratories.

Cailliet R 1980 The Shoulder in Hemiplegia. Philadelphia, FA Davis Co.

Cailliet R 1988 Soft Tissue Pain and Disability, 2nd edn. Philadelphia, FA Davis Co.

Cyriax J 1945 Deep Massage and Manipulation Illustrated. London, Hamish Hamilton Medical Books.

Fuller F 1705 Medicina Gymnastica. R. Knaplock.

Govan ADT, Hodge C, Callander R 1985 Gynaecology Illustrated. Edinburgh, Churchill Livingstone.

Govan AD, Macfarlane PS and Callander R 1991 Pathology Illustrated. New York, Churchill Livingstone.

Greenman P 1989 Principles of Manual Medicine. Baltimore, Williams and Wilkins.

Guyton AC 1961 Textbook of Medical Physiology, 2nd edn. Philadelphia, WB Saunders.

Hart FD (ed.) 1985 French's Index of Differential Diagnosis. Bristol, John Wright.

Hope RA and Longmore JM 1986 Oxford Handbook of Clinical Medicine. Oxford, Oxford University Press.

Janda V 1983 Muscle Function Testing. London, Butterworth.

Juhan D 1987 Job's Body—A Handbook for Bodywork. New York, Station Hill Press Inc.

Kendall FP and Kendall McCreary E 1983 Muscles Testing and Function. Baltimore, Williams and Wilkins.

Madhavan PN, Shwartz N and Shwartz S 1995 Synergistic effect of cortisol and HIV–1 envelope peptide on the NK activities of normal lymphocytes. Brain and Behavior, 9:20–30. National Cancer Institute. Office of Cancer Information, Communication and Education (OCICE) 1999.

Melzek R and Wall P 1988 The Challenge of Pain 2nd edn. Hamondsworth, Penguin.

Mennell J 1920 Massage: Its Principles and Practice. London, J & I Churchill.

Olson TR 1996 ADAM Student Atlas of Anatomy. Baltimore, Williams and Wilkins.

Reid DC 1992 Sports Injury Assessment and Rehabilitation. New York, Churchill Livingstone.

Rich JG (ed.) 2002 Massage Therapy: The Evidence For Practice. Edinburgh, Mosby.

Rolf I 1977 Rolfing: The Integration of Human Structures. New York, Harper and Row.

Stone C 1992 Viscera Revisited. Tigger Publishing.

Stone RJ and Stone J A 1990 Atlas of Skeletal Muscles. WC Brown.

Thomas CL (ed.) 1978 Taber's Cyclopedic Medical Dictionary (13th edn) Philadelphia, FA Davis Company.

Travell JG and Simons DG 1983 Myofascial Pain and Dysfunction, vol. I. Baltimore, Williams and Wilkins.

Wittlinger G and Wittlinger H 1970 Dr Vodder's Manual Lymph Drainage. Heidelberg, Karl F. Haug.

Zatouroff, M. (1985). A Colour Atlas of Physical Signs in General Medicine. London: Wolfe Medical Publications Ltd.

Index